TUMOR CELL HETEROGENEITY: ORIGINS AND IMPLICATIONS

BRISTOL-MYERS CANCER SYMPOSIA

Series Editor
MAXWELL GORDON
Science and Technology Division
Bristol-Myers Company

TUMOR CELL HETEROGENEITY: ORIGINS AND IMPLICATIONS

Edited by

ALBERT H. OWENS, JR.

DONALD S. COFFEY

STEPHEN B. BAYLIN

The Johns Hopkins Oncology Center
The Johns Hopkins University
School of Medicine
Baltimore, Maryland

1982

ACADEMIC PRESS

A Subsidiary of Harcourt Brace Jovanovich, Publishers

New York   London

Paris   San Diego   San Francisco   São Paulo   Sydney   Tokyo   Toronto

ACADEMIC PRESS, INC.
111 Fifth Avenue, New York, New York 10003

United Kingdom Edition published by
ACADEMIC PRESS, INC. (LONDON) LTD.
24/28 Oval Road, London NW1 7DX

Library of Congress Cataloging in Publication Data
Main entry under title:

Tumor cell heterogeneity.

(Bristol-Myers cancer symposia ; v. 4)
Papers presented at the Fourth Annual Bristol-Myers
Symposium on Cancer Research, held at the Johns Hopkins
Oncology Center, Dec. 3-4, 1981.
Includes bibliographical references and index.
1. Cancer cells--Congresses. I. Owens, Albert H.
II. Coffey, Donald S. III. Baylin, Stephen B.
IV. Bristol-Myers Symposium on Cancer Research (4th :
1981 : Johns Hopkins Oncology Center) V. Series.
RC267.T85   1982   616.99'4   82-16255
ISBN 0-12-531520-1

PRINTED IN THE UNITED STATES OF AMERICA

82 83 84 85   9 8 7 6 5 4 3 2 1

Contents

PART I   INTRODUCTION TO THE SYMPOSIUM

Tumor Cell Heterogeneity: A Perspective
ALBERT H. OWENS, JR.

PART II   EVIDENCES OF HETEROGENEITY: CHANGING TUMOR CELL POPULATIONS

Medullary Thyroid Carcinoma: A Model for the
Study of Human Tumor Progression and Cell
Heterogeneity
STEPHEN B. BAYLIN and GEOFFREY MENDELSOHN

Mechanisms for and Implications of the Development of Heterogeneity of Androgen Sensitivity in Prostatic Cancer

JOHN ISAACS

PART III THERAPEUTIC IMPLICATIONS

Drug Resistance and Chemotherapeutic Strategy

JAMES H. GOLDIE

The Heterogeneity of Metastatic Properties in Malignant Tumor Cells and Regulation of the Metastatic Phenotype

ISAIAH J. FIDLER and GEORGE POSTE

PART IV EPIGENETIC MECHANISMS

14 Tumor Subpopulation Interactions

GLORIA H. HEPPNER

15 Cell Differentiation in Neoplasia

CLEMENT L. MARKERT

16 Embryologic Microenvironment in the Regulation of Cancer Cells

G. BARRY PIERCE and ROBERT S. WELLS

PART V   GENETIC MECHANISMS

25 The Role of Genomic Rearrangements in Tumor Cell Heterogeneity

RUTH SAGER

26 The Structure and Function of a Eukaryotic Promoter

STEVEN L. McKNIGHT, MOSES V. CHAO, RAYMOND W. SWEET, SAUL SILVERSTEIN, and RICHARD AXEL

27 Nuclear Structure and DNA Organization

BARRY NELKIN, DREW PARDOLL, SABINA ROBINSON, DON SMALL, and BERT VOGELSTEIN

28 PART VI   Perspectives

What Viruses Tell Us about Tumorigenesis

WALLACE P. ROWE

The Concept of DNA Rearrangement in Carcinogenesis and Development of Tumor Cell Heterogeneity

ANDREW P. FEINBERG and DONALD S. COFFEY

Contributors

Numbers in parentheses indicate the pages on which the authors' contributions begin.

R. ALVAREZ (29), NCI-Navy Medical Oncology Branch, Division of Cancer Treatment, National Cancer Institute, Bethesda, Maryland 20814

KENNETH C. ANDERSON (53), Division of Tumor Immunology, Sidney Farber Cancer Institute, and Department of Medicine, Harvard Medical School, Boston, Massachusetts 02115

S. M. ASTRIN (319), The Institute for Cancer Research, The Fox Chase Cancer Center, Philadelphia, Pennsylvania 19111

RICHARD AXEL (425), Institute of Cancer Research, College of Physicians and Surgeons of Columbia University, New York, New York 10032

MICHAEL P. BATES (53), Division of Tumor Immunology, Sidney Farber Cancer Institute, and Department of Medicine, Harvard Medical School, Boston, Massachusetts 02115

STEPHEN B. BAYLIN (9), The Johns Hopkins Oncology Center and the Department of Medicine, The Johns Hopkins University School of Medicine, Baltimore, Maryland 21205

JOSEPH R. BERTINO (169), Departments of Pharmacology and Medicine, Yale University School of Medicine, New Haven, Connecticut 06510

G. R. BRASLAWSKY (301), Biology Division, Oak Ridge National Laboratory, Oak Ridge, Tennessee 37830

P. A. BUNN, JR. (29), NCI-Navy Medical Oncology Branch, Division of Cancer Treatment, National Cancer Institute, Bethesda, Maryland 20814

PAUL CALABRESI (181), Department of Medicine, Brown University, Roger Williams General Hospital, Providence, Rhode Island 02912

D. N. CARNEY (29), NCI-Navy Medical Oncology Branch, Division of Cancer Treatment, National Cancer Institute, Bethesda, Maryland 20814

MOSES V. CHAO (425), College of Physicians and Surgeons of Columbia University, New York, New York 10032

DONALD S. COFFEY (469), The Johns Hopkins Oncology Center and the Departments of Urology and Pharmacology, The Johns Hopkins University School of Medicine, Baltimore, Maryland 21205

F. CUTTITTA (29), NCI-Navy Medical Oncology Branch, Division of Cancer Treatment, National Cancer Institute, Bethesda, Maryland 20814

JOSEPH E. DE LARCO (205), Laboratory of Viral Carcinogenesis, National Cancer Institute, Frederick, Maryland 21701

DANIEL L. DEXTER (181), Department of Medicine, Brown University, Providence, Rhode Island 02912

BRUCE J. DOLNICK (169), Department of Human Oncology, Wisconsin Clinical Cancer Center, University of Wisconsin Center for Health Sciences, Madison, Wisconsin 53792

ANDREW P. FEINBERG (469), The Johns Hopkins Oncology Center, The Johns Hopkins University School of Medicine, Baltimore, Maryland 21205

ISAIAH J. FIDLER (127), Cancer Metastasis and Treatment Laboratory, NCI-Frederick Cancer Research Facility, Frederick, Maryland 21701

PAUL FISHER (261), Department of Microbiology and Cancer Center/Institute of Cancer Research, Columbia University, New York, New York 10032

CHARLOTTE M. FRYLING (205), Laboratory of Viral Carcinogenesis, National Cancer Institute, Frederick, Maryland 21701

ELISABETH GATEFF (331), Biologisches Institut I (Zoologie), Albert-Ludwigs-Universität, Freiburg, Federal Republic of Germany

SEBASTIANO GATTONI-CELLI (261), Division of Environmental Sciences and Cancer Center/Institute of Cancer Research, Columbia University, New York, New York 10032

A. F. GAZDAR (29), NCI-Navy Medical Oncology Branch, Division of Cancer Treatment, National Cancer Institute, Bethesda, Maryland 20814

DONNA L. GEORGE (399), Department of Medicine, The Johns Hopkins University School of Medicine, Baltimore, Maryland 21205

JAMES H. GOLDIE (115), Division of Advanced Therapeutics, Cancer Control Agency of British Columbia, Vancouver, British Columbia V5Z 3J3, Canada

W. S. HAYWARD (319), The Rockefeller University, New York, New York 10021

GLORIA H. HEPPNER (225), Department of Immunology, Michigan Cancer Foundation, Detroit, Michigan 48201

ANN D. HOROWITZ (261), Division of Environmental Sciences and Cancer Center/Institute of Cancer Research, Columbia University, New York, New York 10032

D. C. IHDE (29), NCI-Navy Medical Oncology Branch, Division of Cancer Treatment, National Cancer Institute, Bethesda, Maryland 20814

JOHN ISAACS (99), The Johns Hopkins Oncology Center and the Department of Urology, The Johns Hopkins University School of Medicine, Baltimore, Maryland 21205

VESNA IVANOVIC (261), Haskell Laboratory, DuPont Company, Newark, Delaware 19711

PATRICIA A. JOHNSON (205), Laboratory of Viral Carcinogenesis, National Cancer Institute, Frederick, Maryland 21701

S. J. KENNEL (301), Biology Division, Oak Ridge National Laboratory, Oak Ridge, Tennessee 37830

PAUL KIRSCHMEIER (261), Division of Environmental Sciences and Cancer Center/Institute of Cancer Research, Columbia University, New York, New York 10032

ROBERT LEONARD (53), Division of Tumor Immunology, Sidney Farber Cancer Institute, and Department of Medicine, Harvard Medical School, Boston, Massachusetts 02115

CLEMENT L. MARKERT (237), Department of Biology, Yale University, New Haven, Connecticut 06511

HANS MARQUARDT (205), Laboratory of Viral Carcinogenesis, National Cancer Institute, Frederick, Maryland 21701

M. J. MATTHEWS (29), NCI-Navy Medical Oncology Branch, Division of Cancer Treatment, National Cancer Institute, Bethesda, Maryland 20814

STEVEN L. MCKNIGHT (425), Department of Biochemical Sciences, Fred Hutchinson Cancer Research Center, Seattle, Washington 98104

GEOFFREY MENDELSOHN (9), Department of Pathology, The Johns Hopkins University School of Medicine, Baltimore, Maryland 21205

J. D. MINNA (29), NCI-Navy Medical Oncology Branch, Division of Cancer Treatment, National Cancer Institute, Bethesda, Maryland 20814

LEE M. NADLER (53), Division of Tumor Immunology, Sidney Farber Cancer Institute, and Department of Medicine, Harvard Medical School, Boston, Massachusetts 02115

B. G. NEEL (319), The Rockefeller University, New York, New York 10021

BARRY NELKIN (441), The Johns Hopkins Oncology Center, The Johns Hopkins University School of Medicine, Baltimore, Maryland 21205

P. NETTESHEIM (301), Laboratory of Pulmonary Function and Toxicology, National Institute of Environmental Health Sciences, Research Triangle Park, North Carolina 27709

GARTH L. NICOLSON (83), Department of Tumor Biology, The University of Texas System Cancer Center, Houston, Texas 77030

PETER C. NOWELL (351), Department of Pathology and Laboratory Medicine, University of Pennsylvania School of Medicine, Philadelphia, Pennsylvania 19104

H. OIE (29), NCI-Navy Medical Oncology Branch, Division of Cancer Treatment, National Cancer Institute, Bethesda, Maryland 20814

ALBERT H. OWENS, JR. (3), The Johns Hopkins Oncology Center, The Johns Hopkins University School of Medicine, Baltimore, Maryland 21205

DREW PARDOLL (441), The Johns Hopkins Oncology Center, The Johns Hopkins University School of Medicine, Baltimore, Maryland 21205

EDWARD K. PARK (53), Division of Tumor Immunology, Sidney Farber Cancer Institute, and Department of Medicine, Harvard Medical School, Boston, Massachusetts 02115

G. BARRY PIERCE (249), Department of Pathology, University of Colorado Health Sciences Center, Denver, Colorado 80262

GEORGE POSTE (127), Smith Kline and French Laboratories, Philadelphia, Pennsylvania 19101, and Department of Pathology and Laboratory

Medicine, University of Pennsylvania School of Medicine, Philadelphia, Pennsylvania 19104

VICKI E. POWERS (399), Department of Medicine, The Johns Hopkins University School of Medicine, Baltimore, Maryland 21205

RICHMOND T. PREHN (73), The Institute for Medical Research, San Jose, California 95128

ELLIS L. REINHERZ (53), Division of Tumor Immunology, Sidney Farber Cancer Institute, and Department of Medicine, Harvard Medical School, Boston, Massachusetts 02115

SABINA ROBINSON (441), The Johns Hopkins Oncology Center and Department of Pharmacology and Experimental Therapeutics, The Johns Hopkins University School of Medicine, Baltimore, Maryland 21205

C. E. ROGLER (319), The Institute for Cancer Research, The Fox Chase Cancer Center, Philadelphia, Pennsylvania 19111

S. ROSEN[1] (29), NCI-Navy Medical Oncology Branch, Division of Cancer Treatment, National Cancer Institute, Bethesda, Maryland 20814

U. G. ROVIGATTI (319), The Institute for Cancer Research, The Fox Chase Cancer Center, Philadelphia, Pennsylvania 19111

WALLACE P. ROWE (461), Laboratory of Viral Disease, National Institute of Allergy and Infectious Disease, National Institutes of Health, Bethesda, Maryland 20205

RUTH SAGER (411), Harvard Medical School, and Sidney Farber Cancer Institute, Boston, Massachusetts 02115

AVERY A. SANDBERG (367), Departments of Genetics and Endocrinology, Roswell Park Memorial Institute, Buffalo, New York 14263

STUART F. SCHLOSSMAN (53), Division of Tumor Immunology, Sidney Farber Cancer Institute, and Department of Medicine, Harvard Medical School, Boston, Massachusetts 02115

SAUL SILVERSTEIN (425), College of Physicians and Surgeons of Columbia University, New York, New York 10032

DON SMALL (441), The Johns Hopkins Oncology Center, The Johns Hopkins University School of Medicine, Baltimore, Maryland 21205

[1]Present address: Division of Oncology, Northwestern University, Chicago, Illinois 60611.

V. E. STEELE (301), Laboratory of Pulmonary Function and Toxicology, National Institute of Environmental Health Sciences, Research Triangle Park, North Carolina 27709

RAYMOND W. SWEET (425), College of Physicians and Surgeons of Columbia University, New York, New York 10032

GEORGE J. TODARO (205), Laboratory of Viral Carcinogenesis, National Cancer Institute, Frederick, Maryland 21701

CLAES TROPÉ (147), Department of Oncology, Gynecology Section, University Hospital of Lund, Lund, Sweden

PAUL O. P. Ts'o (285), Division of Biophysics, The Johns Hopkins University School of Medicine, Baltimore, Maryland 21205

DANIEL R. TWARDZIK (205), Laboratory of Viral Carcinogenesis, National Cancer Institute, Frederick, Maryland 21701

BERT VOGELSTEIN (441), Cell Structure and Function Laboratory, The Johns Hopkins Oncology Center, The Johns Hopkins University School of Medicine, Baltimore, Maryland 21205

I. BERNARD WEINSTEIN (261), Division of Environmental Sciences and Cancer Center/Institute of Cancer Research, Columbia University, New York New York 10032

ROBERT S. WELLS (249), Department of Pathology, University of Colorado Health Science Center, Denver, Colorado 80262

J. WHANG-PENG (29), Medicine Branch, Division of Cancer Treatment, National Institutes of Health, Bethesda, Maryland 20205

Editor's Foreword

This fourth volume of the Bristol-Myers Cancer Symposium Series describes a watershed in cancer research. The degree of heterogeneity of human cancer cells was inferred previously, but the research described here makes it very clear that there is great tumor heterogeneity between patients, and indeed within a given tumor site in a given patient. A given tumor type may also change its characteristics longitudinally over time.

These observations in regard to tumor heterogeneity serve a useful purpose in defining the cancer chemotherapy problem, while at the same time they illustrate the limits of classical cancer chemotherapy with selective cytotoxic agents.

The third volume of this series described the encouraging progress made in recent years in the treatment of leukemias and lymphomas, where contact between individual tumor cells and the blood stream is good and high cytotoxic drug levels at tumor cell targets can be achieved. However, the access of drugs to solid tumors such as those of the breast, lungs, and colorectal systems (the most common tumors) is limited. These tumors are relatively hypoxic and the prognosis for successful treatment, especially in advanced disease, is relatively poor. These facts tend to suggest that selective cytotoxicity is not the total answer to the treatment of solid tumors, and we must look to other modalities to supplement the future treatment of cancer. These modalities will be the subject of future volumes.

Recent progress in immunology and the isolation and study of proteins which stimulate or inhibit cell growth suggests several avenues for future research. The isolation of a plethora of tumor antigens and the finding that monoclonal antibodies can be produced with specific affinities for these antigens suggests that these tumor antibodies might be used as carriers for cytotoxic drugs, or liposomes containing cytotoxic drugs, so that the concentration achievable in the tumor can be high relative to the plasma. In this way we could expect to reduce systemic side effects and enhance the antitumor efficacy of cytotoxic drugs.

Perhaps even more significant than the above are the findings that lymphocytes exhibit cooperativeness in their implementation of cell mediated and humoral defense mechanisms, and that this cooperativeness is mediated in part by specific proteins transmitted by plasma. Much work has been done on the isolation and characterization of proteins that affect cell growth; with newer recombinant DNA techniques, it is now practical to make these proteins available in relatively large amounts for research and, ultimately, therapeutic use. There are certain posttranslational events that involve the differentiation or dedifferentiation of cells bearing a common genome. The involvement of proteins in these phenomena provides the clue that may provide a solution to the problem of tumor cell heterogeneity described so ably in this volume.

Maxwell Gordon
Series Editor

Foreword

When Bristol-Myers established its cancer grant program in 1977, we recognized that anything our company might do could be no more than a modest addition to the government's massive program of support for cancer research.

We suggested to the recipients that the Bristol-Myers grants be applied to research that was promising and potentially significant, but, for whatever reason, unlikely to attract federal funding. The grant institutions were to decide how to allocate the Bristol-Myers funding to their research programs.

The grants have thus supported both basic and clinical research, as well as education and patient care. They have enabled outstanding institutions and individuals to pursue innovative ideas wherever they might lead. In the words of one participating scientist, they have provided "a window on the unexpected."

Five years after the original grants were announced, it has become more important than ever to keep that window open. Reductions in government funding are causing cutbacks in many important programs, including federal support of cancer research.

In 1982, Bristol-Myers again expanded its unrestricted cancer grant program to help take up some of the slack caused by government cutbacks. With new grants to Harvard Medical School/Sidney Farber Cancer Institute and McArdle Laboratory for Cancer Research, total funding through the program has reached $5.34 million, funding 11 institutions in the United States and abroad.

Another part of the program is the annual Bristol-Myers Award for Distinguished Achievement in Cancer Research, which was raised from $25,000 to $50,000 in 1982. Finally, there are the annual Bristol-Myers Symposia on Cancer Research, of which this volume is a part. This three-part program is an integral element in our total commitment to cancer research.

Our program continues to be the largest unrestricted commitment ever made by a corporation to support cancer research. Today more than ever, we believe firmly in the worth and rightness of what we are doing. We intend to keep that "window on the unexpected" wide open.

Richard L. Gelb
Chairman of the Board
Bristol-Myers Company

Preface

The Fourth Annual Bristol-Myers Symposium on Cancer Research was held at The Johns Hopkins Oncology Center in December, 1981. The program was designed to explore the genetic and epigenetic mechanisms underlying tumor cell heterogeneity and their implications for the pathogenesis of neoplastic disorders and their practical clinical management. Outstanding scholars from different fields were invited to participate with a view toward stimulating a productive cross-fertilization of ideas.

Tumor cell heterogeneity proved to be a timely topic in that many contributions of significant new knowledge were forthcoming from several sectors of the cancer research community. Many of these contributions were quite complementary; some were provocative. The investigators enjoyed excellent exchanges during the formal and informal portions of the Symposium. We hope that the prompt publication of this volume will convey some of the spirit of the Symposium as well as its scientific content. Clearly much of the work is fundamental to a more complete understanding of neoplasia.

Many individuals contributed to the success of our Symposium through their expert assistance with the organizational details. We wish to thank them all, especially Dawn Jackson, Kay Joellenbeck, and Eleanor Trowbridge. Further, we wish to express our gratitude to the Bristol-Myers Company for its forthright support of cancer research and its sponsorship of this series of symposia.

Albert H. Owens, Jr.
Donald S. Coffey
Stephen B. Baylin

Abbreviations

AbLV, Abelson virus
ABVD, adriamycin, bleomycin, vinblastine, dacarbazine
ALV, avian leukosis virus
AML, acute myelogenous leukemia
ANLL, acute nonlymphocytic leukemia
APUD, amine precursor uptake and decarboxylation
AT, anaplastic tumors
AVP, arginine vasopressin

BP, benzopyrene

CEA, carcinoembryonic antigen
CGL, chronic granulocytic leukemia
CHEF, Chinese hamster fibroblastic cells
CK-BB, BB isoenzyme of creatine kinase
CML, chronic myelogenous leukemia
CT, calcitonin

DAO, diamine oxidase activity
DDC, dopa decarboxylase
DHFT, dihydrofolate reductase
DMS, double minutes

EF, epithelial focus
EFFU, epithelial focus forming units
EGF, epidermal growth factor
FEL, Friend erythroleukemia

G6PD, glucose 6-phosphate dehydrogenase

HITES, hydrocortisone, insulin, transferrin, estradiol-17β, and
   selenium-containing medium
hTGF, human transforming growth factor
HSR$_s$, homogeneously staining regions

IGF, insulin-like growth factor
L-DDC, L-dopa decarboxylase
LC, large cell
LTR, long terminal repeat sequences

MCA, 3-methyl cholanthrene
MCF, mink cell focus-forming viruses
MNNG, methyl nitroso nitroguanidine
MOMSV, Moloney murine sarcoma virus
MOPP, Mustargen, Oncovin, procarbazine, prednisone
MSV, murine sarcoma virus
MTC, medullary thyroid carcinoma
MTX, methotrexate
MuLV, Maloney strain murine leukemia
MUMTV, murine mammary tumor virus

NGF, nerve growth factor
NRK, normal rat kidney
NSCLC, nonsmall cell lung cancer

PAH, polycyclic aromatic hydrocarbons

RSV, Rous sarcoma virus

SCLC, small cell lung cancer
SGF, sarcoma growth factor

TGF, transforming growth factor
TIF, tumor inhibitory factors
TPA, 12-0-tetradecanoyl phorbol-13-acetate

v-onc, retroviral oncogenes
v-src, oncogene of Rous sarcoma virus
vlp, virus-like particles

TUMOR CELL HETEROGENEITY: ORIGINS AND IMPLICATIONS

PART I

Introduction to the Symposium

1

Tumor Cell Heterogeneity: A Perspective

ALBERT H. OWENS, JR.

Cancers and related disorders have shadowed life since its beginnings. In man, cancers arise most commonly in tissues with self-renewing cell systems. In fact, one might look on neoplastic disorders as caricatures of the normal processes of cell replication and maturation.

As viewed by the clinician, cancers consist of altered cell populations which do not respond normally to physiologic controls. They grow in size because of the relatively unrestrained proliferation of their constituent cells. Further, they invade adjacent normal tissues and spread (metastasize) to distant sites by means of lymphatic and vascular channels.

Over the past century, pathologists have become expert in recognizing neoplastic diseases by means of a microscopic examination of suitably stained tissue biopsies and preparations of exfoliated cells. Among the histologic abnormalities commonly encountered are derangements of the cell nucleus and nucleoli, a high frequency of mitotic figures, alterations of normal tissue architecture and evidences of invasion of adjacent structures, or of distant spread. Further, abnormalities of chromosome number and appearance have been associated with neoplastic behavior.

During recent years, it has become increasingly apparent that cancers are composed of complex subpopulations of cells each of which is likely responsible for the expression of different biologic properties (tumor cell heterogeneity). Thus, despite their often monotonously similar morphologic appearance on routine histopathologic examination, distinct classes of cancer cells are now thought responsible for the relatively unrestrained

cellular proliferation, for the spread to distant sites in the body and for the emergence of tumor cells no longer responsive to therapeutic agents. Further, the biologic characteristics of these cell populations undergo constant change. Indeed, continual biologic change seems to be an essential feature of neoplastic disorders.

The mechanisms that underlie neoplastic cell transformation and the progression of "malignant" clinical diseases are subjects of intensive contemporary research activity. So, too, are the factors that are responsible for the biologic heterogeneity which exists in tumor cell populations and which continues to evolve as the diseases progress. While much evidence exists that genetic events are responsible, other data implicate epigenetic (nongenetic) mechanisms. This apparent paradox has generated its share of argument and speculation.

Perhaps the more popular concept of carcinogenesis is that it is a (point) mutational phenomenon. Mutagenic and carcinogenic chemicals as well as ionizing radiations appear to induce cancers by means of alterations in DNA. Similarly some viruses that can insert genetic material into DNA are capable of transforming normal cells into neoplastic. Further, DNA from cancer cells has been reported to transform normal cells under certain circumstances.

However, much recent evidence indicates that the transition of normal cells into cells which display neoplastic characteristics is not a one-step mutation but rather the result of series of interlocking events which take place over a prolonged period, perhaps many months or years in the case of man. Persuasive data are emerging from studies of viral oncogenesis which suggest that the change to a tumorigenic phenotype is triggered by the expression of a particular cellular gene, perhaps a gene more appropriately expressed during embryonic development. Similarly, experimental results indicate that chemical carcinogenesis is a multistep phenomenon. In fact, much of the epidemiologic evidence in man is compatible with the notion that neoplastic disorders result from a multistep process involving genetic controls.

In established neoplasms, cancer cells divide and produce progeny which are like-appearing on superficial morphologic examination. Chromosomal abnormalities are common and in a few instances specific karyotypic changes are characteristic of a particular disease process. (For example, the abnormal Philadelphia chromosome is characteristic of chronic granulocytic leukemia.) These chromosomal alterations may be linked to the "genetic instability" thought responsible for the biologic variability exhibited by the several populations of cells which exist in a given tumor.

Data from cell hybridization studies indicate that there is chromosomal

control over the neoplastic phenotype. Although the results in various mammalian cell types and species seem somewhat contradictory in detail, it is clear that complete suppression of the neoplastic phenotype can be achieved by the fusion of tumorigenic and non-tumorigenic cells. In certain instances, as these hybrid cells continue to divide, tumorigenic clones again emerge presumably in association with the loss of the chromosome(s) responsible for regulatory control. Likely a family of genes is responsible for the complex regulatory interactions underlying these phenomena.

Further evidence that genetic mechanisms underlie neoplastic disorders lies in the fact that certain heritable diseases transmitted according to Mendelian patterns are associated with an increased incidence of cancers. Similarly, laboratory animals can be bred for an increased (or decreased) incidence of cancers.

On the other hand, cogent arguments have been assembled which indicate that neoplastic disorders may arise by means of nonmutational or epigenetic events. When measured directly, the frequency of transformation following exposure to chemicals or x-rays far exceeds the rates of (point) mutation. Further, chemically inert polymers can induce cancers when implanted subcutaneously.

Many "malignant properties" are manifest by normal cells during some stage of development. For example, lymphocytes, granulocytes and macrophages "invade" tissues as part of their normal functioning and move about to distant parts of the body. Similarly, during embryogenesis, there is movement of various cells to distant sites which leads to implantation and the development of new tissues or organs. Many immature or fetal cells possess phenotypic markers found on certain cancer cells. For example, such markers as carcinoembryonic antigen, α-fetoprotein, and fetal isoenzymes are expressed in immature tissue cells as well as in transformed (cancer) cells.

It seems clear enough that normal cells contain the genetic information for many cancer-like traits. In fact, normal cells in culture may express tumor cell traits when treated with tumor promoters, but revert to normal when the promoter is withdrawn. In selected instances, normal germinal or gonadal tissues when transplanted to an ectopic site may display malignant properties.

There is also evidence for the reversion of cancerous growths to a normally controlled state. For example, crown galls transplanted onto the stems of normal plants may revert; and in frogs, a Lucké adenocarcinoma nucleus may produce a tadpole when transplanted into an enucleated normal egg. Teratocarcinoma cells when injected into the blastocysts of mice can be redirected to normal growth including (competent) germ cells which function normally in a "chimeric" adult animal. Human tumor cells have been shown to develop into a more normal phenotype, also.

In well established tumors, there are evidences of cellular interactions which affect biologic behavior. For example, it appears that certain tumor cell subpopulations can influence the rate of proliferation of other cells, their sensitivity to drugs and their propensity to metastasize. Whether disturbing these cellular interactions by the application of noncurative treatments leads to outcomes adverse to the survival of the tumor-bearing host remains to be investigated.

Thus, there seems to be ample indication that genetic and epigenetic mechanisms are responsible for the initiation and evolution of many types of cancer. Further, it seems quite likely that much of the changing biologic behavior of tumor cells is brought about by means of DNA rearrangements.

Gene rearrangement was postulated some 30 years ago as the mechanism responsible for the color variations encountered in maize kernels. The frequency of occurrence of genetic rearrangement in normal mammalian cells is not known, nor is the precise role of DNA rearrangement in normal cell differentiation. However, rearrangement has been implicated in several important systems including the development of diverse antibody types (specific immunoglobulins) in human B lymphocytes.

DNA rearrangement might reconcile some of the genetic and epigenetic arguments about the pathogenesis of cancers. Rearrangement of the linear order of DNA could be responsible for many of the phenomena generally ascribed to (point) mutation, especially since rearrangement could be caused by chemicals, physical agents, viruses, and a host of physiologic (control) substances.

It is the purpose of this Symposium to review the existing evidence for tumor cell heterogeneity, with emphasis on human tumor systems, and to examine the origins and implications of the ever-changing biologic variability characteristic of tumor cell populations. Current methods for identifying functionally important cancer cell subpopulations are presented and the underlying genetic and epigenetic mechanisms discussed. Particular attention is paid to nuclear structure, to DNA arrangement and to the possible major role of genetic rearrangement in determining tumor cell heterogeneity.

PART II

Evidences of Heterogeneity:
Changing Tumor Cell
Populations

2

Medullary Thyroid Carcinoma: A Model for the Study of Human Tumor Progression and Cell Heterogeneity

STEPHEN B. BAYLIN AND GEOFFREY MENDELSOHN

I. Introduction

Cellular heterogeneity is an increasingly recognized component of neoplastic development. The purpose of the present symposium has been to address the challenges that face investigators in further understanding the

TUMOR CELL HETEROGENEITY
Copyright © 1982 by Academic Press, Inc.
All rights of reproduction in any form reserved.
ISBN 0-12-531520-1

processes by which cellular heterogeneity evolves in tumors and the implications of its existence for tumor behavior and for the treatment of cancer. As one might imagine, the challenge of investigating the dynamics of tumor cell heterogeneity in human neoplasms is especially difficult. There are significant logistical problems in obtaining tissues for the direct study of key developmental stages of a given neoplasm. The great variation in the clinical state of tumors at the time of initial detection and tissue acquisition and the inaccessibility of many tumor lesions for the purposes of laboratory research are particular obstacles. Although morphological heterogeneity within human cancers has long been recognized (and taken into account in diagnostic classifications), much remains to be learned about other important aspects of tumor cell heterogeneity including (1) biochemical characterization of different cell populations; (2) variations in metastatic behavior between cells; (3) variations in drug sensitivity between cell populations; and (4) molecular events that underlie the processes of tumor progression.

In the present chapter, we review studies in a particular human cancer which presents a rather unique opportunity to examine the different stages of development in a human neoplasm. The results suggest that vectorial patterns of change in human tumors can be appreciated; and that dynamic shifts in cell populations can have intimate relationships to the different clinical behavior patterns of a single type of cancer. In addition, the data presented suggest that biochemical classifications of tumor cell populations might form a particularly useful adjunct to routine histological classification in predicting the behavior of a given cancer. Finally, we hope that the information summarized illustrates that human tumors can be a potentially rich source for studies of the molecular events that underlie both normal and neoplastic human cell differentiation.

II. Features of Human Medullary Thyroid Carcinoma (MTC) as a Model for the Study of Tumor Cell Heterogeneity

We have discussed previously (Baylin, 1981; Baylin and Mendelsohn, 1980) the unique characteristics of human MTC which allow investigation of the constituent cell populations at various developmental stages of this neoplasm. It is worthwhile to summarize briefly those characteristics for the purpose of the present chapter. First, the facts that the normal parent cell for MTC has been identified (Williams, 1966) and that a biochemical phenotype for this cell has been established (Foster et al., 1964; Hakanson *et al.*, 1971; Pearse, 1966, 1969) provide an ideal background for studying the biochemistry of the neoplasm; for the majority of common human cancers, such information is not available.

Second, the existence of hereditary forms of this human cancer (Keiser *et al.*, 1973; Schimke and Hartmann, 1965) is another critical feature which makes MTC an excellent model for studying the dynamics of tumor evolution and tumor cell heterogeneity. In this setting, measurements of a circulating marker, calcitonin, allow for extraordinarily early diagnosis of MTC in patients at direct genetic risk for the neoplasm (Melvin *et al.*, 1971; Wolfe *et al.*, 1973). Such early diagnoses have made possible investigation of the earliest lesions in the developmental sequence for this proliferative disorder. Finally, patients with MTC display a tremendous spectrum of tumor behavior (Keiser *et al.*, 1973; Lippman *et al.*, 1982). It has thus been possible to correlate biochemical characteristics of tumor tissue with different degrees of aggressiveness of the disease.

Over the past several years, we have attempted to use all of the above characteristics of MTC in an attempt to systematically examine, morphologically and biochemically, the tumor cell populations characteristic of various stages of tumor development and different types of clinical behavior.

III. The Sequence of Events in the Evolution of Hereditary Human MTC

The ability to identify, with immunohistochemical techniques, the normal calcitonin-secreting C cell in the thyroid gland (DeLellis *et al.*, 1977; Wolfe, *et al.*, 1973) and the recognition that calcitonin synthesis is retained to a high degree in MTC (Tashjian and Melvin, 1968) have allowed a portion of the early developmental events in formation of the hereditary tumor to be established. Patients at direct genetic risk for MTC undergo removal of the thyroid gland when they are found to have low-level abnormalities in calcitonin secretion (Wells *et al.*, 1978a,b; Wolfe *et al.*, 1973). The thyroid glands from many of these individuals contain an apparent premalignant state (Wolfe *et al.*, 1973; Mendelsohn *et al.*, 1978) of abnormal C cell proliferation (Fig. 1). In this setting, abnormal numbers of C cells are seen in multiple locations of the thyroid gland but the full formation of tumor nodules, which would displace and alter normal thyroid architecture, is not present. Presumably, this stage of disease represents the earliest manifestation of a multifocal abnormality in the proliferation of thyroid C cells.

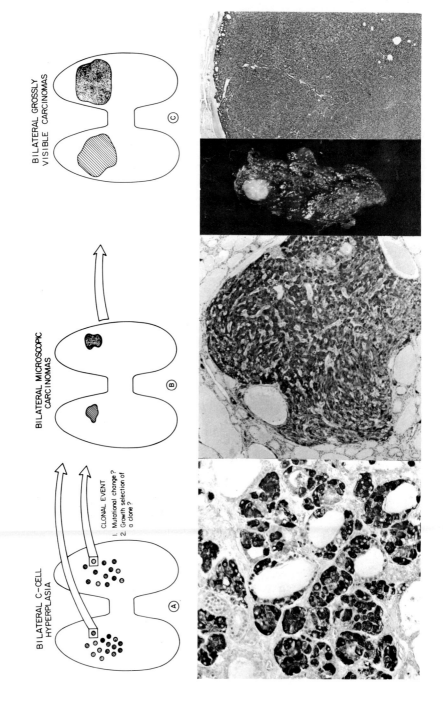

BILATERAL C-CELL
HYPERPLASIA

CLONAL EVENT
1. Mutational change?
2. Growth selection of
a clone?

Ⓐ

BILATERAL MICROSCOPIC
CARCINOMAS

Ⓑ

BILATERAL GROSSLY
VISIBLE CARCINOMAS

Ⓒ

Little is actually known about the exact genetic events that would cause such abnormal proliferation of C cells to begin. In the two-mutational theory of genetic cancer articulated by Knudson *et al.*, (1972, 1975), this multifocal C cell proliferation would represent the inherited defect in patients at risk for developing hereditary MTC. Preliminary evidence that a chromosome alteration is involved has emerged. Karyotypic abnormalities in lymphocytes from patients with the hereditary form of MTC have been preliminarily identified (Van Dyke *et al.*, 1981) and may, if confirmed, represent a genetic event involved in initiating an abnormality in C cell proliferation. In the genetic model of Knudson *et al.* (1972, 1975), this first inherited mutational step would render an increased population of C cells at risk for subsequent steps in malignant transformation which would result in the next stages of MTC.

The next step in tumor formation appears to be the development of microscopic carcinoma from foci of C cell hyperplasia (Fig. 1); again, this often occurs at multifocal points in the thyroid gland. At this stage, larger aggregates of tumor cells can be appreciated which begin to distort the normal architecture of the surrounding thyroid follicles, and which often are seen to contain an extracellular stroma within the tumor lesions (Mendelsohn *et al.*, 1978). Enlargement of these tumor deposits is then responsible for the very small, but grossly visible, multiple tumor deposits which can be found in some patients with early abnormalities of calcitonin secretion (Fig. 1C).

More is known about the apparent sequence of events underlying the formation of these discrete tumor nodules described above. Our own

---

Fig. 1. The early formation of hereditary medullary thyroid carcinoma (MTC). The initial inherited defect results in an increased number of single C cells (C cell hyperplasia) in both lobes of the thyroid (upper panel A). Calcitonin (CT) immunoperoxidase staining (Baylin *et al.*, 1979; Mendelsohn *et al.*, 1978) shows an intense reaction (lower panel A, ×115) in each cell (contrast the dark cytoplasm of the C cells with the light pattern for the surrounding thyroid follicles). The clonal evolution of microscopic carcinoma is shown (upper panel B); the stippled vs. striped pattern for each C cell (panel A) denotes a separate clone and the microscopic tumors on each side of the thyroid (panel B) arise from different clones (see text). As for C cell hyperplasia, CT immunostaining is intense for cells throughout the entire microscopic carcinomas (lower panel B, ×72). Subsequent tumor growth and progression involves enlargement of each microscopic tumor to grossly visible (upper panel C) but still small and not clinically detectable tumor masses. The actual appearance of these lesions is shown in the left lower panel of C; a white nodule is apparent in the upper portion of the thyroid lobe shown and a similar lesion was present in the opposite lobe (not shown). A very low power (×9) photomicrograph of one tumor nodule (lower right panel of C) shows a generalized dark stain in the tumor (contrast to light stain in a small ridge of normal thyroid tissue at the top) reflecting the homogeneous cellular distribution of immunoreactive CT.

work has strongly suggested that each individual carcinoma lesion in a patient with hereditary MTC is formed from a single clone of cells (Baylin *et al.*, 1976). This observation is based on the fact that individual tumor deposits, analyzed for the isoenzyme forms A and B of glucose-6-phosphate dehydrogenase (G6PD) in black females heterozygote for the isozymes, contain only form A or B. In the same individual with multiple tumors, separate clones are involved for each carcinoma since some tumors contain G6PD type A and others type B (Baylin *et al.*, 1978). In the two mutational model of Knudson, our data would suggest that a second mutational event, responsible for eventual carcinoma formation, might occur in a clone of cells rendered susceptible by the inherited defect underlying C cell hyperplasia. Alternatively, final carcinoma formation may result from the selective growth advantage of individual clones among the hyperplastic C cells.

The proven clonal origin of individual carcinomas in patients with hereditary MTC is instrumental to studies of tumor cell heterogeneity in this cancer. As pointed out by Nowell (1976) and in Chapters 9, 15, 16, and 22, the progressive heterogeneity that characterizes many solid tumors can take place in cancers that originally arise from a clonal origin. In human MTC, we can then speculate, with some degree of credibility, that the dynamic changes in tumor cell populations which we describe below represent a time-dependent series of events that take place sequentially in a single clone of tumor cells.

IV. Choice of Biochemical Markers for Study in Human MTC

The C cells of the thyroid gland which give rise to MTC belong to a group of neuroendocrine cells for which some of the sequential steps in development have been outlined. Experimental studies show that these cells arise embryologically in the neural crest (Pearse, 1969) and maintain several neural properties throughout their differentiation. The most prevalent neural property maintained is that of some capability for biogenic amine synthesis (Pearse, 1969) via the enzyme L-aromatic amino acid decarboxylase [L-dopa decarboxylase (DDC)]. It is this ability of many small peptide hormone-secreting endocrine cells to synthesize amines for which Pearse (1969) has coined the term "APUD"; in turn, such APUD properties have now been recognized for the majority of peptide hormone secreting endocrine cells.

The precise sequence of events for the appearance of amine handling properties of endocrine cells versus their capacity, in the terminally differentiated state, to secrete biologically active peptide hormones has not been worked out. However, the work of several investigators in demonstrating a neural origin for some peptide hormone secreting cells (LeDouarin and LeLievre, 1971; Polak *et al.*, 1974) and the work of other investigators in outlining the pathways of differentiation for APUD cells which may not be of neural origin (Cheng and Leblond, 1974; Teitelman *et al.*, 1981) provides clues to events that may occur. We have outlined a working construct for endocrine cell development in Fig. 2 which takes into account some of the findings by these other investigators. This model will be used to illustrate the choice of markers used in our biochemical studies of MTC and to place the findings to be described into perspective.

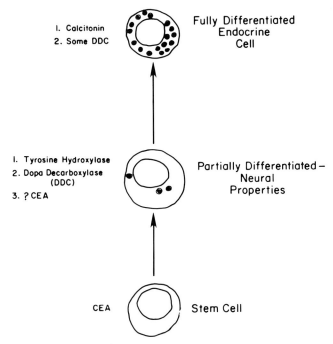

Fig. 2. Possible differentiation events in a peptide hormone secreting neuroendocrine cell (in this case the calcitonin secreting C cell of the thyroid gland). A progressive maturation sequence is shown starting from an undifferentiated stem cell which expresses carcinoembryonic antigen (CEA). The first step in differentiation leads to a cell with a sparse number of neurosecretory granules and predominantly neural features including the presence of the first two enzyme steps in amine synthesizing capacity. The final mature cell is a fully differentiated peptide hormone (calcitonin) secreting cell with a partial capacity for amine synthesis (presence of DDC) and many neurosecretory granules. This temporal sequence of biochemical expression is later related to events in tumor progression for medullary thyroid carcinoma.

In the model, a stem cell is depicted which has relatively undifferentiated features. Since many peptide hormone secreting tumors, now including MTC, have been found at some stages of development (DeLellis et al., 1978; Hamada, 1977) to contain high amounts of carcinoembryonic antigen (CEA), we have depicted this antigen as one possible marker for the stem cell. This postulation takes into account that many normal tissues that give rise to neoplasms containing CEA have been found, on careful examination, to contain some cells capable of producing CEA (Goldenberg et al., 1978).

The stem cell is shown in Fig. 2 giving rise to a more differentiated cell characterized by having some neural properties. This is consistent with the concept of APUD cell development. It is also in keeping with recent data of Teitelman et al. (1981) for the differentiation of rat pancreatic islet cells; during growth of rat embryos, amine biosynthesis activity appeared early during embryonic development and prior to the cellular expression of a specific peptide hormone.

Finally, the terminally differentiated APUD endocrine cell is shown at the top of the Fig. 2 and, in this instance, is depicted as being the C cell of the thyroid gland. This cell is characterized by secretion of a specific polypeptide hormone, calcitonin, and by retention of some neural properties in the form of DDC activity. This stage of development is consistent with findings for normal C cells which are known in most species to contain modest amounts of DDC (Hakanson et al., 1971) as well as having a very high content of the hormone calcitonin.

The markers for study of MTC have largely been chosen to represent the properties of APUD endocrine cells depicted in Fig. 2. These markers are shown in Table I and in three of the four instances represent the spectrum of markers discussed in Fig. 2. The fourth marker shown, diamine oxidase (histaminase) activity, is a known property of human MTC (Baylin et al., 1970). The exact relationship of this enzyme to APUD cells is not known, and our studies were partly designed to place the appearance of this enzyme into perspective for the development of MTC.

V. Cellular Heterogeneity in MTC

We have simultaneously measured the concentrations of three markers, calcitonin (CT), L-dopa decarboxylase activity (DDC), and diamine oxidase activity (DAO), in sections of tumor which represent various clinical stages of MTC (Baylin et al., 1979; Mendelsohn et al., 1978; Lippman et al., 1982; Trump et al., 1979). Immunohistochemical studies of CT and DAO were also performed (Baylin et al., 1979; Mendelsohn et al., 1978).

The results are summarized below and in Table II; the data indicate constantly changing ratios between markers during disease progression and the evolution of cellular heterogeneity.

A. Earliest Stages of MTC

As shown in Table II, slices of thyroid gland containing either premalignant C cell hyperplasia (Fig. 1A) or microscopic carcinoma (Fig. 1B) contained very high amounts of CT relative to the two other markers studied.

TABLE I

Biochemical Parameters Chosen for Study of MTC

1. Calcitonin—The specific polypeptide hormone secreted by normal C cells of the thyroid (Foster et al., 1964; Pearse, 1966).

2. L-Aromatic amino acid decarboxylase [L-dopa decarboxylase (DDC)]— The neurotransmitter synthesis enzyme which represents a neural property of most small polypeptide hormone secreting-endocrine cells (Pearse, 1969).

3. Diamine oxidase [histaminase (DAO)]—An amine (histamine, putrescine) deaminating enzyme activity found in MTC (Baylin et al., 1970).

4. Carcinoembryonic antigen (CEA)—A glycoprotein fetal marker found in tumor tissues (DeLellis, et al., 1978; Hamada, 1977) and the circulation (Wells et al., 1978c) of patients with MTC.

TABLE II

Summary of Biochemical Findings in Progressive Stages of Medullary Thyroid Carcinoma[a]

Stage	Disease vs. normal gland or other tissue[b]			Average ratios— all tissues studied	
	CT	DDC	DAO	DDC/CT	DAO/CT
C cell hyperplasia	+	+	−	0.007	0.006
Microscopic Ca	+	+	+	0.017	0.026
Small tumors	+	+	+	0.003	0.024
Large tumors	+	+	+	0.057	0.094
Metastases	+	+	+	8.50	2.79

[a] Data summarized from Baylin et al. (1979) and Trump et al. (1979).

[b] +, detectable gradient from areas of disease to normal thyroid gland (for primary tumors) and other surrounding normal tissues (for metastic tumor); −, no gradient detected.

These high concentrations of CT were reflected by a homogeneous im-munohistochemistry pattern for the hormone (Fig. 1A). Over 90% of the cells in such lesions manifested strong staining for CT. The high level of CT and the homogeneous cellular distribution for the hormone probably represent a retention of the parent-cell phenotype during the earliest stages of MTC formation.

Only one biochemical parameter suggested a difference between C cell hyperplasia and microscopic carcinoma: the amounts of DAO were signif-icantly higher in microscopic carcinoma and demonstrate a gradient from the areas of diseased thyroid gland to normal thyroid gland (Baylin *et al.*, 1979). Cell heterogeneity for content of DAO was revealed by immunohis-tochemistry studies which detected clusters of cells positive for DAO in these small carcinomas but not in the areas of C cell hyperplasia (Baylin *et al.*, 1979; Mendelsohn *et al.*, 1978).

B. Grossly Visible Primary MTC Lesions

Further biochemical change was apparent when we examined small but grossly visible primary MTC lesions in the thyroid gland. These tumors had a lessening of CT concentration relative to the other two markers so

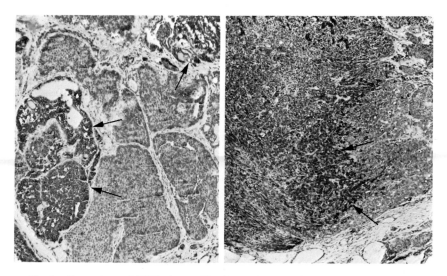

Fig. 3. Two primary MTC lesions with a heterogeneous immunostaining pattern for CT. On the left, separate tumor nodules stain intensely for CT (arrow) while adjacent nodules are negative for the hormone. On the right, clusters of cells stain intensely (arrow) while others are negative within this single nodule. (magnification × 60.)

that ratios of the two enzyme activities to calcitonin were increased as compared to the microscopic lesions discussed above (Table II). This ratio increase was due to two factors: a relative failure of CT concentrations to increase in proportion to the tumor masses and an increase in the specific activities of the other two markers, especially that for DAO.

The relative decrease in CT was even further apparent in large thyroid MTC tumors removed at initial surgery (Table II). Again, both a failure of CT to increase proportional to tumor mass and an increase in specific activities of the other two markers was observed.

In general, the distribution of CT containing cells remained reasonably homogeneous in both small and large grossly visible primary MTC lesions (Fig. 1). Over 90% of the cells stained with an average intensity of approximately 3+. However, a notable exception to this pattern was found in primary thyroid from a small subset of individuals (examples shown in Fig. 3). These tumors had a CT immunostaining pattern similar to that for metastatic lesions discussed below; fewer than 40% of the cells were positive for CT and large areas of CT-negative cells were seen adjacent to cells staining intensely for the hormone (Fig. 3). The clinical implications of this finding for patients with MTC are reviewed in a Section V, D.

C. Metastatic MTC Tissues

During the past two years, we have focused our attention on distant metastatic tumor deposits from patients who have died of widely disseminated MTC (Lippman et al., 1982; Trump et al., 1979). As shown in Table II, a profound reversal of the ratios of CT to the other two markers, as compared to the localized thyroid lesions, can be found. In some instances, as discussed further below, the parent cell hormone, CT, was difficult to detect by the radioimmunoassay procedures. Conversely, specific activities of the two enzyme markers were extremely high in a majority of the tumor desposits tested. Thus, in patients whose disease had progressed to a point where distant metastases dominated the clinical picture, the biochemistry of the tumor tissues appeared to be dramatically altered from that for the phenotype of the parent thyroid C cell and for early tumor lesions developing from it.

A pattern of striking cellular heterogeneity accompanied the biochemical change in metastatic tumor deposits. Nonhomogeneous distribution of CT immunostaining was a characteristic finding in metastatic tumor deposits from patients who have died of MTC (Lippman et al., 1982; Trump et al., 1979). As shown in the example in Fig. 4, all lesions showed less than 40% of cells staining for CT and the intensity of the staining was much diminished from that found for early disease and the typical grossly visible primary thyroid lesions (Fig. 1). In many cases, only a very occa-

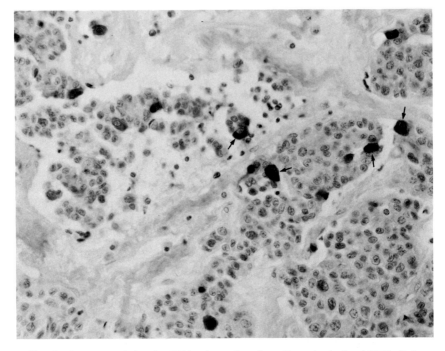

Fig. 4. Immunostaining for CT is shown in a hepatic metastasis of MTC. Only an occasional cell is positive (arrows) while all other surrounding tumor cells fail to stain. × 220.

sional cell stained positive for CT (Fig. 4); metastatic tumor with this staining pattern was present in patients with well-documented familial MTC who had died with an unusually virulent tumor course.

D. Clinical Implications of the Cellular Heterogeneity in MTC

Having identified a series of biochemical changes and evolution of cellular heterogeneity in progressive stages of MTC, we sought to relate the cellular patterns found in primary tumors to the clinical behavior of MTC. Most patients with MTC, especially those with the hereditary form known as multiple endocrine neoplasia type II, have a relatively indolent clinical course. Those patients who have tumor removed at the stages of early microscopic disease have generally remained biochemically free of tumor for periods of 1 to 6 years to date as evaluated by testing of peripheral calcitonin secretion (Lippman *et al.*, 1982; Wells *et al.*, 1978b). The patients presenting with palpable thyroid lesions, which are, of course, grossly visible at the time of surgery, generally retain an abnormality in peripheral calcitonin secretion following surgery (Lippman et al., 1982; Wells et al., 1978b). However, the majority of these patients, despite evidence of residual tumor, do well and may live without signs of clinically evident disease or signs of only slowly progressing disease for many years (Lippman et al., 1982).

We compared the immunohistochemistry findings in 11 patients who presented with palpable thyroid tumors and homogeneous staining patterns for CT (as shown in Fig. 1) to six patients who had primary thyroid tumors with the type of very heterogeneous staining pattern for CT seen in Figs. 3 and 4. As shown in Table III, the presence of cellular heterogeneity for CT in primary MTC tumors appears to have an important correlation with the clinical behavior of MTC. Five of the six patients with heterogeneous staining patterns have died within 1 to 5 years following removal of the primary tumors (Lippman et al., 1982). In contrast, all the 11 patients with homogeneous staining patterns, even those with clear evidence of residual tumor, are alive and doing clinically well during a similar period of follow-up (Lippman et al., 1982).

It is important to note that a number of routine clinical parameters, including age, sex distribution, the presence of familial or sporadic disease, the levels of peripheral CT in the preoperative and postoperative periods, and most importantly, the routine histological examination of the primary tumors, failed to separate the two groups of patients with different CT staining patterns (Lippman et al., 1982). Thus, the type of cellular heterogeneity we are describing in primary MTC tumors could only be appreciated biochemically and through immunostaining procedures. Similarily, the metastatic tumor tissues characterized by altered biochemistry and immunohistochemistry are not distinguished from primary tumors by routine histological procedures.

TABLE III

Survival Analysis in Patients with Homogeneous and Nonhomogeneous Calcitonin Immunostaining Patterns in Primary Medullary Thyroid Carcinoma[a]

CT staining	N	Deaths	Average years of clinical follow-up time (range)
Homogeneous	11	0	3 (0.5–16)
Heterogeneous	6	5[b]	2 (0.5–5)

[a] Data adapted from Lippman et al. (1982).
[b] $p < 0.001$, log rank survival test.

In summary, clinical disease progression in the tumor MTC is correlated with an apparent vectorial change in the biochemistry of the tumor tissue and the distribution of cells which contain the parent cell hormone, CT. In a small group of patients in whom the disease takes an aggressive course, the biochemical abnormalities and cellular heterogeneity for CT distribution can be appreciated in primary tumors at a time prior to clinical evidence for systemic metastases. These observations appear to have immediate clinical relevance in that routine histology of MTC alone may not be sufficient for assessing the clinical status of patients with this tumor. Immunohistochemical studies for CT would seem to be a desirable staging procedure in patients with MTC, especially if further studies of larger groups of patients bear out these initial observations.

E. Biological Considerations for the Changing Biochemistry of MTC

As noted in Section IV, we chose markers for the study of MTC which might be related to the differentiation processes of the type of neuroendocrine cells represented by thyroid C cells and MTC. In the model in Fig. 2, we depicted a working construct of the differentiation sequence of such cells based on information from a number of different investigators. The relative loss of CT in larger MTC tumors, and especially from systemic metastases, with retention of the marker DDC suggested to us that a distinct pattern for change was present in MTC. Furthermore, in the setting of the working construct proposed in Fig. 2, this might indicate the emergence of a more immature phenotype of the neuroendocrine cell with a retention of its amine synthesizing capabilities (an early differentiation event in parent cell formation; Fig. 2) and a loss of synthesis and/or storage capacity for the parent cell peptide hormone, CT (a property that emerges late in terminal differentiation of the parent cell; Fig. 2). Although direct testing for such a hypothesis is difficult in MTC, since the cell does not grow well in culture, we searched for vectorial patterns of biochemical change by analyzing single lesions of systemic metastases from patients who had died of the disease (Lippman et al., 1982). The distribution of the three markers discussed above was systematically tested across regions of these tumor deposits. A distinctly nonrandom pattern was found and regions of tumor where CT concentrations were high were always characterized by low concentrations of the two enzyme activities; the opposite was true for areas of the metastases which were low in CT content. A linear regression analysis of these values showed a highly inverse relationship between the cellular distribution of the two enzyme activities and CT (Lippman et al., 1982).

These above results indicate a highly vectorial pattern to the cellular heterogeneity which is found in MTC. They are most consistent with the hypothesis that the progressive cellular heterogeneity might involve a maturation block in many of the tumor cells; as depicted in Fig. 2, this block would lead to an immature phenotype characterized by reduced capacity for CT secretion and/or synthesis and retention of amine synthesizing capacity via DDC. Interestingly, in studies to be published elsewhere, we have observed in MTC a similar inverse relationship between the appearance of CEA (a marker that might characterize very immature C cells) and CT. In tumor deposits that have a high degree of heterogeneity for CT immunostaining, heavy staining for CEA is generally observed in those areas of tumor that are negative or stain poorly for CT.

The above heterogeneity for CT concentrations and immunostaining in MTC could involve direct changes in the transcriptional processes for expression of the CT gene, but could also involve alterations in posttranslational processing of the hormone which would render it antigenically altered with respect to the antibodies employed in the immunostaining. These alterations, in turn, may again be related to the maturity of the endocrine cell which, in its fully differentiated state, must be capable of cleaving inactive, large molecular precursor forms to smaller biologically active peptide hormones. Investigators have long recognized that endocrine tumors may have altered processing of their parent cell hormones which generally involves a failure to convert the high molecular weight precursor forms to the biologically active products.

Some evidence for alterations in posttranslational processing of CT in both rat and human MTC has already been found by gel chromatography studies (Singer and Habener, 1974; Becker et al., 1978; Roos et al., 1977). We have obtained some preliminary evidence, again, that these abnormalities could be related to progressive alterations which occur during progression of the tumor. In multiple analyses of small MTC lesions by denaturing polyacrylamide gel electrophoresis (Baylin et al., 1981), we have generally found that the small, biologically active form of immunoreactive CT is predominant in extracts of tumor tissue. However, in some larger tumors examined, to date, abnormal accumulation of larger immunoreactive forms has been detected. These larger forms probably represent noncleaved precursor forms of CT (Amara et al., 1980; Jacobs et al., 1979; Moya et al., 1975; Roos et al., 1974). Again, a progressive inability of tumor cells to mature could conceivably alter the precise cleaving of CT precursors to the biologically active form; immaturity of secretory granules and/or other immature characteristics of the cell could be involved in such a process.

VI. Summary

In this chapter, we have presented evidence that progressive cellular heterogeneity, particularly of a biochemical nature, is a concomitant of tumor progression in the human cancer MTC. Through examination of stages of disease ranging from early premalignant lesions to widely disseminated tumor deposits in patients dying of metastatic disease, we have observed alterations in ratios of biochemical markers to one another and distinct alterations in the distribution of cell populations. A vectorial change away from parent cell phenotype is described which is at least partially related to time of tumor growth, and definitely related to the degree of virulence of MTC.

The finding of cellular heterogeneity in MTC is not unexpected since this property of neoplasms is now a widely recognized feature of tumor biology. The challenges for the study of tumor cell heterogeneity in human cancer, which are the major emphasis of this symposium include the need to (1) more fully realize the implications of tumor cell heterogeneity for tumor behavior and treatment; (2) outline further the dynamics of such development in important human cancers; (3) further delineate the parameters that may characterize important types of human tumor cell heterogeneity; and (4) understand the molecular events underlying the changing cell populations in human neoplasms. The information we have obtained in MTC has met some of these challenges and must be studied in far greater detail to accomplish others. First, the changes we have outlined in MTC certainly address the implications of tumor cell heterogeneity for the clinical behavior of tumors. The cellular heterogeneity we have described, particularly for content of the hormone CT, appears to be a concomitant of clinically aggressive behavior in MTC. Second, the dynamics of the heterogeneity presented are partially characterized; certainly, our results strongly suggest that the heterogeneity is progressive with time in MTC and with increasing stages of tumor evolution.

Third, in studying biochemical events in MTC, we have outlined parameters of cellular heterogeneity which would not be recognized by restricting observations to routine histological examination of this tumor. The point that biochemical adjuncts to histological classifications may form an integral part of revising diagnostic categories has now been made for a number of human cancers, including lung carcinomas (Chapter 3) and lymphomas (Chapter 4). A problem in such an approach might arise from the fact that various cell properties that mark evolving cellular heterogeneity in tumors may change totally independent of one another and in a random fashion. If one examines the classic concept of tumor pro-

gression as articulated by Foulds (1954), the variation for the development of cellular heterogeneity within a given type of tumor can be enormous. Thus, one might not expect to recognize observable patterns of
linked events that herald clinically important stages for the natural behavior of a cancer or for the response of the tumor to therapeutic intervention. However, as we have recently stressed for lung cancer (Baylin and
Mendelsohn, 1982) and in the present chapter for MTC, a partial revision
of the tumor progression concept might be warranted. Although there is
certainly variability, over the time of tumor development, in the rate at
which the parameters we have examined in MTC change with relationship
to one another, a distinct pattern clearly is apparent. The individual biochemical markers investigated change in some sequence with respect
to one another and these changes in turn seem to bear some recognizable relationships to the stages of tumor development examined. Thus,
we would suggest that in human cancers a continued rigorous examination of patterns of change in tumor cell characteristics is a worthy goal;
and that such investigations may result in many improvements in our
ability to identify specific stages of individual tumors, to predict their
clinical behavior, and even to monitor the sensitivity of tumor cells to
therapy.

Fourth, and perhaps the biggest challenge addressed by the current
symposium on tumor cell heterogeneity, is the attempt to characterize the
molecular components, both those underlying genetic and epigenetic
changes, which mediate the evolution of the cell heterogeneity. Certainly,
to date, our studies in MTC can only suggest that this tumor model may
be an important one among human cancers for performing such studies.
We have stressed a working concept that depicts the biochemical relationships we have observed within the context of the differentiation process
for the type of neuroendocrine cells from which MTC arises. Some of the
alterations seen in virulent disease appear to represent the emergence of
an immature phenotype relative to the terminally differentiated state of
the parent C cell. This concept would stress the need to examine differentiation sequences in normal human and nonhuman endocrine cells, and
with our advancing technology in study of molecular genetics, to examine
the events in gene expression which might mediate the proper sequence of
biochemical changes which occur over the maturation of the endocrine
cell. In turn, with the use of the ever-increasing battery of genetic probes
available, such studies of human MTC cells at various stages of proliferation and cell growth could prove particularly rewarding in further clarify-
ing the genetic events that may underly the constantly changing ratios of
biochemical markers we have described.

Acknowledgments

The authors express their sincere gratitude to colleagues who have contributed to the data in this chapter (Joseph Eggleston, Donald Gann, Scott Lippman, Donald Trump, and Samuel Wells, Jr.). We also are grateful to Sara Lyles and Gregory Goodwin for technical assistance and Sandra Lund for secretarial services. Portions of these studies were supported by NIH Grants CA-18404, NO1-CB-63994, and Center Grants RR-30, RR-35, and MO1-RR-00722.

References

Amara, S. G., Rosenfeld, M. G., Birnbaum, R. S., and Roos, B. A. (1980). *J. Biol. Chem.* **255**, 2645–2648.

Baylin, S. B. (1981). *In* "Design of Models for Testing Cancer Therapeutic Agents" (I. J. Fidler, and R. J. White, eds.) pp. 50–63. Reinhold, New York.

Baylin, S. B., and Mendelsohn, G. (1980). *Endocrinol. Rev.* **1**, 45–77.

Baylin, S. B., and Mendelsohn, G. (1982). *Semin. Oncol.*, (in press).

Baylin, S. B., Beaven, M. A., Engelman, K., and Sjoerdsma, A. (1970). *N. Engl. J. Med.* **283**, 1239–1244.

Baylin, S. B., Gann, D. S., and Hsu, S. H. (1976). *Science (Washington, D.C.)* **193**, 321–323.

Baylin, S. B., Hsu, S. H., Gann, D. S., Smallridge, R. C., and Wells, S. A., Jr. (1978). *Science (Washington, D.C.)* **199**, 429–431.

Baylin, S. B., Mendelsohn, G., Weisburger, W. R., Gann, D. S., and Eggleston, J. C. (1979). *Cancer* **44**, 1315–1321.

Baylin, S. B., Wieman, K. C., O'Neil, J. A., and Roos, B. A. (1981). *J. Clin. Endocrinol. Metab.* **53**, 489–497.

Becker, K. L., Snider, R. H., Silva, O. L., and Moore, C. F. (1978). *Acta Endocrinol. (Copenhagen)* **89**: 89–99.

Cheng, H., and Leblond, C. P. (1974). *Am. J. Anat.* **141**, 537–562.

DeLellis, R. A., Nunnemacher, G., and Wolfe, H. J. (1977). *Lab. Invest.* **36**, 237–298.

DeLellis, R. A., Rule, A. H., Spiler, I., Nathanson, L., Tashjian, A. H., Jr., and Wolfe, H. J. (1978). *Am. J. Clin. Pathol.* **70**, 587–594.

Foster, G. V., MacIntyre, I., and Pearse, A. G. E. (1964). *Nature (London)* **203**, 1029–1030.

Foulds, L. (1954). *Cancer Res.* **14**, 327–339.

Goldenberg, D. M., Sharkey, R. M., and Primus, F. J. (1978). *Cancer* **42**, 1546–1553.

Hakanson, R., Owman, C., and Sundler, F. (1971). *Biochem. Pharmacol.* **20**, 2187–2192.

Hamada, S., and Hamada, S. (1977). *Br. J. Cancer* **36**, 572–576.

Jacobs, J. N., Potts, J. T., Jr., Bell, N. H., and Habener, J. F. (1979). *J. Biol. Chem.* **254**, 10600–10603.

Keiser, H. R., Beaven, M. A., Doppman, J., Wells, S. A., Jr., and Buja, L. M. (1973). *Ann. Intern. Med.* **78**, 561–579.

Knudson, A. G., Jr., and Strong, L. C. (1972). *Am. J. Hum. Genet.* **24**, 514–532.

Knudson, A. G., Jr., Hethcote, H. W., and Brown, B. W. (1975). *Proc. Natl. Acad. Sci., U.S.A.*, **72**, 5116–5120.

LeDouarin, N. M., and LeLièvre, C. (1971). *CR Assoc. Anat.* **152**, 558–568.

Lippman, S. M., Mendelsohn, G., Trump, D. L., Wells, S. A., Jr., and Baylin, S. B. (1982). *J. Clin. Endocrinol. Metab.* **54**, 233–240.

Melvin, K. E. W., Miller, H. H., Tashjian, A. H., Jr. (1971). *N. Engl. J. Med.* **285,** 1115–1120.

Mendelsohn, G., Eggleston, J. C., Weisburger, W. R., Gann, D. S., and Baylin, S. B. (1978). *Am. J. Pathol.* **92,** 35–52.

Moya, F., Nieto, A., Candela, J. L. R. (1975). *Eur. J. Biochem.* **55,** 407–413.

Nowell, P. C. (1976). *Science (Washington, D.C.)* **194,** 23–28.

Pearse, A. G. E. (1966). *Vet. Rec.* **79,** 587–590.

Pearse, A. G. E. (1969). *J. Histochem. Cytochem.* **17,** 303–313.

Polak, J. M., Pearse, A. G. E., LeLievre, C., Fontaine, J., LeDouarin, N. M. (1974). *Histochemistry* **40,** 209–214.

Roos, B. A., Okano, K., and Deftos, L. J. (1974). *Biophys. Res. Commun.* **60,** 1134–1140.

Roos, B. A., Parthemore, J. G., Lee, J. C., and Deftos, L. J. (1977). *Calcif. Tissue Res.* **22,** 298–302. (Suppl.)

Schimke, R. N., and Hartmann, W. H. (1965). *Ann. Intern. Med.* **63,** 1027–1037.

Singer, F. R., and Habener, J. F. (1974). *Biochem. Biophys. Res. Commun.* **61,** 710–716.

Tashjian, A. H., Jr., and Melvin, K. E. W. (1968). *N. Engl. J. Med.* **279,** 279–283.

Teitelman, G., Joh, T. H., and Reis, D. J. (1981). *Proc. Natl. Acad. Sci. U.S.A.* **78,** 5225–5229.

Trump, D. L., Mendelsohn, G., and Baylin, S. B. (1979) *N. Engl. J. Med.* **301,** 253–255.

Van Dyke, D. L., Jackson, C. E., and Babu, V. R. (1981). *Am. Soc. Hum. Gen., Abstr.* **209,** 69A.

Wells, S. A., Jr., Baylin, S. B., Linehan, W. M., Farrell, R. E., Cox, E. B., and Cooper, C. W. (1978a). *Ann. Surg.* **188,** 139–141.

Wells, S. A., Jr., Baylin, S. B., Gann, D. S., Farrell, R. E., Dilley, W. G., Preissig, S. H., Linehan, W. M., and Cooper, C. W. (1978b). *Ann. Surg.* **188,** 377–383.

Wells, S. A., Haagenson, D. E., Linehan, W. M., Farrell, R. E., and Dilley, W. G. (1978c). *Cancer* **42,** 1498–1503.

Williams, E. D. (1966). *J. Clin. Pathol.* **19,** 114–118.

Wolfe, H. J., Melvin, K. E. W., Cervi-Skinner, S. J., Al Saadi, A. A., Juliar, J. P., Jackson, C. E., and Tashjian, A. H., Jr. (1973). *N. Engl. J. Med.* **289,** 437–441.

Note Added in Proof

Recently, Rosenfeld and colleagues [Rosenfeld, M. G., Lin, C. R., Amara, S. G., Stolarsky, L., Roos, B. A., Ong, E., and Evans, R. M. (1982). *Proc. Natl. Acad. Sci. U.S.A.* **79,** 1717–1721] have obtained evidence for a molecular mechanism in rat medullary thyroid carcinoma cells which may account for the switch from a high to a low calcitonin producing tumor cell. Differential RNA splicing events between the high and low calcitonin synthesizing cells appear to occur. The low calcitonin producing cells contain mRNA encoding a separate region of the calcitonin nuclear RNA transcript.

3

Heterogeneity and Homogeneity of Human Small Cell Lung Cancer

J. D. MINNA, D. N. CARNEY, R. ALVAREZ, P. A. BUNN, JR., F. CUTTITTA, D. C. IHDE, M. J. MATTHEWS, H. OIE, S. ROSEN, J. WHANG-PENG, AND A. F. GAZDAR

TUMOR CELL HETEROGENEITY
ISBN 0-12-531520-1

29

I. Introduction

There will be 110,000 new cases of lung cancer in the United States in 1981 and 25% of these will be histologically typed as small cell lung cancer (SCLC) (Minna *et al.*, 1981c). This type of lung cancer arises from cells of a diffuse neuroendocrine system which is, in part, composed of the amine precursor uptake and decarboxylation (APUD) system (Gazdar *et al.*, 1981a). In the lung, the APUD precursor cell giving rise to SCLC is probably the Kultschitzky cell which in the normal respiratory mucosa expresses APUD properties (Pearse, 1969; Bonikos and Bensch, 1977). SCLC in over 95% of cases is usually beyond the bounds of surgical resection at the time of presentation and the primary treatment is usually with combination chemotherapy with or without radiotherapy (Minna *et al.*, 1981c; Bunn and Ihde, 1981; Bunn *et al.*, 1981). The degree of heterogeneity between SCLC from different patients and within individual patient's tumors may have great clinical relevance. In assessing the homogeneity or heterogeneity of human SCLC, studies in patients are diffficult to do. However, with the advent of successful methods for culturing human SCLC *in vitro* studies can be performed (Gazdar *et al.*, 1980; Carney *et al.*, 1980a; Carney *et al.*, 1981a). The analysis of both clinical and *in vitro* data pertaining to tumor cell heterogeneity is the subject of this presentation.

II. Histology of Small Cell Lung Cancer

A. Homogeneity of Histological Subtypes

From analysis of autopsy material, bronchial biopsies, bronchial washings, sputum cytology, and biopsies of lymph nodes, liver, bone marrow, soft tissue masses, and resected pulmonary tumors there is general acceptance of light microscopic criteria for the histological diagnosis of

SCLC (Matthews and Gazdar, 1981; Carney *et al.*, 1980b). The World Health Organization Lung Cancer Classification divides SCLC into (1) an oat-cell (lymphocyte-like) subtype; (2) an intermediate subtype (including fusiform, polygonal, and "other" subtypes); and (3) a "combined" subtype, composed of small cell carcinoma combined with frank adenocarcinoma or squamous cell carcinoma. In all cases, cytoplasm is sparse, nuclei hyperchromatic, prominent nucleoli are rare, host chronic inflammatory response and desmoplasia are often minimal, and there often is marked DNA staining of elastic fibrils in areas of necrosis (Matthews and Gazdar, 1981). The lymphocyte-like type is characterized by cells with uniform nuclei, over twice the size of a lymphocyte, with the nuclei being round, oval, or spindled but always hyperchromatic while the cytoplasm is sparse and by light microscopic criteria appears to be absent. The cells may be arranged in loose clusters, ribbons, or pseudorosettes supported by a thin vascular fibrous stroma. The intermediate type is characterized by cells with nuclei 2–3 times the size of a lymphocyte, the chromatin being distributed uniformly throughout the nucleus, and the cytoplasm, although sparse, is more distinct than in the lymphocyte-like type, and the cells are arranged in sheets, pseudoductal structures, ribbons, tubules, or trabecular pattern.

B. Heterogeneity of Histological Subtypes

The WHO "intermediate" subtype includes two examples of histological heterogeneity within individual tumors. The first is where mixtures of lymphocyte-like tumor cells are combined with the fusiform or polygonal intermediate subtypes. In prior nomenclature used by the Working Party for the therapy of lung cancer (WPL) the lymphocyte-like type (oat cell) was called WPL-21, the fusiform and polygonal intermediate types were called WPL-22, and the mixed type was referred to as WPL-21/22. The mixture of cell types occurs in about 7% of diagnostic biopsy specimens of SCLC. (Table I). In addition, when multiple biopsies are available from an individual patient, there will be concordance between the SCLC histological subtype of the primary diagnostic specimens (e.g., bronchial biopsy) and other specimens (e.g., bone marrow biopsy) in 74% of cases and discordance (multiple SCLC subtypes) in 26% (Carney *et al.*, 1980b).

Another example of histological heterogeneity within an individual patient's tumor and included in the WHO "intermediate" subtype are tumors with a mixture of characteristics of the fusiform or polygonal subtype, and large cells with abundant cytoplasm and prominent large nuclei, prominent nucleoli, and distinct cytoplasmic borders (WPL 22/40) (Fig. 1). This latter subtype occurs in 5–15% of tumors at the time of diagnosis

TABLE I

Histological Subtypes of Small Cell Lung Cancer Found in Pretreatment Specimens[a]

Classification[b]		(%)
WHO	WPL	Frequency
		(N = 156)
Oat cell	Lymphocyte-like (WPL-21)	44
Intermediate	Fusiform, polygonal, tubular (WPL-22)	34
Oat cell	Mixed lymphocyte, fusiform, polygonal (WPL-21/22)	7[c]
Intermediate	Fusiform, polygonal, lymphocyte-like mixed with large cell cancer (WPL-22/40)	12
Combined	Small cell with squamous cell or adenocarcinoma (WPL-22/12 or 22/32)	<1

[a] Adapted from Carney et al. (1980b) and Radice et al. (1981).
[b] WHO, World Health Organization; WPL, Working Party for therapy of lung cancer.
[c] In patients thought to have no histological heterogeneity on the diagnostic biopsy specimen, 26% will have a different histological subtype of pure SCLC (e.g., lymphocyte-like, fusiform, polygonal) if multiple biopsies are examined from different sites within individual patients.

and, as will be discussed, is the best studied in clinical and experimental systems. The "combined" subtype of the WHO classification includes small cell tumors with squamous carcinoma or adenocarcinoma and occurs in <1% of SCLC cases at presentation. However, this combined type is seen in over one-third of treated cases at autopsy (Matthews, 1979; Abeloff et al., 1979).

C. Response and Survival Characteristics of Histological Subtypes

We have conducted a detailed analysis of response to combination chemotherapy and survival of the different histological subtypes of SCLC (Carney et al., 1980b; Radice et al., 1981; Matthews and Gazdar, 1981) (Table II). There are essentially no significant response or survival differences between the oat cell (lymphocyte-like, WPL-21), and the intermediate types of SCLC that have "pure" SCLC histology (fusiform, polygonal, and mixtures of these, WPL-22, WPL21/22). The slight differences in overall response rate between the homogeneous (WPL-21, or WPL-22) subtypes and the patients with mixtures of these (WPL-21/22) (75% vs. 90%) are not statistically significant. In contrast, those patients showing mixtures of small cell and large cell cancer (WPL-22/40) have significantly diminished response to combination chemotherapy and median survival

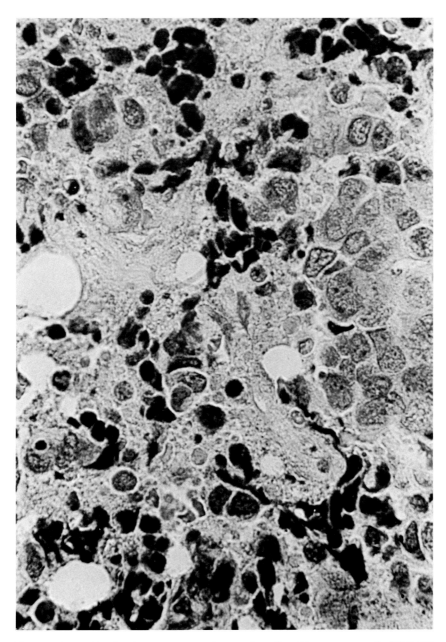

Fig. 1. Biopsy showing heterogenous mixture of small and large tumor cells (WPL-22/40).

TABLE II

Response and Survival Characteristics of Small Cell Lung Cancer Histological Subtypes[a]

Classification			Therapy response[b] (%)			Median survival[b]
WHO	WPL	N	Complete	Partial	None	(weeks)
Oat cell	WPL-21	54	47	39	4	43
Oat cell	WPL-21/22	8	50	25	25	44
Intermediate	WPL-22	41	49	42	9	43
Intermediate	WPL-22/40	19	16	42	42	26

[a] Adapted from Carney et al. (1980b) and Radice et al. (1981).

[b] Significant differences for response to therapy and survival: $p < 0.001$ for response to therapy between WPL-22/40 group and other "pure" SCLC groups; $p = 0.008$ for survival between WPL-22/40 and other "pure" SCLC groups. Differences between other groups are not statistically significant.

(Table II). Although not presented here, there were no significant differences in other factors that could account for these response and survival differences such as performance status, age, sex, or stage of disease (Carney et al., 1980b; Radice et al., 1981). We conclude that the presence of histological heterogeneity of the small cell plus large cell (WPL 22/40) type in the initial biopsy specimens has a significantly inferior clinical prognosis compared to the other SCLC histological subtypes. However, in the NCI registry of long-term survivors of SCLC it is interesting to note that 10% of the patients were of the small cell plus large cell (WPL 22/40) histological subtype (Matthews et al., 1980). Thus, the presence of this type does not preclude potential cure.

III. Clinical Aspects of Small Cell Lung Cancer

The homogeneity of the clinical aspects of SCLC has been reviewed in detail elsewhere (Minna et al., 1981c; Bunn and Ihde, 1981; Ihde et al., 1981). The tumor presents as a primary lesion in the chest, is metastatic to regional (mediastinal) lymph nodes in over 70% of cases, and has distant, extrathoracic metastases in over 70% when carefully staged. In 4% of cases, histologically, typical small cell carcinomas can present as an extrapulmonary neoplasm (Levenson et al., 1981). Presumably these tumors arose from APUD cells known to be located outside the chest (Pearse, 1969).

There is a vast literature of data concerning responsiveness of SCLC to combination chemotherapy or radiotherapy (Minna et al., 1981c; Bunn and Ihde, 1981). With appropriate treatment, over 90% of patients demonstrate an objective tumor response to combination chemotherapy with or without radiotherapy, with significant increases in survival compared to no or lesser treatments. Approximately 50% of all patients obtain a complete clinical regression of tumor and these patients have significantly better survival than patients with lesser (partial) responses. In addition, all of the long-term survivors come from the complete responding group. In fact, 5–10% of all patients are potentially cured, being alive and free of clinical evidence of disease 4 or more years from the start of therapy (Minna *et al.*, 1981c; Bunn *et al.*, 1981).

The majority of available evidence suggests that the ability to obtain a complete response and long-term survival are related to pretreatment stage and particularly total bulk of tumor, and pretreatment performance status, rather than to differences (heterogeneity) between tumors (Ihde *et al.*, 1981). Whether the propensity to develop multiple sites of extrathoracic metastastic disease or liver or brain mestastases (all poor prognostic signs) (Ihde *et al.*, 1981) is related to biological differences between individual small cell tumors or tumor subpopulations within individual patients remains to be determined.

Within individual patients, with the exception of sanctuary sites in the central nervous system, and liver metastases, other sites of tumor appear to respond equally well to combination chemotherapy. The reason for the lesser response of liver metastases is unknown. While drug resistance ultimately develops in 90% of patients, this appears to occur in the prior sites of bulk disease. However, this has not been documented extensively.

The hypothesis that patients achieving a complete response may have received a chemotherapy regimen which by chance contains drugs to which they are very sensitive, while other patients treated with the same regimen who only achieve a partial response may have tumors with lesser sensitivity to that combination remains to be proved. In fact, clinical trials have not suggested that patients showing a partial response to one regimen are extremely sensitive to another regimen (Bunn and Ihde, 1981). If this sensitivity could be worked out through *in vitro* drug and radiation sensitivity testing significant clinical treatment advances would occur.

IV. Chromosomal Aspects of Small Cell Lung Cancer

A. Homogeneity: del(3)(p14-23) Is a Specific Marker of Small Cell Lung Cancer

Chromosome banding studies have been carried out on continuous, clonable cell lines, and on 2- to 3-day short-term cultures of SCLC tumors which revealed a specific chromosomal defect associated with human small cell lung cancer (Whang-Peng *et al.*, 1982a,b). We found that all of the metaphases of all of the SCLC tumors studied had a deletion involving a portion or all of the short arm of chromosome 3 (Table III). Shortest region of overlap analysis showed that the common region deleted was del(3)(p14-23) often expressed as an interstitial deletion. This deletion was found in small cell tumors biopsied before any chemotherapy, and in tumors relapsing on chemotherapy. It was seen in tumors derived from males and females, in tumors from a variety of metastatic sites, in tumor cell lines started directly from patients, or from nude mouse heterotransplantation, in short-term (2-day) cultures, or direct preparations of tumor cells from bone marrow, and was preserved in continuously growing SCLC lines for periods of over 97 months. This was seen in a tumor obtained from Shimosato from Japan (NCI-N230), and another from the Johns Hopkins Cancer Center (NCI-H175, also called OH-1). It was not seen in B lymphoblastoid lines autologous to the tumors (for example, in B lymphoblastoid lines NCI-H128BL, or NCI-H209BL autologous to SCLC lines NCI-H128 and NCI/H209), or in diploid cells in the peripheral blood or bone marrow or patients whose aneuploid tumor cells demonstrated the abnormality (e.g., NCI-P220, NCI-P329, NCI-P340). Thus, the 3p abnormality is an acquired somatic cell defect that is tightly associated with the continued replication of the tumor cells. Of great interest, lines derived from SCLC that contained mixtures of small cells and large cells (e.g., NCI-H175, NCI-H196), or which had converted to large cells entirely (e.g., NCI-H82) exhibited 100% of metaphases with the del 3p. While defects in chromosome 3 were occasionally seen in 5 non-small lung cancer lines (including a large cell lung cancer) the del(3)(p14-23) was not consistently seen. Thus, the defect appears to be specific for SCLC.

In many cases, a normal appearing chromosome 3 (often in several copies) was seen in addition to the del(3). Similarly, often multiple copies of the del(3) were also present. (Whang-Peng, 1981b). Whether the del 3p is causally related to the malignant behavior of SCLC or only associated remains to be determined. Likewise, whether the deleted portion of 3 is translocated to another chromosomal site or loss from the cell is unknown. Thus, the possibilities for mechanism of action include a deletion with expression of a recessive gene on the normal appearing chromosome 3, or insertion of the deleted region somewhere else in the genome to disrupt normal cell functions.

B. Heterogeneity of Other Chromosomal Changes in Small Cell Lung Cancer

Numerical abnormalities were found in nearly every SCLC. There was considerable heterogeneity of chromosome numbers between SCLC lines

TABLE III

Homogeneity of Abnormalities of Chromosome 3 in Small Cell Lung Cancer[a]

Cell line	Sex	Source	Cytology	Time	3p abnormalities[b]
Small cell tumors with no prior chemotherapy					
NCI-P220	M	BM	SCLC	2 days	del(3)(p14-23),del(3)(p14q13)
NCI-H220	M	PE	SCLC	8 months	del(3)(p11),del(3)(p13q13)
NCI-H187	M	PE	SCLC	4 months	del(3)(p14q13),del(3)(p14-23)
NCI-H250	M	Brain	SCLC	5 months	del(3)(p14-23)
NCI-H182	F	LN	SCLC	8 months	del(3)(p14-23)
NCI-H209	M	BM	SCLC	11 months	del(3)(p14)
NCI-N230	M	Lung	SCLC	97 months	del(3)(p14q13)
Small cell tumors relapsing on chemotherapy					
NCI-P329	M	BM	SCLC	2 days	del(3)(p14-23)
NCI-P340	M	BM	SCLC	Direct	del(3)(p14q21),del(3)(p14-23)
NCI-P340	M	PB	SCLC	3 days	del(3)(p14q21),del(3)(p14-23)
NCI-H211	F	BM	SCLC	4 months	del(3)(p14-23),t(3;19)(p13qter:p11 qtr)
NCI-H175 (OH-1)	M	PE	SCLC + LC	6 months	del(3)(p23q26)
NCI-H82	M	PE	LC	10 months	del(3)(p21),inv(3)(p14-23)
NCI-H146	M	BM	SCLC	11 months	del(3)(p14q24)
NCI-H140	M	LN	SCLC	12 months	del(3)(p13),del(3)(p14-23)
NCI-H69	M	PE	SCLC	13 months	del(3)(p21-24),del(3)(p23q26)
NCI-H196	M	PE	SCLC + LC	14 months	del(3)(p13-23),del(3)(p13)
NCI-H64	M	LN	SCLC	14 months	del(3)(p14-23)
NCI-H60	F	PE	SCLC	17 months	del(3)(p14-21),t(3;4) (p23 q11:q11 qter)
NCI-H128	M	PE	SCLC	26 months	del(3)(p14q23),del(3)(p14)

[a] Adapted from Whang-Peng et al. (1982b). Cell line prefixes: H, cell line started directly from human tumor; N, cell line started from nude mouse heterotransplant; P, short-term (2-day) culture or direct preparation from the patient. Source of tumors: M, male; F, female; PE, pleural effusion; BM, bone marrow; LN, lymph node. Cytology: SCLC, small cell lung cancer; LC, large cell cytology; SCLC + LC = mixture of cells, some with small cell and some with large cell cytology. Time = months or days in culture. Direct = spreads made directly from patient tumor sample without intervening culture.

[b] At least one 3p abnormality present in 100% of the metaphases studied for each cell line.

including hypodiploid, near diploid, hyperdiploid, tetraploid, and bimodal tumors (Table IV). Thus, the expression of malignancy and the biochemical APUD program (to be discussed) was indepenedent of the modal number of chromosomes. Several tumors had bimodal chromosome numbers (each mode containing the specific 3p deletion abnormality) and represent dramatic examples of heterogeneity within individual tumors. We have performed a clonal analysis on one of the SCLC lines (NCI-H128) which has a bimodal number of chromosomes. Both tumor cells obtained from the original pleural effusion, and in the continuously growing tissue culture line had two DNA content peaks (one at 1.3 and the other at a DNA content of 1.5 relative to a normal diploid DNA content of 1.0). This line was cloned in soft agar and the subclones assayed for DNA content by flow cytometry. Three clones had a single DNA content peak of 1.3, while nine clones had a DNA content peak of 1.5. None of the clones had a bimodal DNA content indicating that the heterogeneity of DNA content in the original tumor reflected clonal heterogeneity, and also confirmed the clonal nature of the isolates. As will be discussed later, all 12 clones had biochemical markers (e.g., L-dopa decarboxylase) and cytomorphology typical of SCLC.

Every chromosome except 18 was involved in a structural aberration. However, the most frequently involved chromosomes in structural aberrations in different tumors are listed in Table V. In these cases not all of the tumor cell metaphases [documented by the presence of a del(3p)] had the indicated structural aberration. Thus, there was heterogeneity (mosaicism) within SCLC lines in the large majority of cases for structural abnormalities of chromosomes 1, 2, 9, 10, and 14. Whether certain structural

TABLE IV

Heterogeneity of Chromosome Number between Small Cell Lung Cancer Lines[a]

Chromosome number	No. of cell lines
Hypodiploid	3
Near diploid	1
Hyperdiploid	7
Tetraploid	4
Bimodal	3
Hypodiploid + near tetraploid	
Two hyperdiploid peaks	
Hyperdiploid + hypertetraploid	
Total	18

[a] Adapted from Whang-Peng et al. (1982b).

TABLE V

Most Frequently Involved Chromosomes in Structural Aberrations Creating Heterogeneity (Mosaicism) within Small Cell Lung Cancer Tumors[a]

Structurally aberrant chromosome	No. of cell lines with abnormality ($N = 18$)
1	13
2	11
9	10
10	12
14	10

[a] Adapted from Whang-Peng et al. (1982b). All lines had del(3)(p14-23) or greater deletion of 3p in 100% of the metaphases and the indicated structural aberration in less than 100% of the metaphases, thus creating heterogeneity for these chromosomal aberrations within individual tumors.

abnormalities are associated with different clinical or biological behavior remains to be determined.

V. Biochemical Markers Associated with Small Cell Lung Cancer

A. Homogeneously Expressed Markers

Using the established SCLC tissue culture cell lines as well as biopsy and autopsy samples from patients, we have studied the expression of a variety of biochemical markers, particularly those related to the APUD cell origin of SCLC (Table VI). We have found the expression of high specific activities of L-dopa decarboxylase (L-DDC, EC 4.1.1.28), formaldehyde induced fluorescence, dense core ("neurosecretory") granules, neuron specific enolase (EC 4.2.1.11), and the BB isozyme of creatine kinase (CK-BB) (EC 2.7.3.2) all to be characteristic of SCLC and expressed at levels 100-fold or higher than in non-small cell lung cancer (NSCLC) types (epidermoid, adenocarcinoma, large cell carcinoma, and mesothelioma). These markers thus provide biochemical footprints of the differentiation of SCLC (Gazdar et al., 1980, 1981a, b, c).

To search for heterogeneity, we have conducted a clonal analysis of SCLC lines for the expression of L-DDC and cytomorphology. Several lines (NCI-H128, NCI-H60, NCI-H69) with typical SCLC cytology which expressed significant levels of L-DDC were cloned in soft agar and the

TABLE VI

Homogeneous Expression of Biochemical Markers in Small Cell Lung Cancer Tumors and Cell Lines Demonstrating "Pure" Small Cell Cytology (Lymphocyte-Like, Fusiform, Polygonal)[a]

Marker	Range of expression in lung cancer types	
	Small cell	Non-small cell
Dense core granules	clusters	absent
Formaldehyde induced fluorescence	+	−
L-dopa decarboxylase (Units/mg protein/hour)	22–646	<0.1
CK-BB (ng/mg protein)	2,490–17,555	0–420
Neuron-specific enolase (ng/mg protein)	280–5,017	11–137
Bombesin (pmol/mg protein)	0.02–12.7	<0.01

[a] Adapted from Gazdar et al. (1980, 1981a,b,c), Moody et al. (1981), and unpublished data. Data from 18-19 SCLC and 9-10 NSCLC tissue culture lines. All the SCLC lines had "pure" small cell cytology.

clonal progeny assayed for cytology and L-DDC specific activity. While there were up to eight-fold variations in L-DDC special activities, all of 48 subclones expressed high specific L-DDC activities. In contrast, large cell variants (NCI-N231/417 and NCI-H82) expressing low activities of L-DDC but having the 3p deletion, were cloned and all the progeny expressed low specific activities of L-DDC (Table VII). As will be discussed later, these large cell variants were either derived from a line with typical small cell cytomorphology (NCI-N231) which expressed high specific activities of L-DDC, or from a primary tumor (NCI-H82) with mixtures of small and large cells (WPL-22/40). In addition, there was perfect correlation in the clones between the expression of the typical SCLC cytology with high levels of L-DDC. Thus, there appears to be clonal stability of expression of L-DDC and cytomorphology. Recently, we have discovered that a new polypeptide hormone, bombesin, is often expressed in very high levels in SCLC (Moody et al., 1981). We were prompted to look for this peptide hormone because of the recently described presence of "bombesinergic cells" in the fetal lung (presumably the fetal Kultschitzky cell) (Wharton et al., 1978). We have not yet performed a clonal analysis for the expression of this peptide hormone. We are presently trying to develop immune histochemical assays for all the APUD markers so that a much larger number of individual cells may be scored to see if infrequent phenotypic reversion (e.g., L-DDC + to −) may be detected.

TABLE VII

Clonal Analysis of L-Dopa Decarboxylase Expression and Cytomorphology in Small Cell Lung Cancer (SCLC) and Large Cell (LC) Variants

			L-Dopa decarboxylase units	
Line	Cytology	No. clones tested and cytology	Uncloned parent	Range in clones
NCI-H69	SCLC	16 all SCLC	240	194–390
NCI-H249	SCLC	14 all SCLC	111	109–665
NCI-H60	SCLC	6 all SCLC	280	111–573
NCI-H128	SCLC	12 all SCLC	377	51–403
NCI-N231/417	Large cell variant	11 all LC	0.23	0.07–0.48
NCI-H82	Large cell variant	12 all LC	0.86	<1.0

We have also studied the expression of membrane receptors for the peptide hormones nerve growth factor (NGF) and epidermal growth factor on SCLC and NSCLC cell lines (Shwerin *et al.,* 1981). We have found that the SCLC lack EGF receptors while the NSCLC lines all have significant levels of these receptors. In contrast, some SCLC lines express significant but low levels of NGF receptors while these were not detected on NSCLC lines. At present we do not have information concerning the clonal variation of these peptide hormone receptors.

B. Heterogeneity of Expression of Some Peptide Hormones

The group at Dartmouth working on SCLC tissue culture lines have published extensively on the expression of various peptide hormones by SCLC lines (Pettingill *et al.,* 1980; Sorenson *et al.,* 1981). We have also collaborated with several investigators (Dermody, Moody, Pert, Eiden, Brownstein, Becker, Weintraub) and found that adrenocorticotropic hormone (ACTH), arginine vasopressin (AVP), calcitonin, met-enkephalin, CCK/gastrin, and luteinizing hormone were expressed in a few SCLC lines (data in preparation). While calcitonin was the most frequently expressed peptide hormone of this group it was also found in NSCLC lines. Thus, we find considerable heterogeneity of expression of these peptide

TABLE VIII

Clonal Heterogeneity of the Expression of Some Peptide Hormones in Small Cell Lung Cancer Line NCI-H128[a]

Cell line	DNA content	Expression of		
		ACTH	AVP	Calcitonin
Tissue culture line	2 peaks	+	+	+
Nude mouse heterotransplant	2 peaks	+	+	+
Clones of NCI-H128				
1	1 peak	+	−	−
2	1 peak	+	+	−
3	1 peak	+	+	+

[a] Adapted from Radice and Dermody (1980).

hormones in contrast to the uniform expression of bombesin in SCLC.

We have conducted a limited clonal analysis of three of the peptide hormones ACTH, AVP, and calcitonin in the SCLC line (NCI-H128) (Radice and Dermody, 1980). We use this line not only because it produced all three hormones but also because we could verify the clonal nature of the sublines by reassaying for DNA content. Thus, the parent line (tissue culture or nude mouse heterotransplant) expressed significant levels of ACTH, AVP, and calcitonin and two DNA content peaks. In contrast, analysis of clonal derivatives revealed either one or the other of the DNA peaks and several different hormone production phenotypes in the clones (Radice and Dermody, 1980) (Table VIII). Some clones expressed all three hormones while others only expressed one or two of the hormones. This heterogeneity of peptide hormone expression has clinical and biological implications. The clinical implications are that these peptide hormone levels cannot be used alone as indicators of tumor response or progression because subpopulations of tumor lacking in expression of hormones may develop. The biological implications arise from the possible "cross feeding" of tumor cells within a population by these hormones if they act in an autostimulatory or "autocrine" fashion. Thus, we suggest the possibility that a subclone within a tumor population may make a peptide hormone (such as AVP) which is required for the growth of all the cells in the tumor while another subclone may not make this hormone. However, the second subclone may make another hormone required for tumor cell growth (e.g., bombesin) which the first subclone does not make. Thus, the heterogeneity of peptide hormone production within a tumor may act as an important growth regulatory mechanism.

VI. Monoclonal Antibody Defined Antigenic Markers on Small Cell Carcinoma

Using hybridoma cell fusion techniques we have prepared a series of mouse and rat monoclonal antibodies that have specificity for human small cell lung cancer (Cuttitta *et al.*, 1981; Minna *et al.*, 1981b). To prepare these, we immunized mice and rats with human SCLC tissue culture lines, and then made hybrids between mouse myeloma cells and the rodent spleen cells. The hybrid culture fluids were screened for antibody activity that would react with two different SCLC lines but not with B lymphoblastoid, or skin fibroblast lines that were autologous to these. These hybrids were then stabilized for antibody production by repeated recloning and then tested against a number of normal and neoplastic human tissues. The stable antibody producing hybrids with the initial screening characteristics represent less than 1% of all the hybridomas screened. We have found that many of these antibodies react with human SCLC tumors taken directly from patients, but not with normal adult lung or liver. Whether or not they react with a small subfraction of normal adult or fetal pulmonary cells remains to be determined. Of interest, one of the antibodies (534F8) reacts with some NSCLC lines, neuroblastoma,

TABLE IX

Monoclonal Antibody Binding Phenotypes[a]

Target cell type	Monoclonal antibody binding	
	534F8	604A9
Small cell lung cancer	+	+
B lymphoblastoid cells	−	−
Skin fibroblasts	−	−
Normal adult lung, liver	−	−
Epidermoid lung cancer	+	−
Adenocarcinoma, lung	+	−
Large cell lung cancer	+	−
Breast cancer	+	+
Neuroblastoma	+	−
Melanoma	−	−
Glioblastoma	−	−
Osteogenic sarcoma	−	−
B cell lymphomas	−	−
T cell lymphomas	−	−

[a] Adapted from Cuttitta *et al.* (1981) and Minna *et al.* (1981b). 534F8 is a mouse IgM χ while 604A9 is a rat IgM χ.

and breast cancer while the other line (604A9) reacts with SCLC, and breast cancer but not with a variety of NSCLC lines (Table IX). These two antibodies thus define different determinants.

A. Homogeneity of Monoclonal Antibody Binding between Tumors

Several of the antibodies, such as mouse antibody 534F8 or rat antibody 604A9, react with nearly all of the large panel of SCLC lines we have tested demonstrating homogeneity. However, there are some SCLC tumor or cell lines which appear classic SCLC by all other criteria which show little or no binding of these antibodies.

B. Heterogeneity of Monoclonal Antibody Binding within Tumors

Because antibodies permit assays for the expression of determinants on individual cells we have tested for heterogeneity of expression of these antigens on SCLC cell lines (Table X). The SCLC lines differed in the percentage of cells which bound monoclonal antibody 534F8 ranging from approximately 10 to 90%. This expression appeared to be cell cycle independent (data not shown). We also tested clonal derivatives for the fraction of cells that would bind monoclonal antibodies and have found conflicting results. Using the cell sorter assays we have found that the clones do not contain cells that are either all positive or all negative for 534F8 binding, but instead clones with various fractions of positive cells are found much as was seen in the primary SCLC lines. In radiobinding assays, in contrast, we have isolated at least some clones that either give a strong binding signal or fail to show binding above background levels (Table X). Thus, we have evidence for both a clonal basis for antigen expression or lack of expression (radiobinding data), and for more complex regulation of antigen expression where clones differ in the fraction of cells expression antigen. In addition, in immunohistochemical studies of autopsy material we have seen strong antibody staining of some tumor nodules, but failure of other closely located tumor nodules to bind antibody (Minna et al., 1981b). Thus, we conclude that while most SCLC lines bind the monoclonal antibody there is strong evidence for heterogenity of antigen expression on tumor cells within individual patients. Such evidence must be taken into account in planning diagnostic or therapeutic use of the monoclonal antibodies.

TABLE X

Heterogeneity of Monoclonal Antibody 534F8 Binding within Small Cell Lung Cancer Cell Lines[a]

Cell line	Cell sorter assays (% cells positive for antibody binding)
NCI-H209	95
NCI-H187	35
NCI-H146	12
NCI-H128	39
Clone 1	20
Clone 8	44
Clone 11	79
NCI-H128 B lymphoblastoid	<1

	Radiobinding assays (binding ratio)
NCI-H128, NCI-H60	30–45
NCI-H128 Clone 1	20
Clone 5	50
NCI-H60 Clone 4	<1

[a] Cell sorter assays were performed by incubating live cells with monoclonal antibody 534F8, washing, then incubating with fluorscein-labeled goat anti-mouse immunoglobulin, washing, and then counting the positive cells in a TPSII Cell Sorter. Radiobinding assays were performed by incubating glutaraldehyde solid phase fixed cells with 534F8, then incubating with rabbit anti-mouse IgM, followed by ^{125}I-labeled protein A. Binding ratio = cpm experimental minus background divided by background.

VII. Growth of Small Cell Lung Cancer *in Vitro*

A. Clonogenic Assays

Of fundamental importance to designing new forms of clinical treatment is a determination of what fraction of tumor cells within a patient before and after treatment are capable of continued replication. Cells with these properties are referred to as "clonogenic" cells and/or "stem" cells. The answer to this fundamental problem has not yet been resolved. We have taken a large number of SCLC bearing tumor samples from patients and cloned them in soft agarose (Carney *et al.*, 1980a, b) (Table XI). We have found there is little variation between different patients' tumors ability to form colonies since 85% of all tumors do this. There is, however, a 10- to 30-fold difference in the number of colonies formed per plated tumor cell in soft agarose, determined by using aneuploid DNA content as an inde-

TABLE XI

Evidence for Heterogeneity of Agarose Clonogenicity within and between Small Cell Lung Cancers[a]

Assay for tumor cell growth	
Soft agarose colony formation of primary tumors	51/60 (85%)
Colony forming efficiency of tumor cells:	
Primary tumors using DNA content as a tumor cell marker (N = 56 tumors)	0.05–1.5%
Established SCLC cell lines (N = 12)	0.1–2.5%
Ability of agarose colonies to continue to replicate when transferred to microwells:	
Primary agarose colonies from patients (10–20 colonies per patient's tumor)	1/15 tumors
Agarose colonies from established cell lines	10/10 cell lines
Ability of primary agarose colonies to continue to replicate when transferred intracranially to nude mice	8/10 tumors
Clonal analysis of colony forming efficiency of SCLC lines:	
Agarose colony forming efficiency of	
NCI-H128 parent line	1.3%
12 clones	0.5–2.0%

[a] Adapted from Carney et al. (1981b) and Gazdar et al. (1980).

pendent tumor cell marker. We do not yet know if there is a difference in clinical course between patients with the lower and the higher cloning efficiency.

Of much greater importance is the small fraction of tumor cells which form colonies in soft agarose (1–2% in the best cases). We have also cloned the established SCLC tissue culture lines in agarose, and again the cloning efficiencies range from 0.1 to 2.5% (Gazdar et al., 1980). Similar results have been seen with cloning the cell lines in liquid medium in microwells. When the clones are themselves retested for colony forming ability the same cloning forming efficiencies (0.5–2%) are seen. This indicates that the defect in colony formation is a clonally inherited trait. Thus, in both the primary tumor specimens and established cell lines 95–99% of the cells do not demonstrate clonogenicity and this difference represents a major type of heterogeneity seen within SCLC tumors. At present, we do not know if this heterogeneity is caused by a true epigenetic difference between the clonable and nonclonable tumor cells, a reflection in heterogeneity of tumor cells, or only a technical problem with the culture conditions caused by damage of the cells. We also note that epigenetic differences between tumor cells could either be an indication of cells in or out of the replicative cell cycle (cells in G_0), or a difference in the growth factor requirements between the cells. In the latter case, the clonable tumor cells have their growth factor requirements met by the culture conditions we use, while the "nonclonable" ones do not. We are studying this problem further.

We have also asked whether or not the tumor cells capable of forming colonies in soft agarose are themselves capable of unlimited replication *in vitro* (i.e., are "stem cells"). To this end we have picked 10–20 colonies from several different patients' primary cultures in soft agarose and attempted to propagate them in liquid medium (Table XI). To our surprise, in all cases but one, the cells were not able to continue to replicate in culture. In contrast, clones derived from the established SCLC cell lines all were able to replicate when subcultured. Thus, there is a fundamental difference between the agarose clonogenic cells of the established cell lines and the primary tumor specimen colonies. Whether the *in vitro* cell lines represent a selection of more primitive stem cells remains to be determined. The one patient whose tumor was able to be replicated from agarose colonies (NCI-N592) appears to make a factor that will allow the cloning of SCLC lines in serum free medium (Carney *et al.*, in preparation; Minna *et al.*, 1981a). Thus, there is heterogeneity between SCLC patients for the ability of initial clonal isolates to continue to grow *in vitro*.

B. Assays for Growth Factor Requirements

We have found that the established SCLC lines could replicate in medium without serum that was supplemented with hydrocortisone, insulin, transferrin, estradiol-17β, and selenium (HITES medium) (Simms *et al.*, 1980). This medium also allowed the selective replication of SCLC tumor cells but not normal stromal cells in 77% of tumors from 37 different patients (Carney *et al.*, 1981a). In fact, we only saw tumor cell growth in fetal calf serum containing medium in 44% of the same tumor samples indicating there is either something inhibitory or lacking in fetal calf serum compared to HITES medium. This HITES medium was also selective for SCLC and did not allow the continued replication of other types of primary tumors including adenocarcinoma of the lung.

While all established SCLC lines replicated in HITES medium some did so better than others. We thus began to test for the ability of other factors added to HITES to stimulate the replication of the SCLC lines. In tests of a large number of other known hormones and growth factors we found the addition of 1% bovine serum albumin, arginine vasopressin (10 ng/ml), bombesin ($10^{-7}M$), and $10^{-5}M$ ethanolamine-phosphorylethanolamine when added singly to HITES stimulated the growth of some SCLC lines. We thus added these factors together to give a new serum free medium which we call SCLC-2 medium. This medium was tested and compared to

TABLE XII

Heterogeneity of Growth Factory Requirements of Small Cell Lung Cancer Lines in Serum Free Medium[a]

RPMI-1640 medium supplemented with	Cell line (relative cell number day 8)	
	NCI-H209	NCI-H69
HITES	1.0	1.0
10% fetal calf serum	43	2.7
SCLC-2 medium	60	2.7

[a] Adapted from Minna *et al.* (1981a) and Oie *et al.* (in preparation). SCLC-2 medium contains RPMI-1640 medium (GIBCO) supplemented with HITES (hydrocortisone (10^{-8} M), bovine insulin (5 μg/ml), human transferrin (5 ng/ml), 10% bovine serum albumin (crystalline RIA grade, Sigma), arginine vasopressin (10 ng/ml), bombesin (10^{-7} M), ethanolamine-phosphorylethanolamine (10^{-5} M).

HITES and fetal calf serum supplemented medium on several of the established SCLC lines. (Table XII). We found that there was heterogeneity between the lines, with the replication of some lines stimulated compared to that in HITES by the addition of fetal calf serum, or SCLC-2 medium. In fact, in all cases SCLC-2 gave better growth than serum supplemented medium. We are now testing to see if primary patient tumor samples also differ in their ability to replicate in HITES versus SCLC-2 medium. Similarly, we are interested to find out if there is clonal heterogeneity within SCLC tumors for the growth factor requirements. We predict this because of the requirement of AVP for growth, and the other data (Table VIII) demonstrating clonal heterogeneity of AVP expression.

VIII. Heterogeneity of Tumorigenicity in Nude Mice

The established SCLC lines are tumorigenic when 5×10^6 cells are injected subcutaneously into athymic nude mice (Gazdar *et al.*, 1980). Parent, uncloned SCLC line NCI-H128 causes tumors with a latency of 4–5 weeks. When clones of NCI-H128 were tested for nude mouse tumorigenicity we found considerable heterogeneity (Table XIII). Some clones formed tumors in 4 weeks, some required 10 weeks, while others never formed tumors during the life-span of the inoculated nude mice. The clones that failed to form tumors had similar cloning efficiencies as those that formed tumors. We conclude from these experiments that there is clonal heterogeneity in the ability of SCLC to form tumors in nude mice.

TABLE XIII

SCLC Clones Demonstrate Heterogeneity of Nude Mouse Tumorigenicity[a]

Cell line	Tumor latency (Weeks)
NCI-H128 parent	4–5
Clones	
7 clones	4
2 clones	10
3 clones	>24

[a] 5×10^6 cells inoculated/mouse; 5 mice tested/clone.

IX. Transformation from a Small Cell to a Large Cell Carcinoma

We have already discussed the occurrence of tumor cells with typical small cell histology with those of cells with a "large cell" histology (WPL-22/40) occurring in up to 12% of pretreatment SCLC biopsy specimens. In addition, Matthews (1979) described 35 cases out of 97 SCLC at autopsy which showed morphological changes deviating from SCLC and in 15 of these large cell components were seen. The other 20 had squamous, adeno, giant cell, and carcinoid components. Abeloff *et al.*, (1979) also described six cases of mixed SCLC and large cells as well as five cases of non-small cell lung cancer histology in a series of 40 autopsies performed on patients thought initially to have SCLC. Thus, this histological heterogeneity is a common finding. Whether it develops as a result of therapy or the underling tumor cell biology remains to be determined.

Because of these clinical findings we were very interested to note the development of tumor cells with transitional and large cell morphology in our continuously growing established SCLC lines and in the SCLC lines undergoing nude mouse heterotransplantation (Gazdar *et al.*, 1981c). So far, we have seen seven samples of this phenomenon (Gazdar *et al.*, in preparation). These seven lines have been compared and contrasted to cell lines derived from SCLC tumors which retain classic small cell histology including the SCLC lines from which they were derived (Table XIV). In one case the large cell line (NCI-H82) was derived from a primary tumor that contained mixtures of small cells and large cells and no small cell line was established from this tumor. We first point out that these large cell and transitional morphology variants differ from non-small cell lung cancer tumors including large cell tumors by virtue of the presence of the del(3)(p14-23) chromosomal marker; the expression of high specific activities of the BB isozyme of creatine kinase; and expression of inter-

TABLE XIV

Comparisons between Properties of Established SCLC Tissue Culture Lines with Typical Small Cell Histology with Those That Have Undergone a Transition to a Large Cell Variant[a]

Characteristics	Histological type	
	Small cell	Large cell or transitional
Growth morphology in culture	Compact	Loose
Doubling time	Slow	Faster
Colony forming efficiency	1%	10–20%
Presence of del(3)(p14-23)	Present	Present
CK-BB isozyme	High levels	High levels
Neuron-specific enolase	High levels	Intermediate levels
L-Dopa decarboxylase	High levels	Low or undetectable
Dense core granules	Present	Absent
Bombesin	Present	Usually absent
Monoclonal antibody binding rations		
534F8	30–100	3–5
604A9	10–80	<1
Radiation sensitivity		
D_0	70–140	101–112
Extrapolation number ($\bar{n}$)	1	4

[a] Adapted from Gazdar et al. (1981c), unpublished and Carney et al. (1982).

mediate levels of neuron-specific enolase. Thus, there are several markers relating them to SCLC. Their growth morphology in culture is different, and they exhibit potentially more "malignant" behavior by having shorter population doubling times and higher cloning efficiencies than lines with typical small cell histology. Of interest, they fail to express markers of APUD cell differentiation such as L-DDC, dense core granules, or bombesin. Also, they exhibit either reduced or absent binding of monoclonal antibodies with specificity for SCLC. Some of their radiobiological characteristics are of great interest (Carney et al., 1982). The slope (D_0) of their radiation survival curve as a function of radiation dose is very similar to the typical small cell carcinomas. However, their extrapolation value ($\bar{n}$) is increased fourfold. This probably indicates the development of some form of radiation repair system. We conclude from this data that the conversion from a small cell histology to a large cell or transitional morphology variant is accompanied by a large number of significant biological and biochemical changes. In sum, these changes would indicate the "dedifferentiation" of the lines, the development of potentially more malignant behavior, and possibly the development of resistance to therapy such as radiation therapy. We suggest that such a mechanism of generating heterogeneity will have profound clinical consequences as well as giving new biological variants to study the differentiation of APUD tumors. While the mechanism of this conversion is not known, it has been associated with the development of a homogeneously staining chromosomal region in at least two cases (lines NCI-H82, and NCI-N231/417) (Whang-Peng, 1981b, c). In addition, in other cases that we are watching enter this transition phase (lines NCI-H60 and NCI-H69), we have seen the development of double minute chromosomes. It is thus possible that gene amplification may be one mechanism associated with the transition from a small cell to a large cell type.

Acknowledgments

We wish to acknowledge all the NCI clinical associates who aided us in the care of the patients, and the collection of the tumor specimens. We also thank E. Russell, V. Bertness, H. Simms, A. Simmons, S. Stephenson, J. Fedorko, T. Gregorio, and B. Wright for technical assistance, and E. Meyer for preparation of the manuscript. H. Oie is sponsored by the Litton Bionetics Frederick Cancer Research Center.

References

Abeloff, M. D., Eggleston, J. C., Mendelsohn, G., Ettinger, D., and Baylin, S. B. (1979). *Am. J. Med.* **66**, 757–764.

Bonikos, D. S., and Bensch, K. G. (1977). *Am. J. Med.* **63**, 765–771.

Bunn, P. A., Jr., and Ihde, D. C. (1981). *In* "Lung Cancer" (R. B. Livingston, ed.), Vol. 1, pp. 169–208. Nijhoff, The Hague.

Bunn, P. A., Jr., Lichter, A. S., Glatstein, E., and Minna, J. D. (1981). *In* "Small Cell Lung Cancer" (F. A. Greco, R. K. Oldham, and P. A. Bunn, Jr., eds.), pp. 413–446. Grune & Stratton, New York.

Carney, D. N., Gazdar, A. F., and Minna, J. D. (1980a). *Cancer Res.* **40**, 1820–1823.

Carney, D. N., Matthews, M. J., Ihde, D. C., Bunn, P. A., Jr., Cohen, M. H., Makuch, R. W., Gazdar, A. F., and Minna, J. D. (1980b). *J. Natl. Cancer Inst.* **65**, 1225–1230.

Carney, D. N., Bunn, P. A., Jr., Gazdar, A. F., Pagan, J. A., and Minna, J. D. (1981a). *Proc. Natl. Acad. Sci. U.S.A.* **78**, 3185–3189.

Carney, D. N., Gazdar, A. F., Bunn, P. A., Jr., and Guccion, J. G. (1981b). *Stem Cells Renewing Cell Popul. Proc. Symp.* (in press).

Carney, D. N., Mitchell, J., and Kinsella, T. (1982). *Proc. Am. Assoc. Cancer Res.* (in press).

Cuttitta, F., Rosen, S., Gazdar, A. F., and Minna, J. D. (1981). *Proc. Natl. Acad. Sci. U.S.A.* **78**, 4591–4595.

Gazdar, A. F., Carney, D. N., Russell, E. K., Sims, H. L., Baylin, S. B., Bunn, P. A., Jr., Guccion, J. G., and Minna, J. D. (1980). *Cancer Res.* **40**, 3502–3507.

Gazdar, A. F., Carney, D. N., Guccion, J. G., and Baylin, S. B. (1981a). *In* "Small Cell

Lung Cancer" (F. A. Greco, R. Oldham, and P. A. Bunn, Jr., eds.), pp. 145–175. Grune & Stratton, New York.

Gazdar, A. F., Zweig, M. H., Carney, D. N., Van Steirtegh, A. C., Baylin, S. B., and Minna, J. D. (1981b). *Cancer Res.* **41**, 2773–2777.

Gazdar, A. F., Carney, D. N., and Minna, J. D. (1981c). *Yale J. Biol. Med.* **54**, 187–193.

Ihde, D. C., Makuch, R. W., Carney, D. N., Bunn, P. A., Cohen, M. H., Matthews, M. J., and Minna, J. D. (1981). *Am. Rev. Respir. Dis.* **123**, 500–507.

Levenson, R. M., Jr., Ihde, D. C., Matthews, M. J., Cohen, M. H., Gazdar, A. F., Bunn, P. A., Jr., and Minna, J. D. (1981). *J. Natl. Cancer Inst.* **67**, 607–612.

Matthews, M. J. (1979). *Prog. Ther. Res.* **9**, 155–165. *In* "Lung Cancer" (F. Muggia and M. Rozencweig, eds.). Raven, New York.

Matthews, M. J., and Gazdar, A. F. (1981). *In* "Lung Cancer" (R. B. Livingston, ed.), Vol. I, pp. 283–306. Nijhoff, The Hague.

Matthews, M. J., Rozencweig, M., Staquet, M. J., Minna, J. D., and Muggia, F. M. (1980). *Eur. J. Cancer* **16**, 527–531.

Minna, J. D., Carney, D. N., Oie, H., Bunn, P. A., Jr., and Gazdar, A. F. (1981a). *In* "Growth of Cells in Defined Medium" (A. Pardee and G. Sato, eds.), Vol. 6. Cold Spring Harbor Press, New York (in press).

Minna, J. D., Cuttitta, F., Rosen, S., Bunn, P. A., Jr., Carney, D. N., Gazdar, A. F., and Krasnow, S. (1981b). *In Vitro* **17**, 1058–1070.

Minna, J. D., Higgins, G. A., and Glatstein, E. J. (1981c). Cancer of the lung. *In* "Principles and Practice of Oncology" (V. T. DeVita, S. Hellman, and S. A. Rosenberg, eds.). pp. 396–473. Lippincott, Phildadelphia, Pennsylvania.

Moody, T. W., Pert, C. B., Gazdar, A. F., Carney, D. N., and Minna, J. D. (1981). *Science (Washington, D.C.)* **214**, 1246–1248.

Pearse, A. G. (1969). *J. Histochem. Cytochem.* **17**, 303–313.

Pettengill, O. S., Sorenson, G. D., and Wurster-Hill, D. H. (1980). *Cancer* **45**, 906–918.

Radice, P. A., and Dermody, W. C. (1980). *Proc. Am. Assoc., Cancer Res.* **21**, 41.

Radice, P. A., Matthews, M. J., Ihde, D. C., Gazdar, A. F., Carney, D. N., Bunn, P. A., Cohen, M. H., Fossieck, B. E., Makuch, R. W., and Minna, J. D. (1981). *Cancer* (in press).

Sherwin, S. A., Minna, J. D., Gazdar, A. F., Todaro, G. J. (1981). *Cancer Res.* **41**, 3538–3542.

Simms, E., Gazdar, A. F., Abrams, P. G., and Minna, J. D. (1980), *Cancer Res.* **40**, 4356–4363.

Sorenson, G. D., Pettergill, O. S., Brinck-Johnson, T., Gate, C. C., and Maurer, L. H. (1981). *Cancer* **47**, 1789–1796.

Whang-Peng, J., Kao-Shan, C. S., Lee, E. C., Bunn, P. A., Carney, D. N., Gazdar, A. F., and Minna, J. D. (1982a). *Science* (in press).

Whang-Peng, J., Bunn, P. A., Jr., Kao-Shan, C. S., Lee, E. C., Carney, D. N., Gazdar, A., and Minna, J. D. (1982b). *Cancer Gen. Cytogen.* (in press).

Whang-Peng, J., Kao-Shan, C. S., Lee, E. C., Bunn, P. A., Carney, D. N., Gazdar, A. F., Portlock, C., Minna, J. D. (1981c). *In* "Gene Amplification," The Banbury Report. Cold Spring Harbor Laboratory Press, New York (in press).

Wharton, J., Polak, J. M., Bloom, F. R., and Pearse, A. G. E. (1978). *Nature (London)* **273**, 769–770.

4

Immunologic Heterogeneity of Human T and B Cell Lymphoid Malignancies

LEE M. NADLER, KENNETH C. ANDERSON, EDWARD K. PARK, MICHAEL P. BATES, ROBERT LEONARD, ELLIS L. REINHERZ, AND STUART F. SCHLOSSMAN

I. Introduction

Human leukemias and lymphomas have long been recognized as heterogeneous diseases on the basis of their morphologic appearance, clinical presentation, and response to therapy (*1-3*). In recent years, this heterogeneity has been further elucidated by the development of immunologic markers which have permitted the definition of the lineage of the malignant lymphocyte (*4-8*). More recently, attempts have been made to relate the malignant lymphocyte to normal stages of hematopoietic differentiation. Utilizing markers that identify B cells, T cells, and myeloid cells, it is now possible to identify clinical subgroups of patients with leukemia and lymphoma not previously distinguishable by standard morphologic or histochemical techniques (*9-12*).

Historically, the classical immunologic markers to define B and T cells were cell surface immunoglobulin (sIg) and the receptor for sheep erythrocyte (E), respectively (13). Receptors for the Fc portion of human immunoglobulin (Fc) (*14-16*), the third component of the complement system (C3) (17), and the HLA-D related Ia-like antigens (Ia) (*18, 19*) are also found on both B and T cells but have had limited utility since they are not uniquely expressed on cells of a single lineage. Due to the technical difficulties inherent in their identification and the lack of specificity of these cell surface markers, considerable attention has been directed in the last several years toward defining cell surface antigens uniquely expressed on normal T or B cells which might therefore be used to identify and classify human leukemias and lymphomas.

Several laboratories have been successful in preparing heteroantisera which identify cell surface antigens expressed on populations of normal lymphoid and myeloid cells. Although these heteroantisera proved to be useful in defining subpopulations of cells, their limited supply and requirement for extensive absorption significantly limited their utility in biologic or clinical investigation. With the development of the hybridoma technique to produce monoclonal antibodies, many of these difficulties have now been overcome (*20*). As will be detailed below, a number of distinct cell surface antigens expressed on cells of T and B cell lineage have now been identified and characterized. These antigens have proved useful in defining both the lineage and state of differentiation of the neoplastic B and T cell. Moreover, the expression of these antigens on leukemias and lymphomas has permitted us to relate the malignant cell to normal stages of differentiation. It now seems clear that our understanding of the heterogeneity of lymphoid and myeloid cells is in its infancy. A complete understanding of the heterogeneity of leukemias and lymphomas will only be possible when we understand more precisely the subpopulations, ontogeny, and function of normal hematopoietic cells.

II. Heterogeneity of Human T Cell Leukemias and Lymphomas

A. Normal Physiology and Ontogeny

In human and murine systems the T lymphocyte has clearly been shown to be functionally heterogeneous. The first major evidence of heterogeneity of human T lymphocytes was the demonstration of functionally distinct subpopulations of human T cells which could be defined and isolated by heteroantisera (21-26). More recently, several laboratories have developed monoclonal antibodies against human T cell antigens in an attempt to study both differentiation and function of normal T lymphocytes (27-38). These monoclonal antibodies have, in addition, been used to study states of abnormal T cell function and to classify T cell leukemias and lymphomas.

In our laboratory, Reinherz and colleagues have developed a series of monoclonal antibodies which define antigens expressed on T lymphocytes at varying stages of differentiation (27-34). Table 1 summarizes the cellular expression and approximate molecular weight of the antigens defined by these antibodies. As depicted in this table, the first three antibodies, termed anti-T1, anti-T3, and anti-T12, define molecularly distinct antigens which are all similarly expressed on 100% of peripheral T cells and a small subpopulation of thymocytes (27-29). The second series of antigens termed anti-T4, anti-T5, and anti-T8 define the phenotype of the helper inducer cell (T4) and the cytotoxic/suppressor cell (T5/8) (30-32). The anti-T6 antigen is unique in that it is expressed only on thymocytes and is not expressed on more mature T lymphocytes (29, 33). The T9 and T10 antigens, although not T cell specific, are useful in that they are expressed on early thymocytes and are helpful in delineating thymic differentiation (29). Anti-T11, which identifies the E rosette receptor, is ex-

TABLE I

Monoclonal Antibodies to Human T Cell Surface Antigens

Monoclonal antibodies	Cell surface expression (% reactivity with antibodies)			Approximate molecular weights of antigens	
	Thymocytes	T cells	Non-T cells	Nonreduced	Reduced
Anti-T1	10	100	0	69,000	69,000
Anti-T3	10	100	0	19,000	19,000
Anti-T12	10	100	0	120,000	—
Anti-T4 A,B,C	75	60	0	62,000	62,000
Anti-T5	80	25	0	76,000	30,000 + 32,000
Anti-T8 A,B,C	80	30	0	76,000	30,000 + 32,000
Anti-T6	70	0	0	49,000	49,000
Anti-T9	10	0	0	190,000	94,000
Anti-T10	95	5	10	37,000	45,000
Anti-T11	100	100	<5	55,000	55,000
Anti-TQ1	5	50	10	—	—

pressed on 100% of thymocytes and 100% of T cells and is clearly distinct from these other T cell antigens (*34*).

These T cell specific antigens have been used to postulate a model for T cell differentiation (*29*). As seen in Fig. 1, the prothymocyte is thought to originate in normal human bone marrow and migrate to the thymus. Considerable evidence exists that many more prothymocytes enter the thymus than the number of mature T cells exported. The earliest antigens expressed within the thymus are T10 followed in time by T9 and T10 together. The T9-T10 cell accounts for approximately 10% of thymic lymphocytes. In the process of maturation, thymocytes lose T9, retain T10, and acquire a thymocyte distinct antigen, T6. Concurrently, these cells express antigens defined by monoclonal antibodies anti-T4 and anti-T5/8. These "common" thymocytes express T4, T5/8, T6, and T10, account for approximately 70% of the total thymic population, and are primarily cortical in location. With further maturation, thymocytes lose T6, acquire T1 and T3 found on mature T cells, and segregate into either T4+ or T5/8+ subsets. This late functional stage accounts for approximately 10% of the thymic population and these thymocytes are found primarily in the medullary region. Immunologic competence is acquired at this stage of differentiation but is not developed fully until thymic lymphocytes are exported. At exportation, these cells lose T10, resulting in circulating T cells of either T1+, T3+, T4+, or T1+,T3+,T5/8+ phenotype. In normal peripheral blood, the helper inducer cell (T1+,T3+,T4+) is twice as common as the cytotoxic/suppressor cell (T1+,T3+,T5/8+).

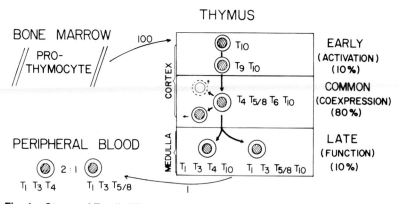

Fig. 1. Stages of T cell differentiation in humans. Three discrete stages of thymic differentiation can be defined on the basis of reactivity with monoclonal antibodies. The cell surface antigens expressed during T cell ontogeny are shown.

B. T Cell Leukemias and Lymphomas

The identification of discrete stages of T cell maturation suggested that it might be possible to relate leukemias and lymphomas of T cell origin to these discrete stages of differentiation. Our studies over the last several years and more recently those of others have confirmed the hypothesis that the T cell malignancies reflect the same degree of heterogeneity and maturation as is seen in normal T cell ontogeny. As is seen in Table II, by identifying the T cell surface phenotype of the malignant cell, it is possible to relate these stages of T cell differentiation to normal thymic maturation.

Tumor cells from approximately 20% of patients with acute lymphoblastic leukemia (ALL) and from almost all patients with lymphoblastic lymphoma (LL) have been shown to be of T cell lineage (39-41). Patients with either T cell, lymphoblastic malignancy are typically adolescent males. The lymphoma is characterized by mediastinal lymphadenopathy at presentation, whereas the leukemia is defined by the presence of malignant lymphoblasts in the bone marrow or peripheral blood. Patients with LL rapidly progress to a leukemic picture indistinguishable from T-ALL, suggesting that LL may represent an early stage of T-ALL. Patients with LL have a significantly prolonged survival compared to T-ALL patients treated with similar therapeutic strategies (42). This difference in survival between patients with T-ALL and LL suggests that there

TABLE II

**Cell Surface Antigens Expressed on
T Cell Derived Human Leukemias and Lymphomas**[a]

T cell differentiation	T cell antigen by stage	T cell malignancies
Early thymocyte	T9, T10, or T10	Majority of T-All
Common thymocyte	T6, T4, T5⁄8, T10	Majority of T-LL; minority of T-ALL
Mature thymocyte	T4, T5⁄8, T10, T1, T3	Minority of T-LL; Rare T-ALL
Mature peripheral T (inducer)	T1, T3, T4	All Sezsary and mycosis fungoides, majority of T-CLL, T-cell NHL (DH and DPDL)
Mature peripheral T (cytotoxic/suppressor)	T1, T3, T5⁄8	T-CLL rare; T-cell NHL

[a] Lineage specific ERR (T11) or A99.

may either be distinct biologic differences between the T lymphoblasts characterizing these diseases or that the treatment at an earlier stage of disease favors survival.

It is now possible, utilizing our model for thymic differentiation, to relate the T cell ALL's and the T LL's to stages of thymic maturation (43-45). As seen in Table II, the majority of patients with T-ALL have a cell surface phenotype identical to an early thymocyte or pro-thymocyte. In a minority of patients, the tumor cells have a cell surface phenotype which corresponds to the common thymocyte or mature thymocyte. The observation that the T-ALL tumor cell corresponds to a pro-thymocyte or early thymocyte is consistent with the clinical presentation of massive bone marrow infiltration in T-ALL. In contrast to T-ALL, the majority of patients with T-LL share the phenotype of the common thymocyte. As seen in the T-ALLs, a few patients with T-LL have the phenotype of a late or more mature thymocyte. The clinical observation that T-LL clinically presents with minimal or no bone marrow involvement and massive mediastinal involvement is consistent with the notion that this tumor has an intrathymic origin. These results suggest that T-ALL and T-LL are probably not different clinical stages of a single neoplastic process. The differences noted in clinical presentation, survival, and response to therapy may well result from the specific thymic pool, the differentiative stage, or the drug susceptibility of the distinct malignant T lymphoblast.

In addition to T-ALL and LL, several other T cell malignancies were studied to correlate these diseases with stages of T cell differentiation. Patients with Sezary syndrome, T cell CLL, and T cell non-Hodgkin's lymphoma are quite distinct, yet every patient studied had a phenotype identical to a mature T cell subset (46). As seen in Table II, patients with Sezary syndrome were always T1,T3,T4+, whereas patients with T cell CLL or T cell non-Hodgkin's lymphoma were either T1,T3,T4+ or T1,T3,T5/8+. These cells did not express or coexpress antigens associated with earlier stages of thymic maturation.

Although the cellular phenotype of the malignant T cell of most patients studied corresponded to normal stages of T cell ontogeny, a number of cases of T cell ALL and lymphoblastic lymphoma clearly appeared to be anomalous. It is not clear at this time whether these anomalous presentations are due to aberrations of the neoplastic state or whether they represent alternate lines of differentiation which are yet to be delineated. Clearly, it will require much further study and a significantly larger number of patients to determine whether these "anomolous" cases have a normal cellular counterpart and will be useful in understanding normal cellular differentiation.

III. Heterogeneity of Human B Cell Leukemias and Lymphomas

A. Ontogeny and Normal Differentiation

The human B lymphocyte has traditionally been defined as a cell which expresses either cytoplasmic or integral cell surface immunoglobulin (47-49). In addition to immunoglobulin, other markers expressed on normal B cells include Ia-like antigens and Fc and C3 receptors. The precise stages of human B cell differentiation have been difficult to define since most of these cell surface determinants are expressed throughout B cell differentiation (Fig. 2). The earliest known stage of B cell differentiation is termed the pre-B cell and these cells contain cytoplasmic μ heavy chain (50-52). B cell differentiation then proceeds by the acquisition of cell surface immunoglobulin and the development of isotype diversity. Initially the expression of immunoglobulin, C3, and Fc is faint and with maturation, the intensity of these antigens on the cell surface increases. As seen in Fig. 2, all stages of B cell differentiation prior to the virgin B cell are antigen independent. When the B cell interacts with antigen, the virgin B cell transforms into a lymphoblast. This transformed B cell, although morphologically distinct, still has the identical phenotype of the virgin B cell in regard to sIg, Fc, and C3 (53). These transformed B cells proceed along the secretory pathway to the plasma cell. During this maturation, cell surface immunoglobulin C3 and Ia are lost and a new antigen, T10, is acquired on the surface of the plasma cell (54).

Except for integral cell surface immunoglobulin and its isotypes, the other cell surface determinants expressed on B lymphocytes are not restricted in their expression to B cells. Cell surface markers limited in their expression to B lymphocytes would therefore be extremely useful in enumeration and functional analysis of normal and malignant B cell populations. We have recently developed two B cell specific monoclonal antibodies which appear to be expressed at discrete stages of B cell differentiation. The first antigen, B1, is expressed on surface immunoglobulin positive B lymphocytes isolated from peripheral blood and lymphoid organs and is not found on resting or activated T cells, monocytes, null cells, granulocytes, erythrocytes, or platelets (55-58) (Fig. 3A-C). In lymphoid tissues, the B1 antigen is primarily localized in the lymphoid follicles, i.e., B cell regions (58). When surface immunoglobulin bearing B cells are stimulated with pokeweed mitogen to secrete immunoglobulin, the B1 antigen is lost on the cell surface (57). The loss of the B1 is accompanied by the development of presecretory cytoplasmic IgG and the ap-

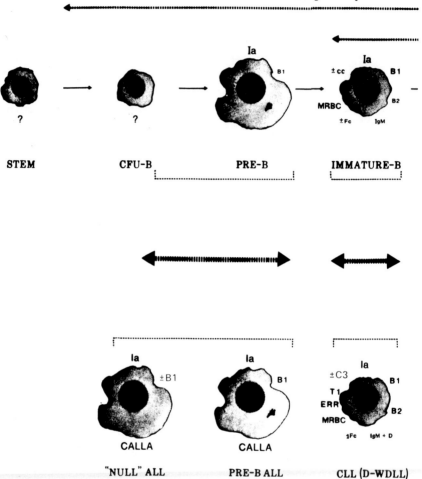

TUMOR CELL SURFACE

Fig. 2. Hypothetical model of human B cell differentiation. Discrete stages of B cell differentiation are proposed. In murine and human systems, the first phase of B cell differentiation occurs in the absence of antigen (antigen independent), whereas the second phase requires antigen (antigen dependent). These stages can be identified by the presence and degree of expression of markers including cytoplasmic immunoglobulin, surface immunoglobulin isotype, mouse erythrocyte receptors (MRBC), receptors for Fc and C3, and the presence of Ia antigen. The proposed expression of B1 and

DIFFERENTIATION

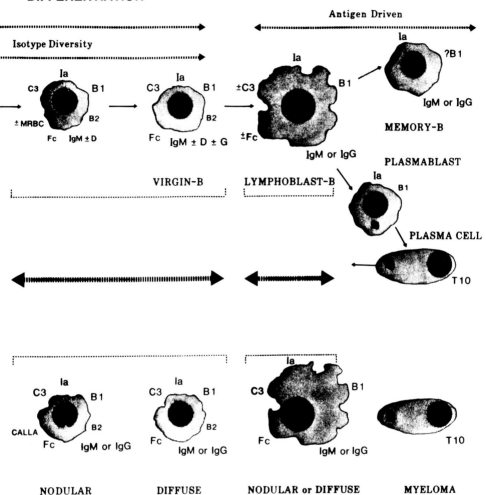

NODULAR	DIFFUSE	NODULAR or DIFFUSE	MYELOMA
PDL		TRANSFORMED (HISTIOCYTIC)	

PHENOTYPE

B2 is based on the results of *in vitro* experiments with normal cells and the differential expression of B1 and B2 on leukemia and lymphoma cells. In the upper panel, the intensity of expression of the individual antigens is represented by the size of the lettering. The correlation of the phenotype of the B cell leukemias and lymphomas with their normal cellular counterpart is attempted in the lower level. Although there are differences between the malignant and normal B cell differentiative stages (see text), a relative correlation appears to be possible. Again, the size of the lettering represents the intensity of antigen expression.

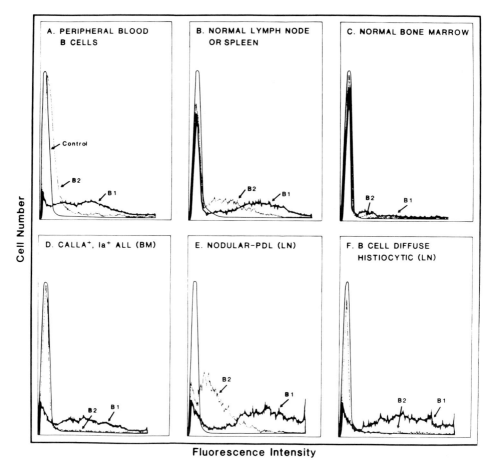

Fig. 3. Expression of B1 and B2 on normal and malignant tissues. The flow cytometric fluorescence histogram profiles of peripheral blood B cells (A), normal lymph node or spleen cells (B), normal bone marrow cells (C), CALLA+Ia+ non-T cell ALL cells (D), nodular PDL cells (E), and B cell diffuse histiocytic lymphoma cells (F) with anti-B1 and anti-B2 is depicted in this figure. Background staining was obtained by incubating cells with an isotype identical unreactive monoclonal antibody.

pearance of plasma cells suggesting that B1 is a pan-B cell differentiation antigen (57).

A second human B cell specific antigen, B2, has also been identified (56). By indirect immunofluorescence and quantitative absorption, B2 like B1 is expressed exclusively on immunoglobulin positive B cells isolated from peripheral blood and lymphoid tissue. In contrast to the B1 antigen, the B2 antigen is expressed weakly on peripheral blood B cells but is expressed strongly on B cells isolated from lymph node, tonsil and spleen (Fig. 3A and B). Chemical characterization indicated that the B1 and B2 antigens were unique. The B2 antigen migrates as a single band of molecular weight of approximately 140,000 under both reducing and non-reducing conditions (56). The B1 antigen, in contrast, is a protein of approximately 30,000 MW (56). Like B1, only anti-B2 reactive B cells could be induced to differentiate under the stimulus of pokeweed mitogen to plasma cells.

Recent experiments have provided evidence that B1 and B2 are B cell differentiation antigens (57). This evidence has been derived from studies employing a pokeweed mitogen driven model of B cell differentiation. Pokeweed mitogen induces differentiation of B cells to antibody secreting cells, a function that is T cell dependent in man (59). In a series of experiments, either peripheral blood B cells or splenic B cells were stimulated with pokeweed mitogen and followed over time for the disappearance of B1 and B2. The B2 antigen was lost on the cell surface by 4 days and B1 was lost by day 6 or 7 of stimulation. When B2 was lost from the cell surface, the cells had transformed into lymphoblasts, many of which contained cytoplasmic IgM. Moreover, when the B1 antigen was lost, cytoplasmic IgG was noted. As is depicted in Fig. 2, a hypothetical model of B1 and B2 expression is shown. The B1 antigen may begin as early as the pre-B cell, increases in intensity, and disappears at the stage of the plasma cell. The B2 antigen seems to appear later than B1, increases in intensity, and disappears when the virgin B cell becomes a lymphoblast.

Application of these B cell associated antigens to lymphoid tissue sections demonstrated that these antigens were compartmentalized within the secondary lymphoid follicle (58). Specifically, the majority of cells in the primary follicle and mantles of the secondary follicle express cell surface antigen similar to those of circulating B cells, mainly IgM, IgG, Ia, B1, and B2. In contrast, the germinal center cells of the secondary follicle stained with IgM, IgG, B1, B2, and Ia, but not IgD. The germinal center stained much more intensely than the mantle zones with anti-B2, whereas no such striking difference in staining intensity was observed with anti-B1. These results indicated that the generation of the germinal centers in the primary lymphoid follicle involved phenotypic changes that correspond largely to those observed after antigenic and mitogenic activation of B lymphocytes.

B. Human B Cell Leukemias and Lymphomas

With the *in vitro* evidence that the B1 and B2 antigens are expressed on distinct stages of B cell differentiation, we investigated the expression of these antigens on tumor cells isolated from patients with leukemias and lymphomas. These cell tumors have been defined historically by their expression of monoclonal k or γ light chain. Previously we have shown that

TABLE III

Reactivity of Anti-B1 and Anti-B2 Antibodies with Leukemias and Lymphomas

		Number reactive	
Tumor	Number of patients	Anti-B1	Anti-B2
Lymphomas			
B cell	96	96	36
T cell	15	0	0
Null cell	10	4	0
	121	100	36
Leukemias			
CLL—B cell	73	73	61
CLL—T cell	5	0	0
ALL—Non-T	81	38	5
ALL—T	24	0	0
CML—stable phase	15	0	0
CML—blast crisis	19	7	0
AML/AMoL	91	0	0
	308	118	66

tumors of B cell origin uniformly express monoclonal immunoglobulin and Ia-like antigens. As seen in Table III, tumor cells isolated from patients with B cell lymphomas and B cell chronic lymphocytic leukemia were uniformly reactive with the anti-B1 antibody (60). Moreover, a few patients with null cell lymphoma and approximately half of the patients with non-T cell ALL and CML in blast crisis also expressed B1. The B1 antigen was not found on T cell lymphomas, T cell CLL's, and T cell ALL's. In addition, tumors of myeloid origin including stable phase CML and acute myeloblastic leukemias, were similarly unreactive with anti-B1. These results confirmed that the B1 antigen was expressed uniquely on tumor cells of B cell lineage and suggested that the non-T cell ALL's and CML's in blast crisis might share a common B cell lineage.

Although all B cell lymphomas except myelomas express the B1 antigen, the expression of B2 on leukemias and lymphomas appeared to be more restricted (56). Only one-third of patients with B cell lymphoma and most patients with B cell CLL expressed the B2 antigen. In contrast to the expression of B1 on non-T cell ALL and CML in blast crisis, only a handful of patients with non-T cell ALL reacted with anti-B2. Moreover, the B2 antigen was not expressed on T cell tumors including T cell CLL, T cell ALL, and T cell lymphomas. The B2 antigen was unreactive with any tumors of myeloid origin including stable phase CML, CML in blast crisis, or AML.

The limited expression of the B2 antigen on B cell non-Hodgkin's lymphomas permits one to correlate more precisely the malignant lymphocyte with its normal cellular counterpart. As seen in Table IV, the non-Hodgkin's lymphomas have been subdivided according to the Rappaport histopathologic classification. The B1 antigen was reactive with all B cell tumors and approximately half of null cell diffuse histiocytic lymphomas but was unreactive with myelomas. In contrast, the B2 antigen appeared to be found on B cell tumors from the immature B cell (CLL) to the virgin B cell (nodular or diffuse PDLs) (Table IV, Fig. 2). The B2 antigen was not found on tumors isolated from patients with either nodular or diffuse histiocytic lymphomas which corresponded to the transformed or lymphoblastic B cell. The tumors which correspond to the secretory phase of B cell differentiation included Waldenstrom's macroglobulinemia and myeloma. These were unreactive with anti-B2 also. Examination of Table IV suggests that B cell tumors which have been thought to correspond to later stages of differentiation lack the B2 antigen. These observations on the heterogeneous expression of the B2 antigen on B cell non-Hodgkin's lymphomas confirmed the *in vitro* evidence that the B2 antigen is lost at approximately the time of transformation of the virgin B cell into the B lymphoblast (Fig. 2).

We have recently had the opportunity to study approximately 100 pa-

TABLE IV

Reactivity of Anti-B1 and Anti-B2 Antibodies with B Cell Non-Hodgkin's Lymphomas

Histology	Number of patients	Number reactive	
		Anti-B1	Anti-B2
Nodular			
PDL	21	21	18
Histiocytic	6	6	0
Mixed	10	10	6
Diffuse			
PDL	21	21	17
Histiocytic—B	19	19	2
Histiocytic—"Null"	10	4	0
Mixed	4	4	1
Undifferentiated	4	4	4
Burkitt's	11	11	0
Waldenstrom's	4	4	0
Myeloma	6	0	0
	116	104	48

tients with B cell chronic lymphocytic leukemia (*61*). As seen in Fig. 2, most CLL cells weakly express cell surface IgM and/or IgD. The expression of Ia and B1 is considerably stronger than the faint expression of cell surface immunoglobulin. The concomittant expression of B2 antigen and sIg, Ia, and B1 on most cells suggests that these cells may correspond to the immature B cell (Fig. 2). Of great interest is the finding that the T1 antigen, which is normally expressed on all peripheral blood T cells and a fraction of thymocytes, is also expressed on B cell CLL cells. Moreover, another antigen found on all peripheral T cells and thymocytes (T11) is also found on some CLL's. The precise meaning of the expression of T1 on CLL cells is unknown, but the absence of T1 on normal peripheral blood B cells provides one line of evidence that B cell CLL is not the neoplastic counterpart of this cell. It is therefore possible that the CLL cell is derived from a small subpopulation within normal bone marrow which coexpresses the B1 and T1 antigens.

The cellular origin of poorly differentiated lymphocytic lymphomas has been studied recently also (*62*). The cell surface phenotype of approximately 40 patients with nodular lymphoma revealed a moderate expression of monoclonal immunoglobulin, strong expression of B1 and Ia, and weaker expression of B2 (Figs. 2 and 3E). Of great interest is the recent observation that the nodular PDLs also expressed a common acute lymphoblastic leukemia antigen (CALLA) (*63*). This observation is in distinct contrast to the diffuse PDL's which have an identical phenotype but do not express CALLA. These observations suggest that the nodular and diffuse PDL's may be derived from distinct populations of B cells. Moreover, preliminary data suggest that the CALLA antigen may be found in very small amounts on germinal center B cells (*62*) and may provide further evidence that these tumors are derived from germinal center B cells.

In contrast to the poorly differentiated lymphomas, the transformed or histiocytic lymphomas almost never express B2 (Figs. 2 and 3F). These cells appear to be the neoplastic counterpart of the B lymphoblast. The nodular histiocytic lymphomas also express the CALLA antigen as did the nodular PDL's, but the diffuse histiocytic lymphomas do not (*62*). The expression of B1, cell surface immunoglobulin, and Ia-like antigens is quite strong on these tumor cells. Examination of the CLL's, PDL's and histiocytic lymphomas therefore supports the hypothesis that the malignant lymphomas are heterogeneous and correspond to distinct stages of B cell differentiation.

Leukemic cells from approximately 80% of patients with acute lymphoblastic leukemia (ALL) lack both cell surface immunoglobulin and T cell antigens. Although these cells are devoid of conventional B or T cell antigens, they express a variety of cell surface markers including the common acute lymphoblastic leukemia antigen (CALLA) (*64-69*) and the Ia-

TABLE V

Reactivity of Anti-B1 and Anti-B2 Antibodies with Calla Positive (J5) and Negative Leukemic Cells

Tumor	Number of patients	Number reactive with antisera		
		Ia+	B1+	B2+
Non-T cell ALL, CALLA+	68	68	44	5
Non-T cell ALL, CALLA−	17	17	0	0
CML—Blast crisis, CALLA+	13	10	8	1
CML—Blast crisis, CALLA−	6	3	0	0
	104	98	52	6

like antigens (Ia) (Fig. 2). The cellular origin of these non-T ALL's has been the subject of numerous studies which, for the most part, suggest that they are of B cell origin. Several laboratories have demonstrated that tumor cells from approximately 20–30% of patients with non-T ALL have a pre-B cell phenotype since they express intracytoplasmic μ chain but lack cell surface immunoglobulin (70–72). We have shown previously that approximately 50% of non-T cell ALLs and CML in blast crisis were reactive with anti-B1 (Fig. 2). As seen in Table V, the non-T cell ALL's and CML in blast crisis can be divided into the following subgroups: (1) Ia+CALLA+B1+; (2) Ia+CALLA+B1−; and (3) Ia+CALLA−B1−. A small number of non-T cell ALL's also coexpress the B2 antigen, suggesting that they are more differentiated. These studies provided evidence for the heterogeneity of non-T cell ALL and the reactivity of these tumors with anti-B1 provided evidence that they are of B cell lineage.

The cellular origin of the Ia+CALLA+B1− non-T cell ALL's has been investigated recently (73). Non-T cell ALL lines and tumor cells isolated from patients with non-T cell ALL which are Ia+CALLA+B1− were studied *in vitro* with a variety of agents known to promote cellular differentiation. Phorbol diester (TPA) or phytohemagglutinin conditioned lymphocyte culture media (PHA-LCM) were capable of inducing the expression of B1 on the four non-T cell ALL lines tested. Moreover, leukemia cells from nine patients with Ia+CALLA+B1− cytoplasmic μ negative ALL could be induced *in vitro* with TPA to express both B1 and cytoplasmic μ. In contrast, five patients with Ia+CALLA−B1− cytoplasmic μ− non-T cell ALL could not be induced with TPA to express CALLA, B1, or cytoplasmic μ. These studies suggest that the non-T cell ALL's are heterogeneous and represent a spectrum of early B cell differentiation including the pre-pre-B cell (Ia+CALLA+B1−cμ−), the intermediate pre-B cell (Ia+CALLA+B1+cμ−) and, finally, the "true" pre-B cell

$(Ia+CALLA+B1+c\mu+)$. The cellular origin of the remaining Ia$-$CALLA$-$B1$-$ form of non-T cell ALL (20%) is still unknown.

Cell surface markers have identified considerably greater heterogeneity within the human T and B cell lymphoid neoplasms than was evident by standard morphologic and histochemical techniques. Utilizing markers specific for lineage and state of differentiation, it is now possible to correlate the malignant lymphocyte with its normal cellular counterpart. Considering the complexity of the immune system in regard to ontogeny, differentiation, function, and migration, it is not surprising that the lymphoid malignancies reflect this degree of diversity. Moreover, the biologic and clinical heterogeneity of these diseases is clearly greater than has been identified by presently employed classification schemes. The challenge of the next several years is to integrate our understanding of the diversity of the immune system with the clinical heterogeneity of the leukemias and lymphomas in an attempt to devise a more rational classification scheme. Hopefully, this scheme will not only be biologically accurate but, more importantly, will identify clinically relevant subgroups of patients.

Acknowledgments

This manuscript was supported by National Institutes of Health grants AI 12069, CA 19589, and CA 25369.

Dr. Nadler is a research Fellow of the Medical Foundation, Inc., Boston, Massachusetts.

References

1. Hayhoe, R. G. I., and Flemans, R. J. (1970). "An Atlas of Haematological Cytology." pp. 110–265. Wiley (Interscience), New York.
2. Galton, D. A. G., Catovsky, D., and Wiltshaw, E. (1978). Clinical spectrum of lymphoproliferative diseases. *Cancer* **42,** 901–910.
3. Frei, E. III, and Sallan, S. E. (1978). Acute lymphoblastic leukemia: treatment. *Cancer* **42,** 828–838.
4. Aisenberg, A. C., and Bloch, K. J., (1972). Immunoglobulins on the surface of neoplastic lymphocytes. *N. Engl. J. Med.* **287,** 272–276.
5. Borella, L., and Sen, L. (1973). T cell surface markers on lymphoblasts from acute lymphocytic leukemia. *J. Immunol.* **111,** 1257–1260.
6. Brouet, J. C., and Seligmann, M. (1978). The immunological classification of acute lymphoblastic leukemias. *Cancer* **42,** 817–827.
7. Siegal, F. P. (1978). Cytoidentity of the lymphoreticular neoplasms. *In* "The Immunopathology of Lymphoreticular Neoplasms" (J. J. Twomey and R. A. Good, eds.), pp. 281–324. Plenum, New York.
8. Mann, R. B., Jaffe, E. S., and Berard, C. W. (1979). Malignant lymphomas: a conceptual understanding of morphologic diversity. *Rev. Am. J. Pathol.* **94,** 104–191.

9. Nadler, L. M., Stashenko, P., Reinherz, E. L., Ritz, J., Hardy R., and Schlossman, S. F. (1981). Expression of normal differentiation antigens on human leukemia and lymphoma cells. *In* "Malignant Lymphoma: Etiology, Immunology, Pathology, Treatment" (H. Kaplan, and S. Rosenberg, eds.), pp. 187–225. Academic Press, New York.

10. Bloomfield, C. D., Kersey, J. H., Brunning, R. D., and Gajl-Peczalska, K. J. (1976). Prognostic significance of lymphocyte surface markers in adult non-Hodgkin's malignant lymphoma. *Lancet* **ii**, 1330–1333.

11. Chessells, J. M., Hardisty, R. M., Rapson, N. T., and Greaves, M. F. (1977). Acute lymphoblastic leukemia in children: classification and prognosis. *Lancet* **ii**, 1307–1309.

12. Bloomfield, C. D., Gajl-Peczalska, K. J., Frizzera, G., Kersey, J. H., and Goldman, A. I. (1979). Clinical utility of lymphocyte surface markers combined with the Lukes-Collins histologic classification in adult lymphoma. *N. Engl. J. Med.* **301**, 512–518.

13. Chess, L., and Schlossman, S. F. Human lymphocyte subpopulations. *Adv. Immunol.* **25**, 213–247.

14. Huber, H., Douglas, S. D., and Fudenberg, H. H. (1969). The IgG receptor: an immunological marker for the characterization of mononuclear cells. *Immunology* **17**, 7–21.

15. Bianco, C., Patrick, R., and Nussenzweig, V. (1970). A population of lymphocytes bearing a membrane receptor for antigen-antibody complement complexes. *J. Exp. Med.* **132**, 70–720.

16. Dickler, H. B., and Kunkel, H. G. (1972). Interaction of the aggregated γ-globulin with B lymphocytes. *J. Exp. Med.* **136**, 191–196.

17. Ross, G. D., Rabellino, E. M., Polley, M. J., and Grey, H. M. (1973). Combined studies of complement receptor and surface immunoglobulin bearing cells in normal and leukemic human lymphocytes. *J. Clin. Invest.* **52**, 377–385.

18. Winchester, R. J., Fu, S. M., Wernet, P., Kunkel, H. G., Dupont, B., and Jerslid, C. (1975). Recognition by pregnancy serum of non-HLA alloantigen selectivity on B lymphocytes. *J. Exp. Med.* **141**, 924–929.

19. Schlossman, S. F., Chess, L., Humphreys, R. E., and Strominger, J. L. (1976). Distribution of Ia-like molecules on the surface of normal and leukemic human cells. *Proc. Natl. Acad. Sci. U.S.A.* **73**, 1288–1292.

20. Kohler, G., and Milstein, C. (1975). Continuous cultures of fused cells secreting antibody of predefined specificity. *Nature (London)*, **256**, 495–497.

21. Chechik, B. E., Pyke, K. W., and Gelfand, E. W. (1976). Human thymus/leukemia associated antigen in normal and leukemic cells. *Int. J. Cancer* **18**, 551–556.

22. Borella, L., Sen, L., Dow, L. W., and Casper, J. T. (1977). Cell differentiation antigens versus tumor related antigens in child acute lymphoblastic leukemia (ALL). Clinical significance of leukemia markers. *Haematol. Blood Transfusion* **20**, 77–85.

23. Boumsell, L., Bernard, A., Coppin, H., Richard, Y., Penit C., and Rouget, P. (1979). Human T cell differentiation antigens and correlation of their expression with various markers of T cell maturation. *J. Immunol.* **123**, 2063–2067.

24. Evans, R. L., Breard, J. M., Lazarus, H., Schlossman, S. F., and Chess, L. (1977). Detection, isolation, and functional characterization of two human T cell subclasses bearing unique differentiation antigens. *J. Exp. Med.* **145**, 221–233.

25. Evans, R. L., Lazarus, H., Penta, A. C., and Schlossman, S. F. (1978). Two functionally distinct subpopulations of human T cells that collaborate in the generation of cytotoxic cells responsible for cell-mediated lympholysis. *J. Immunol.* **120**, 1423–1428.

26. Reinherz, E. L., Schlossman, S. F. (1979). Con A inducible suppression of MLC: evidence for mediation by the TH_2+ T cell subset in man. *J. Immunol.* **122**, 1335–1341.

27. Reinherz, E. L., Kung, P. C., Goldstein, G., and Schlossman, S. F. (1979). A monoclonal antibody with selective reactivity with functionally mature thymocytes and all peripheral human T cells. *J. Immunol.* **123**, 1312–1317.

28. Reinherz, E. L., Hussey, R. E., and Schlossman, S. F. (1980). A monoclonal antibody blocking human T cell function. *Eur. J. Immunol.* **10,** 758–762.
29. Reinherz, E. L., Kung, P. C., Goldstein, G., Levey, R., and Schlossman, S. F. (1980). Discrete stages of human intrathymic differentiation: analysis of normal thymocytes and leukemic lymphoblasts of T lineage. *Proc. Natl. Acad. Sci. U.S.A.* **77,** 1588–1592.
30. Reinherz, E. L., Kung, P. C., Goldstein, G., and Schlossman, S. F. (1979). Separation of functional subsets of human T cells by a monoclonal antibody. *Proc. Natl. Acad. Sci. U.S.A.* **76,** 4061–4065.
31. Reinherz, E. L., Kung, P. C., Goldstein, G., and Schlossman, S. F. (1979). Further characterization of the human inducer T cell subset defined by monoclonal antibody. *J. Immunol.* **123,** 2894–2896.
32. Reinherz, E. L., Kung, P. C., Goldstein, G., and Schlossman, S. F. (1980). A monoclonal antibody reactive with the human cytotoxic/suppressor T cell subset previously defined by a heteroantiserum termed TH_2. *J. Immunol.* **124,** 1301–1307.
33. Reinherz, E. L., and Schlossman, S. F. (1980). The differentiation and function of human T lymphocytes: A review. *Cell* **19,** 821–827.
34. Reinherz, E. L., and Schlossman, S. F. (1981). The characterization and function of human immunoregulatory T lymphocyte subsets. *Immunol. Today,* pp. 69–75.
35. McMichael, A. J., Pilch, J. R., Galfre, G., Mason, D. Y., Fabre, J. W., and Milstein, C. (1979). A human thymocyte antigen defined by a hybrid myeloma monoclonal antibody. *Eur. J. Immunol.* **9,** 205–210.
36. Ledbetter, J. A., Evans, R. L., Lipinski, M., Cunningham-Rundles, C., Good, R. A., and Herzenberg, L. A. (1981). Evolutionary conservation of surface molecules that distinguish T lymphocyte/inducer and cytotoxic/suppressor subpopulations in mouse and man. *J. Exp. Med.* **153,** 310–323.
37. Boumsell, L., Coppin, H., Pham, D., *et al.* (1980). An antigen shared by human T cell subset and B cell chronic lymphocytic leukemic cells. *J. Exp. Med.* **152,** 229–234.
38. Engleman, E. G., Warnke, R., Fox R. I., and Levy, R. (1981). Studies on a human T lymphocyte antigen recognized by a monoclonal antibody. *Proc. Natl. Acad. Sci. U.S.A.* **78,** 1791–1795.
39. Borella, L., and Sen, L. (1973). T cell surface markers on lymphoblasts from acute lymphocytic leukemia. *J. Immunol.* **111,** 1251.
40. Sen, L., and Borella, L. (1975). Clinical importance of lymphoblasts with T markers in childhood acute leukemia. *N. Engl. J. Med.* **292,** 828.
41. Kersey, J. H., Nesbit, M. E., Hallgreen, H. M., Sabad, A., Yunis, E. J., and Gajl-Peczalska, K. (1975). Evidence for origin of certain childhood acute lymphoblastic leukemias and lymphomas in thymus-derived lymphocytes. *Cancer* **36,** 1348.
42. Weinstein, H. J., Vance, Z. B., Jaffe, N., Buell, D., Cassady, J. R., and Nathan, D. G. (1979). Improved prognosis for patients with mediastinal lymphoblastic lymphoma. *Blood* **53,** 687.
43. Reinherz, E. L., Nadler, L. M., Sallan, S. E., and Schlossman, S. F. (1979). Subset derivation of T cell acute lymphoblastic leukemia in man. *J. Clin. Invest.* **64,** 392–397.
44. Nadler, L. M., Reinherz, E. L., Weinstein, H. J., D'Orsi, C. J., and Schlossman, S. F. (1980). Heterogeneity of T cell lymphoblastic malignancies. *Blood* **55,** 806–810.
45. Bernard, A., Boumsell, L., Reinherz, E. L., Nadler, L. M., Ritz, J., Coppin, H., Richard, Y., Valensi, F., Dousset, J., Flandrin, G., Lemerle, J., and Schlossman, S. F. (1981). Malignant T cells from acute lymphoblastic leukemia and from malignant lymphomas exhibit different patterns of surface antigens. *Blood* **57,** 1105–1110.
46. Boumsell, L., Bernard, A., Reinherz, E. L., Nadler, L. M., Ritz, J., Coppin, H., Richard, Y., Dubertret, L., Valensi, F., Degos, L., Lemerle, J., Flandrin, G.,

Dousset, J., and Schlossman, S. F. (1981). Surface antigens on malignant Sezary and T-CLL cells correspond to those of mature T cells. *Blood* **57**, 526–530.

47. Gathings, W. E., Lawton, A. R., Cooper, M. D. (1977). Immunofluorescent studies of the development of pre-B cells, B lymphocytes and immunoglobulin isotype diversity in humans. *Eur. J. Immunol.* **7**, 804–810.

48. Froland, S. S., and Natvig, J. B. (1970). Effect of polyspecific rabbit anti-immunoglobulin antisera on human lymphocytes in vitro. *Int. Arch. Allerg. Appl. Immunol.* **39**, 121–132.

49. Froland, S. S., Natvig, J. B., and Berdal, P. (1971). Surface-bound immunoglobulin as a marker of B lymphocytes in man. *Nature New. Biol. (London)* **134**, 251–252.

50. Owen, J. J. T., Raff, M. C., and Cooper, M. D. (1975). Studies on the generation of B lymphocytes in the mouse embryo. *Eur. J. Immunol.* **5**, 468.

51. Pearl, E. R., Vogler, L. B., Okos, A. J., Crist, W. M., Lawton, A. R., and Cooper, M. D. (1978). B lymphocyte precursor in human bone marrow. An analysis of normal individuals and patients with antibody deficiency states. *J. Immunol.* **120**, 1169.

52. Cooper, M. D. (1981). Pre-B cells: Normal and abnormal development. *J. Clin. Immunol.* **1**, 81–89.

53. Cooper, M. D., and Lawton, A. R. Development of lymphoid tissues. *In* "The Immunopathology of Lymphoreticular Neoplasms" (J. J. Twomey and R. A. Good, eds.), pp. 1–22. Plenum, New York.

54. Poppema, S., Bhan, A. K., Reinherz, E. L., McCluskey, R. T., and Schlossman, S. F. (1979). Distribution of T cell subsets in human lymph nodes. *J. Exp. Med.* **153**, 30.

55. Stashenko, P., Nadler, L. M., Hardy, R., and Schlossman, S. F. (1980). Characterization of a human B lymphocyte specific antigen. *J. Immunol.* **125**, 1678–1685.

56. Nadler, L. M., Stashenko, P., Hardy, R., van Agthoven, A., Terhorst, C., and Schlossman, S. F. (1981). Characterization of a human B cell specific antigen (B2) distinct from B1. *J. Immunol.* **126**, 1941–1947.

57. Stashenko, P., Nadler, L. M., Hardy, R., and Schlossman, S. F. (1981). Expression of cell surface markers following human B lymphocyte activation. *Proc. Natl. Acad. Sci. U.S.A.* **78**, 3848–3852.

58. Bhan, A. K., Nadler, L. M., Stashenko, P., and Schlossman, S. F. (1981). Stages of B cell differentiation in human lymphoid tissues. *J. Exp. Med.* **154**, 737–749.

59. Fauci, A. S., Pratt, K. R. K., and Whalen, G. (1976). Activation of human B lymphocytes. II. Cellular interactions in the PFC response on human tonsillar and peripheral blood B lymphocytes to polyclonal activation by pokeweed mitogen. *J. Immunol.* **117**, 2100–2104.

60. Nadler, L. M., Stashenko, P., Ritz, J., Hardy, R., Pesando, J. M., and Schlossman, S. F. (1981). A unique cell surface antigen identifying lymphoid malignancies of B cell origin. *J. Clin. Invest.* **67**, 134–140.

61. Nadler, L. M., Bates, M. B., Park, E. K., Anderson, K. C., Leonard, R., and Schlossman, S. F. (1982). Unique stages of early B cell differentiation defined by a B cell specific monoclonal antibody (B4) (in preparation).

62. Nadler, L. M., Bhan, A. K., Harris, N., Ritz, J., and Schlossman, S. F. (1982). Nodular lymphomas correspond to discrete stages of B cell differentiation (submitted).

63. Ritz, J., Nadler, L. M., Bhan, A. K., Notis-McConarty, J., Pesando, J. M., and Schlossman, S. F. (1981). Expression of common acute lymphoblastic leukemia antigen (CALLA) by lymphomas of B cell and T cell lineage. *Blood* **58**, 648.

64. Greaves, M. F., Grown, G., Rapson, N. T., and Lister, T. A. (1975). Antisera to acute lymphoblastic leukemia cells. *Clin. Immunol. Immunopathol.* **4**, 67–84.

65. Pesando, J. M., Ritz, J., Lazarus H., Baseman-Costello, S., Sallan, S. E., and Schloss-

man, S. F. (1979). Leukemia-associated antigens in ALL. *Blood* **54,** 1240–1248.

66. Billing, R., Minowada, J., Cline, M., Clark, B., and Lee, K. (1978). Acute lymphocytic leukemia associated cell membrane antigen. *J. Natl. Cancer Inst.* **61,** 423–429.

67. Ritz, J., Pesando, J. M., Notis-McConarty, J., Lazarus, H., and Schlossman, S. F. (1980). A monoclonal antibody to human acute lymphoblastic antigen. *Nature (London)* **283,** 583–585.

68. Greaves, M. F. (1981). Monoclonal antibodies as probes for leukemic heterogeneity and hemapoietic differentiation. *In* "Leukemia Markers" (W. Knapp, ed.), p. 19. Academic Press, New York.

69. Roberts, M., Greaves, M. F., Janossy, G., Sutherland, R., Pain, C.(1978). Acute lymphoblastic leukemia (ALL) associated antigen. I Expression in different hematopoietic malignancies. *Leuk. Res.* **28,** 105.

70. Vogler, L. B., Crist, W. M., Bockman, D. E., Pearl, E. R., Lawton, A. R., and Cooper, M. D. (1978). Pre-B cell leukemia: a new phenotype of childhood lymphoblastic leukemia. *N. Engl. J. Med.* **198,** 872–878.

71. Brouet, J. C., Preud homme, J. L., Penit, C., Valensi, F., Rouget, P., and Seligmann, M. (1979). Acute lymphoblastic leukemia with pre-B cell characteristics. *Blood* **54,** 269–273.

72. Greaves, M. F., Verbi, F. W., Vogler, L. B., Cooper, M. D., Ellis, R., Ganeshguru, K., Hoffbrand, V., Janossy, G., and Bollum, F. J. (1979). Antigenic and enzymatic phenotypes of the pre-B subclass of acute lymphoblastic leukemia. *Leuk. Res.* **3,** 353–362.

73. Nadler, L. M., Ritz, J., Bates, M. P., Park, E. K., Anderson, K. C., Sallan, S. E., and Schlossman, S. F. (1982). Induction of human B cell antigens in non-T cell acute lymphoblastic leukemia. *J. Exp. Med.,* in press.

Antigenic Heterogeneity:
A Possible Basis for Progression

RICHMOND T. PREHN

Introduction

It is now widely believed, perhaps with an element of wishful thinking, that most and perhaps all tumors are at least potentially immunogenic in the original host. The fact that spontaneous tumors of rodents are seldom immunogenic when tested in syngeneic animals (Prehn and Main, 1957) tends to be attributed to a lack of sensitivity of the tests or to be simply ignored. It is certainly true that among chemically induced tumors, of which most are clearly immunogenic (Prehn and Main, 1957), the percentage that are demonstrably so is dependent on the sensitivity of the tests. Thus, the assumption that all tumors are immunogenic, albeit some only very weakly, is tenable.

Even if one assumes that immunogenicity, as judged by the *in vivo* immunization challenge test (Lawler *et al.*, 1981), is a widespread attribute of tumors, it is nonetheless evident that it is not, in most situations, the sole determiner of tumor behavior. For example, when the chemical oncogen 3-methylcholanthrene (MCA) is given subcutaneously in uniform

TUMOR CELL HETEROGENEITY

dosage to a series of inbred animals, there is great variation in the latencies of tumor formation and the growth rates of the tumors. Although there is a marked tendency for the more highly immunogenic tumors to have relatively short latencies, weakly or even nonimmunogenic tumors are found throughout the distribution (Bartlett, 1972).

The tendency of the more immunogenic tumors to have relatively short latencies in the primary host could have an explanation unrelated to the effects of immunity. One possibility, for example, might be that the effectiveness of the MCA may vary among the animals and that those most affected are likely to develop tumors with greater changes from the normal, i.e., be faster growing and, incidentally, more immunogenic. This hypothesis is consistent with the observation that mice of an inbred strain do indeed differ in their metabolism of a hydrocarbon oncogen (Niebert *et al.*, 1975) and in their innate susceptibility to oncogenesis (Prehn, 1975). However, it has been shown that the immune reaction is not just incidental, since the differences in susceptibility do not occur among immuno-crippled mice (Prehn, 1979). Also, tumors induced in the immune-free environs of diffusion chambers show a completely random relationship between immunogenicity and latency (Bartlett, 1972). These observations establish the fact that an immune response is absolutely essential to the coupling between the immunogenicity and the latency of primary tumors. Tumors of short latency tend to be relatively immunogenic, but it is the immune reaction that, either by stimulating some to grow faster and/or by killing those that grow slower, imposes the relationship between immunogenicity and latency.

II. Hypotheses Relating Tumor Immunogenicity and Growth Rates

The hypothesis that any highly immunogenic tumors that also happen to be slow growers, i.e., have long latent periods, are killed, grows out of the surveillance hypothesis and is buttressed by the indubitable fact that an immune response, especially in a specifically immunized animal, can be lethal to tumor cells. One could simply postulate that if a tumor is, for any reason, very rapidly growing, it might literally outgrow the immune response even if the tumor were highly immunogenic.

The alternative hypothesis, that the more immunogenic tumors may be stimulated to more rapid growth by exposure to the immune response, is supported by Winn test data with transplanted tumors. Specifically immune spleen cells, mixed in varying proportions with target tumor cells, resulted in accelerated tumor growth when the mixtures were injected into immunocrippled mice and when the proportion of spleen cells to tumor cells was about 1:1. Larger proportions of spleen cells failed to stimulate or actually inhibited the tumors (Prehn, 1972). Similar evidence of stimulation of tumor has been seen with antibody (Heidrick *et al.*, 1978; Shearer *et al.*, 1974). Data analogous to the Winn test data, but in oncogenesis experiments, have also been obtained (Prehn, 1977). In these experiments the immunological capacities of the mice were titrated, typically by restoring radiated thymectomized mice with varying numbers of normal syngeneic spleen cells, and the animals were then challenged with MCA. Tumors appeared most rapidly in partially restored animals and much more rapidly than they appeared in the maximally immunodepressed.

The data suggesting immunostimulation of tumor growth by modest to low levels of immune reaction are quite extensive and congenial with many biological observations (Prehn and Lappe, 1971; Prehn, 1977; Prehn and Outzen, 1980); however, these data could be reconciled, at least in part, to the surveillance explanation by postulating that spleen populations contain mixtures of cells of varying function, in particular suppressors as well as effectors, and that these varying populations have differing growth rates and/or thresholds so that their proportional effect might vary greatly depending on the dosage of spleen cells. In this way one might be able to retain the concept of an immune response that, if it works at all, is only inhibitory to tumor and give up the idea that immunity might, at one level (low level) be stimulatory, and at another (high level) be inhibitory to tumor growth.

In summary, the immunostimulation hypothesis suggests that the optimal immune reaction for tumor growth, i.e., the reaction associated with the shortest latencies, should be significant but not too strong, i.e., it should be at some intermediate level of reactivity. This level of reactivity would, on average, best be supplied by tumors of an intermediate level of immunogenicity. The surveillance explanation predicts, in contrast, that the shortest latencies would be associated with the least host immune reaction. The least host immune reaction would provide the least surveillance and therefore would provide tumors of the highest average immunogenicity as well as of the shortest latency. In the surveillance theory, the highest immunogenicities would be among tumors that occur when surveillance fails, and the tumors are consequently growing most rapidly.

The possibility of distinguishing between these hypotheses provoked me to reexamine and reinterpret my own published work concerning the relationship between tumor latency and immunogenicity (Prehn, 1969).

III. Relationship between Tumor Latency and Immunogenicity

Ninety tumors were examined for the relationship between latency and immunogenicity when animals were given a constant dose of MCA. Because of the large size of the study, some features not seen in studies of lesser size were apparent. In particular, reconsideration of the data (Fig. 1) shows that the tumors with the shortest latencies had, on average, intermediate rather than very high levels of immunogenicity. The immunogenicities of the 22 tumors of shortest latency (latencies shorter than 13 weeks) were high as compared with those of the 21 tumors of longest latency (over 23 weeks), but not nearly as high as those of many of the 23 tumors that arose with intermediate latencies of from 13 to 15 weeks. Thus, the data relating tumor immunogenicity to latent period conform to the expectations of the immunostimulation hypothesis. They do not fit the

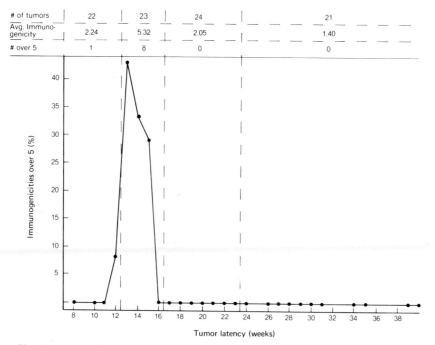

Fig. 1. The relationship between tumor latency (the time in weeks between MCA administration and a tumor of 5 mm average diameter) and tumor immunogenicity over 5. [Immunogenicity is the ratio of average tumor size in controls/average tumor size in immunized mice (Lawler et al., 1981).] The raw data has been published (Prehn, 1969).

predictions of the surveillance theory, at least not without a further assumption: If one assumed that immunodepression by the MCA were a significant factor, as it might be (Prehn, 1963), the time course could be such that the maximal depression would occur at the very time when tumors of the highest immunogenicity were occurring. In this manner the data, showing that the greatest average immunogenicity did not occur in tumors of the shortest latency, could be reconciled to the surveillance hypothesis. However, according to this formulation, one would have expected the maximum tumor incidence, as well as the maximum immunogenicity, to have coincided clearly with the time of maximum immunodepression. This did not happen; the high peak of immunogenicity in the second tumor quartile was not matched by a corresponding peak of incidence. The incidence in the first quartile appears to be comparable to the incidence in the second.

It should be noted that, while the surveillance hypothesis demands that the maximum immunogenicity occur at the time of maximum tumor incidence, and so does not seem to fit the data, the alternative immunostimulation hypothesis demands that the maximum incidence coincide with an intermediate average immunogenicity and with minimal latency. At first glance, it is not clear from the data, as I already noted, that the tumor incidence in the first quartile was different from that in the second. However, the result is actually in accord with prediction because the immunostimulation hypothesis assumes that the shortest latencies will be associated with an intermediate level of immune reaction; the tumors of the second quartile would therefore, in actuality, be divided between two populations, those of very high immunogenicity, presumably associated with mice of less than optimal immune reactivity, and those of quite low immunogenicity, presumably associated with mice of greater than optimal reactivity. The highest tumor incidence would therefore be associated with the intermediate level of immune reactivity in the first tumor quartile and the result thus conforms very well to the predictions of the immunostimulation hypothesis.

These data fit the immunostimulation better than the surveillance hypothesis and imply that the relationship between latency and immunogenicity of primary tumors is most probably due to stimulation, by the immune response, of those tumors of intermediate immunogenicity. However, these data do not bear on the possibility that some facet of the leukocytic system, a facet unrelated to the results of immunization-challenge type tests, may serve a surveillance function. They imply only that the type of immune reaction that is measured by immunization-challenge type tests is much more stimulatory than inhibitory in MCA oncogenesis.

IV. Immunogenic Heterogeneity within Tumors

Thus far, I have discussed immunogenic heterogeneity among tumors; now I would like to turn to immmunogenic heterogeneity within tumors. That tumors are hetergeneous by a number of parameters has been known for many years and was formalized in the histological studies of Henderson and Rous (1962). They showed that histologically variant, but relatively stable, sublines could be isolated from single primary tumors. This type of work led to the observations of Foulds on the nature of tumor progression (Foulds, 1954, 1969).

If tumor immunogenicity plays the biological role I have been suggesting, and if there is antigenic, or better, immunogenic heterogeneity within a tumor, it follows that the immunogenic heterogeneity should play a role in tumor progression. I investigated the possible immunogenic heterogeneity of MCA-induced sarcomas by a method similar in principle to that used by Henderson and Rous. Small fragments of tumor were separated from opposite poles of primary or transplanted sarcomas and sublines called "pseudo-clones" were established from each. Two pseudo-clones were established from each tumor and each pair was subsequently, in transplantation-challenge type experiments, compared for, among other things, its antigenic specificity, immunizing capacity, and response to immunity (Prehn, 1970). A bewildering array of variations between the pseudo-clones was discovered in a high percentage of cases. In some cases one member of a pair could immunize better than the other and this property might or might not be related to a greater or lesser response to immunity. The variations between the pairs were no more or less frequent in primary than in subsequent tumor generations (with one exception), suggesting that new variants were constantly being formed. In other words, I was apparently observing the immunological counterpart of the histological variations seen by Henderson and Rous and which helped to mold Foulds's conclusions concerning progression.

The difference between the primary and secondary tumors was that a difference in antigenic specificity between the paired sublines was detected in only one case, a pair of clones from a primary tumor. In that instance, each clone was able to immunize against itself, but not against the other subline. This result suggests that, while antigenic specificity is very stable, the primary MCA induced tumor may be a mixture of several independent primaries. This conclusion, that the primary carcinogen-induced tumor may not be monoclonal, has been confirmed by Fialkow using the isozyme chimera technique (Reddy and Fialkow, 1979).

Apart from specificity, the very great heterogeneity of the sublines in immunological properties suggests that transplanted tumors should not be very stable in their quantitative immunological parameters. Indeed, Globerson and Feldman showed that highly immunogenic benzopyrene-induced sarcomas would quite regularly lose immunogenicity within three transplant generations; they also showed that an early transplant generation could successfully immunize against a later generation that had itself lost the power to immunize (Globerson and Feldman, 1964). Bubenik also showed that tumor antigens were subject to immunological selection (Bubenik *et al.*, 1965).

Despite the observations listed above, I have been impressed with how stable tumor immunogenicity, as measured by immunization-challenge type experiments, has proved to be among MCA-induced tumors in my laboratory. Although immunogenicities appear to rise or fall in successive transplant generations without any apparent reason, the more general observation has been that highly immunogenic MCA induced tumors usually remain highly immunogenic for many generations and weakly or non immunogenic tumors tend to retain that characteristic. I do take the routine precaution of transplanting tumors into immunocrippled recipients, but I am not convinced this is necessary. While a more systematic examination of the question is obviously demanded, I am impressed with the rather surprising immunogenic stability of these tumors. Similar observations were made by Old (Old *et al.*, 1962).

If this impression of stability despite internal heterogeneity is correct, there are at least two possible explanations. The first derives from the observations of Heppner (Chapter 14) that, in a mammary tumor, four different tumor sublines with distinct morphological and behavioral characteristics were maintained ad infinitum in the original tumor in definite and stable proportions; there was obviously some type of symbiotic interaction among the sublines. Perhaps this type of behavior is a general phenomenon and occurs among immunologically variant sublines of MCA induced sarcomas. However, the fact that the sublines, in my experiments, came from physically separated areas of tumor suggests to me that such an explanation is unlikely.

The other explanation for stability of immunogenicity may lie in the possible functional effects of tumor immunogenicity that I described previously. If a considerable degree of tumor immunogenicity is helpful to tumor growth, there would be selective pressure to maintain an optimal immunogenicity. The optimal level might be different in, and characteristic of, each separate tumor. Obviously more extensive studies of the type described by Bubenik would be in order to examine this hypothesis.

One other comment concerning immunogenic progression: It is quite possible that the mechanisms and especially the rates of immunogenic progression may be very different upon transplantation than they are in the primary host. Not only is the host's immunological environment different, but the sampling involved in transplantation will probably alter the rate of apparent progression.

Finally, I do not know at this point whether immunogenic progression would be expected to lead to greater or lesser degrees of immunogenicity. From the observations that suggest a competitive advantage for tumors that arouse an intermediate level of immune reaction, one might predict that highly immunogenic and lowly immunogenic tumors would both progress toward a common end point of intermediate immunogenicity. This prediction has not yet been adequately tested, but I would guess that this prediction will not be supported by observation; I have already suggested that, while it is true that an intermediate level of immunogenicity appears to be advantageous on average, it is probable that each individual tumor has its own unique optimal level of immunogenicity. In any event, the transplanted MCA tumors, with their apparent immunogenic stability, may not be good models in which to study immunogenic progression. Perhaps they complete their progressions in the primary host or within the first one or two transplant generations. Slower growing tumors, such as those induced with lower concentrations of MCA (L. M. Prehn, unpublished), may be better experimental material.

Acknowledgments

Supported by Public Health Service (PHS) grants CA31837 and CA31836 from the National Cancer Institute and an American Cancer Society, Inc., grant.

References

Bartlett, G. L. (1972). *J. Nat. Cancer Inst.* **49**, 493–504.
Bubenik, J., Adamcova, B., and Koldovsky, P. (1965). *In* "Genetic Variations in Somatic Cells." *Proc. of Symposium on the mutational process Praha,* pp. 403–408. Academia Publ. House of Czechoslovak Acad Sci., Praha.
Foulds, L. (1954). *Cancer Res.* **14**, 327–339.
Foulds, L. (1969). *In* "Neoplastic Development" (Leslie Foulds, ed.), pp. 69–75. Academic Press, New York.
Globerson, A., and Feldman, M. (1964). *J. Natl. Cancer Inst.* **32**, 1229–1243.
Heidrick, M. L., Ryan, W. L., and Curtis, G. L. (1978). *J. Natl. Cancer Inst.* **60**, 1419–1425.
Henderson, J. S., and Rous, P. (1962). *J. Exp. Med.* **115**, 1211–1230.
Lawler, E. M., Outzen, H. C., and Prehn, R. T. (1981). *Cancer Immunol. Immunotherapy* **11**, 87–91.
Niebert, D. W., Robinson, J. R., Niva, A., Kumaki, K., and Poland, A. P. (1975). *J. Cell Physiol.* **85**, 393–414.
Old, L. J., Boyse, E. A., Clarke, D. A., and Carswell, E. A. (1962). *Ann. N. Y. Acad. Sci.* **101**, 80–106.

Prehn, R. T. (1963). *J. Natl. Cancer Inst.* **31,** 791–805, 1095–1096.
Prehn, R. T. (1977). *Int. J. Cancer* **20,** 918–922.
Prehn, R. T. (1977). *J. Natl. Cancer Inst.* **59,** 1043–1049.
Prehn, R. T. (1979). *Int. J. Cancer* **24,** 789–791.
Prehn, R. T., and Main, J. M. (1957). *J. Natl. Cancer Inst.* **18,** 769–778.
Prehn, R. T., and Outzen, H. C. (1980). *Prog. Immunol.* **80,** 651–658.
Reddy, A. L., and Fialkow, P. (1979). *J. Exp. Med.* **150,** 878–887.
Shearer, W. T., Philpott, G. W., and Parker, C. W. (1974). *J. Exp. Med.* **139,** 367–379.

Cell Surface Antigen Heterogeneity and Blood-Borne Tumor Metastasis

GARTH L. NICOLSON

I. Introduction

Normal cells almost always maintain proper tissue positioning and appropriate interactions with other normal cells: The loss of these characteristics is one of the most indicative signs of malignancy (Nicolson and Poste, 1976). *In vivo* malignant cells elude the normal controls which govern proper tissue positioning and cellular interactions and escape from the primary tumor mass to invade and metastasize to near and distant host sites (reviews: Fidler *et al.,* 1978; Sugarbaker, 1979; Poste and Fidler, 1980; Fidler and Nicolson, 1981). Although in some cases the movements

TUMOR CELL HETEROGENEITY
Copyright © 1982 by Academic Press, Inc.
All rights of reproduction in any form reserved.
ISBN 0-12-531520-1

of malignant cells mimic the characteristic movements of embryonic cells at specific stages of development and differentiation (Franks, 1978), this is not an absolute determinant of malignancy or metastasis. Once the malignant cells have invaded surrounding tissues, detached, and spread to other sites, they have the *potential* to form new metastatic colonies; however, only a very few cells within a malignant tumor apparently have the capacity to successfully survive at each step of the metastatic process (Fidler, 1976; Poste and Fidler, 1980). This suggests that the metastatic cells possessed unique characteristics that allowed them to metastasize.

As a tumor progresses in its host, it is thought that rare variant cell subpopulations arise within the lesion. Since these variant cells are thought to be subject to host selection pressures, the resulting tumor diverges to a heterogeneous population of various cell types. Foulds (1956a,b,c,d) studied the changes that occurred in mammary tumors during their evolution and found that malignant tumors often achieve autonomy from host controls while acquiring or losing certain tumor characteristics. This phenomenon has been termed tumor progression, and it can result in the emergence of tumor cell subpopulations with enhanced malignant and metastatic potentials (Nowell, 1976.).

The successful selection *in vivo* of highly metastatic tumor cell sublines is generally attributed to the existence of heterogeneous tumor cell subpopulations. Several systems exist where tumor cell subpopulations have been selected for enhanced abilities to metastasize or colonize specific organs. For example, Fidler (1973) was one of the first to select for enhanced organ colonization properties. Using the murine B16 melanoma he selected sublines for their abilities to implant, survive, and grow in the lung to form gross tumor nodules or experimental metastases. Several additional B16 selections have been conducted and these selections have yielded sublines that show enhanced abilities to colonize brain (Brunson *et al.*, 1978; Nicolson *et al.*, 1981), liver (Tao *et al.*, 1979) or ovary (Brunson and Nicolson, 1979). In addition, other animal tumor models for metastasis have been similarly established for fibrosarcoma (Kripke *et al.*, 1978), sarcoma (Nicolson *et al.*, 1978; Yogeeswaran *et al.*, 1980), lymphoma (Schirrmacher *et al.*, 1979; Shearman and Longenecker, 1981), carcinoma (Fogel *et al.*, 1979; Hart *et al.*, 1981; Neri *et al.*, 1982), and lymphosarcoma (Brunson and Nicolson, 1978).

The derivations of highly metastatic tumor cell sublines by selection are probably dependent on the heterogeneity of the original tumors used for the selections. That tumors contain subpopulations of highly metastatic cells even before selection *in vivo* has been shown by cell cloning. Fidler and Kripke (1977) demonstrated that highly metastatic subpopulations exist in tumors by cloning the parental B16 melanoma and comparing the experimental metastatic potentials of several clones in fluctuation assays. They found that B16 cell clones varied widely in their metastatic properties, and this heterogeneity was not caused by the techniques used for cell cloning (Fidler and Kripke, 1977). The heterogeneity of metastatic subpopulations has now been established in a number of tumor systems by cell cloning techniques (Nicolson *et al.*, 1978; Suzuki *et al.*, 1978; Kripke *et al.*, 1978; Reading *et al.*, 1980b; Shearman and Longenecker, 1981; Fidler and Nicolson, 1981; Chambers *et al.*, 1981; Kerbel *et al.*, 1981; Neri *et al.*, 1982). Although the cell clones obtained by these techniques appeared to be stable during short-term culture *in vitro*, they can eventually diverge with time and generate phenotypic heterogeneity within the originally clonal cell populations (Talmadge *et al.*, 1979; Chow and Greenberg, 1980; Fidler and Nicolson, 1981; Neri and Nicolson, 1981; Nicolson *et al.*, 1982).

We have used the RAW117 tumor system to examine phenotype variability *in vitro* and *in vivo*. This system is based on the RAW117 lymphosarcoma or large cell lymphoma. This is a parental tumor line of recent origin (Raschke *et al.*, 1975) that colonizes or metastasizes to lung, liver and lymph nodes at low frequencies in BALB/c mice. We have selected for metastatic variants in this population by repeatedly selecting for the ability to colonize liver and have obtained sublines with enchanced liver metastatic potentials (Brunson and Nicolson, 1978; Reading *et al.*, 1980b). In addition, this system has also been used to generate cell clones (Reading *et al.*, 1980b) and subpopulations with altered cell surface and/ or metastatic properties by sequential selection for lack of binding to immobilized lectins *in vitro* (Reading *et al.*, 1980a). We have examined the stabilities of some of these RAW117 sublines (Nicolson *et al.*, 1982) and have asked questions concerning the type(s) of cell surface alterations that are important in metastasis and the phenotypic heterogeneity of such properties.

II. Materials and Methods

A. Cells

RAW117 lymphosarcoma cells were grown as described (Brunson and Nicolson, 1978). Methods for sequential *in vivo* selection of sublines with enhanced abilities to form solid tumors in the livers of BALB/c mice, and the procedures for *in vitro* selection of lectin-binding variant sublines are reported elsewhere (Brunson and Nicolson, 1978; Reading *et al.*, 1980a).

Clones were established from the parental cell line RAW117-P, from the *in vivo*-selected subline RAW117-H10 (selected sequentially 10 times for liver colonization) and from the *in vitro*-selected subline RAW117-P · Con A[a10] (selected sequentially 10 times for lack of binding to immobilized concanavalin A) and RAW117-H10 · WGA[a10] (selected sequentially 10 times for lack of binding to immobilized wheat germ agglutinin) as described by Reading *et al.* (1980a). For *in vitro* stability tests several clones of RAW117-P and RAW117-H10 were passaged *in vitro* and assayed *in vivo* at various passage numbers by harvesting of cells and injection intravenously into groups of BALB/c mice.

B. Tumor Colonization Assays

RAW117 sublines were assayed for organ colonization (experimental metastasis) after intravenous injection of $0.5-1 \times 10^4$ viable lymphosarcoma cells as described by Brunson and Nicolson (1978). Experiments continued until death, or they were terminated at approximately 10–12 days after injection, whereupon visible tumor nodules were counted in all major organs. Organ colonization assays were confirmed by histology.

C. Binding of Radiolabeled Lectins

Affinity purified concanavalin A and wheat germ agglutinin were prepared and radiolabeled with ^{125}I according to Reading *et al.* (1980a) and Nicolson *et al.* (1980).

D. Competition Radioimmune Assays

Quantitative analysis of viral antigens was performed by competition radiommune assay as described (Reading *et al.*, 1980b). Antigen content was determined by a comparison of sample curves and those obtained with purified antigens.

E. Analysis of Cell Surface Proteins and Glycoproteins

Cells were labeled by lactoperoxidase-catalyzed ^{125}I-iodination techniques (Reading *et al.*, 1980a,b). Cell samples were solubilized and run on 7.5% polyacrylamide slab gels. Surface proteins were identified by autoradiography. Alternatively, cell glycoproteins were identified in the slab gels by the binding of ^{125}I-labeled concanavalin A or wheat germ agglutinin (Reading *et al.*, 1980a,b).

F. Antibody-Mediated Inhibition of Metastasis

In some of the experiments RAW117-H10 cells were treated with purified IgG F(ab')$_2$ antibody fragments, washed, and then injected intravenously into animals. Antibodies used included rabbit IgG anti-H-2 and IgG anti-murine embryonic liver antigen (anti-EML). H-2 K glycoprotein was affinity purified from RDM4 AKR lymphoma by the procedures of Herman and Mescher (1979). The antigen was injected in complete Freund's adjuvant into rabbit footpads once, and then biweekly at intramuscular sites. After five injections the rabbits were bled and serum assayed for anti-H-2 activity. The antisera (a gift from Dr. R. Kubo, National Jewish Hospital, Denver) used to make IgG antibody preparations reacted with public specificities of H-2 α chains and β_2-microglobulin and was not haplotype specific. Anti-EML was produced against stage-specific mouse embryonic liver cells according to Grady et al. (1981). Briefly, 1×10^7 dissociated mouse embryo liver cells were injected intravenously into rabbits at weekly intervals. After the third injection, sera were collected on alternative weeks following booster injections and were stored at -20°C. The serum was thawed, heated at 56°C for 40 minutes to destroy complement, and tested for reactivity with mouse embryonic liver cells. Divalent F(ab')$_2$ antibody fragments were prepared from purified IgG fragments according to Nisonoff et al. (1960, 1961). The F(ab')$_2$ preparation was further treated with formalin-fixed S. aureus bacteria to remove any residual F$_c$-containing components. RAW117-H10 cells were washed three times by centrifugation and resuspension in phosphate-buffered saline, and 1×10^6 cells were suspended in 0.4 ml phosphate-buffered saline containing 1 mg/ml of the appropriate F(ab')$_2$ antibody fragment preparation. Control cells were washed and incubated in phosphate-buffered saline. The incubations were performed in sealed tubes with agitation (tube rotator) for 2 hours at 4°C. After the incubation period, the cells were washed three times by centrifugation and resuspension in phosphate-buffered saline, and viability was determined by Trypan blue dye exclusion. Groups of BALB/c mice were injected (5×10^3 cells/0.2 ml inoculum) intravenously, and tumor nodules determined at day 10–14 in different experiments. In some experiments the assays were terminated at death (McGuire et al., 1982).

III. Results

A. Selection of Sublines and Cell Cloning

Using the RAW117 lymphosarcoma, cell sublines have been obtained by in vivo selection for their abilities to colonize liver or lung (Table I). Alternatively, cell sublines have been selected in vitro for their lack of

TABLE I

Selection and Biologic Properties of *in Vivo* and *in Vitro* Selected Sublines of RAW117 Lymphosarcoma

Subline	Selection	Average No. (range) visible tumor nodules[a]		
		Liver	Lung	Other sites
RAW117-P (parental)	—	0.5 (0–5)	0.4 (0–1)	2/10 spleen
RAW117-P·Con A[a10]	10× immobilized-Con A	112 (0–250)	1 (0–4)	6/10 spleen
RAW117-H5	5× liver colonization	25 (9–42)	0.6 (0–2)	3/10 spleen
RAW117-H10	10× liver colonization	230 (92–>250)	1.5 (1–5)	9/10 spleen; 6/10 lymph nodes
RAW117-H10·WGA[a10]	10× liver colonization; 10× immobilized-WGA	20 (0–>250)	1 (0–4)	4/10 spleen; 2/10 lymph nodes
RAW117-L15 cl. 2	15× lung colonization	3 (0–20)	23 (2–33)	2/10 spleen

[a] 5×10^3 viable RAW117-lymphosarcoma cells were injected intravenously into groups of 10 BALB/c mice and the numbers of visible tumor nodules determined after 10–21 days.

binding to immobilized lectins such as concanavalin A or wheat germ agglutinin (Table I). These selected sublines showed either an increase or decrease in metastatic properties when assayed *in vivo* by injection intravenously (Brunson and Nicolson, 1978; Reading *et al.*, 1980a) or subcutaneously (Reading *et al.*, 1980b). When we selected sequentially for enhanced liver colonization, sublines were obtained that colonized liver more efficiently but showed colonization of lung that was not significantly different from the parental line used to start the selections. Even though the assay in Table I was performed by tail vein injection where the tumor cells must stop initially in the lung, there was no increase in lung colonization with each liver selection. In contrast, selection for lung colonization eventually yielded sublines with enhanced lung tumor colony formation. Selection *in vitro* for reduced adherence to immobilized concanavalin A yielded after 10 sequential selections subline RAW117-P · Con A[a10] which was distinctly more malignant compared to the parental RAW117 line, while 10 selections of RAW117-H10 for lack of adherence to immobilized wheat germ agglutinin produced subline RAW117-H10 · WGA[a10] which was less malignant than the H10 subline (Table I).

Cell clones have been obtained from the *in vivo* and *in vitro* selected RAW117 sublines (for example, see Reading *et al.*, 1980b). In general, these clones show differences in metastatic potential indicative of the heterogeneous nature of this neoplasm. Since the selection process probably resulted in a simple enrichment in cell clones with the appropriate properties, it was reasonable that the selected sublines still showed heterogeneity. Indeed, when the data for 16–41 individual clones of RAW117-P, RAW117-H10, RAW117-P · Con A[a10] and RAW117-H10 · WGA[a10] were pooled and presented together, they were comparable to or mimicked the polyclonal cell populations of each line or subline (Fig. 1). These data also indicated that selections for more metastatic phenotypes result in an enrichment in individual cell clones with enchanced metastatic properties (cf. Fig. 1d with 1b).

The stabilities of line RAW117-P and subline RAW117-H10 have been examined by subcloning during long-term growth *in vitro*. Although the parental cell line and the selected sublines were relatively stable during *in vitro* growth (Brunson and Nicolson, 1978), several clones obtained from these were phenotypically unstable (Nicolson *et al.*, 1982). After approximately 20-40 passages in tissue culture, some of these clones diverged in their metastatic properties (Nicolson *et al.*, 1982).

B. Cell Surface Analysis of RAW117 Sublines and Clones

We have examined certain cellular properties of the parental RAW117 line and selected sublines including doubling time in culture, lectin agglu-

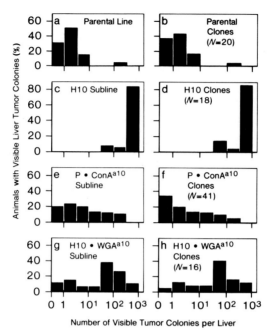

Fig. 1. Biological properties of RAW117 parental line and selected sublines compared to their cell clones. Animals in groups of 10 were injected intravenously with 5 × 10$_x$ lymphosarcoma cells, and the numbers of visible experimental liver tumor colinies counted approximately 10–12 days later. (a), Parental RAW117 line; (b) pooled data for 20 clones of parental RAW117; (c) RAW117-H10 subline; (d) pooled data for 18 clones of RAW117-H10; (e) RAW117-P Con A [a10] subline; (f) pooled data for 41 clones of RAW117-P ConA [a10]; (g) RAW117-H10 WGA [a10] subline; (h) pooled data for 16 clones of RAW117-H10 WGA [a10]. (Data, in part, is from Reading et al., 1980b, and Nicolson et al., 1981.)

tinability, numbers of lectin-binding sites per cell, amounts of viral antigens per cell, and exposures of cell surface proteins and glycoproteins (Reading et al., 1980a,b; Nicolson et al., 1980, 1982). Some of these properties are summarized in Table II. Of the cellular properties examined for their relationship to metastasis only the amounts of viral envelope glycoprotein gp70 and the exposure of an approximately 70,000 molecular weight glycoprotein correlated well with metastatic potential; both of these were lost or dramatically reduced in cells of high metastatic potential (Table II; Reading et al., 1980b). The gp70 is detected in cell surface labeling experiments as an approximately 70,000 molecular weight component, and the amounts and exposures of cell surface gp70 related inversely with metastatic potential in this system. Upon examination of sev-

TABLE II

Summary of Phenotypic Properties of *in Vivo* and *in Vitro* Selected Sublines of RAW117 Lymphosarcoma

Subline	Doubling time *in vitro* (h)	Property			
		Con A binding (ng/10^6 cells)[a]	WGA binding (ng/10^6 cells)[a]	gp70 Content (ng/10^6 cells)[b]	70,000 Surface component[c]
RAW117-P (parental)	12–14	2.42 ± 0.2	4.12 ± 0.3	407 ± 10	+ +
RAW117-P·Con A[a10]	12–14	1.72 ± 0.3	4.31 ± 0.2	309 ± 5	+
RAW117-H5	12–14	1.81 ± 0.3	3.91 ± 0.3	120 ± 22	+
RAW117-H10	12–14	1.54 ± 0.2	3.59 ± 0.2	65 ± 13	−
RAW117-H10·WGA[a10]	12–14	2.16 ± 0.3	3.82 ± 0.4	575 ± 26	+
RAW117-L15 cl. 2	12–14	ND[d]	ND[d]	209 ± 15	+

[a] Amounts of [^{125}I]concanavalin A or [^{125}I]wheat germ agglutinin bound minus control containing 0.1 M inhibitory saccharide. Data are the mean values for three separate experiments ± standard deviation.

[b] Amounts of gp70 determined by competition radioimmune assays. Date are the mean values for three experiments ± confidence levels for standard error of prediction of antigen value from linear regression analyses of radioimmunoassay curves.

[c] Absence (−) or presence at low (+) or high (++) levels of an approximately 70,000 MW cell surface component identified by lactoperoxidase-catalyzed [^{125}I]iodination or binding of [^{125}I]concanavalin A to sodium dodecylsulfate polyacrylamide gels.

[d] Not determined.

eral cell clones from the parental line and selected sublines, this relationship was confirmed further such that there was a high correlation ($r = 0.93$) between metastatic potential and loss of gp70 (Fig. 2).

C. Antigens and Liver Colonization of RAW117 Cells

Although the loss of gp70 correlated well with the overall metastatic potential of RAW117 cells, this cell surface change did not explain the specificity of colonization of the *in vivo* selected sublines. This latter property has been associated with the display of an oncofetal antigen on the RAW117 cells. Liver-colonizing RAW117 sublines expressed an antigen that was related to and cross reacts with an embryonic liver antigen involved in fetal liver cell adhesion (Grady *et al.*, 1981). For example, liver-colonizing RAW117-H10 cells contained more of this antigen compared to the parental RAW117 line or the lung-selected RAW117-L14 subline (McGuire, *et al.*, 1982). Treatment of high liver-colonizing metastatic subline RAW117-H10 with F(ab')$_2$ or Fab' antibody fragments against the oncofetal antigen blocked colonization of liver by these cells and resulted in long-term survival of the lymphosarcoma-injected animals (Nicolson *et al.*, 1982; McGuire, *et al.*, 1982). However, treatment of the same

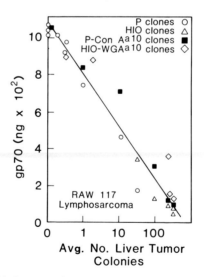

Fig. 2. Relationship between the content of viral envelope glycoprotein gp70 determined by competition radioimmune assay and the ability to form visible experimental liver tumor colonies for several cell clones obtained from RAW117-P, RAW117-H10, RAW117-P·ConA[a10], and RAW117-H10·WGA[a10]. (Data, in part is from Reading *et al.*, 1980b; for details see Section II.)

RAW117 cells with anti-H-2 $F(ab')_2$ or Fab' reagents had no effect on these parameters, though the anti-H-2 antibody fragments bound to almost the same numbers of antigen sites compared to the antibody fragments against the oncofetal antigen(s). Quantitatively, BALB/c mice injected intravenously with 5×10^3 RAW117-H10 cells all had greater than 200 visible liver tumor colonies by 12 days postinjection and died at a median of 14 days (range 14–18 days). Injection of RAW117-H10 cells treated with anti-H-2 antibody fragments did not change these values, but injection of H10 cells after treatment with the antibody fragments against the oncofetal liver antigen resulted in a median of 0 (range 0–50) liver tumor nodules, and in another experiment, all animals survived greater than 31 days postinjection with no evidence of liver involvement (Nicolson et al., 1982). Since the lung colonizing subline tested had less of the liver oncofetal antigen in quantitative absorption assays (McGuire, et al., 1982) these results suggest that specific cell surface receptors may be involved in organ-specific metastasis.

IV. Discussion

Our RAW117 metastatic system appears to be similar to human large cell lymphoma or lymphosarcoma. The RAW117 cells are of non-thymus-derived, B cell lineage (Raschke et al., 1975), and they colonize lungs, liver, spleen and lymph and lymph nodes like the human counterpart disease (Mollander and Pack, 1964) of similar origin (Lukes and Collins, 1974). We have utilized sequential selection and/or cloning techniques to obtain the rare, highly metastatic cells in this tumor (Brunson and Nicolson, 1978; Reading et al., 1980a,b). Although these RAW117 sublines were relatively stable in tissue culture, we found many individual RAW117 cell clones to be unstable when propagated alone in culture (Nicolson et al., 1982). Analogous findings have been made recently using B16 melanoma (Fidler and Nicolson, 1981; Poste et al., 1981), IAR6 hepatocarcinoma (Talmadge et al., 1979), and 13762 adenocarcinoma (Neri and Nicolson, 1981). Several sequential selections in vivo or in vitro were required to obtain the highly malignant RAW117 cell subpopulations; this was probably necessary because of the unstable nature of most of the highly malignant clones in the original tumor.

The mechanisms governing tumor cell clonal instability are unknown, but they could be important in tumor evolution or progression by ensuring the frequent generation of some highly malignant cells in the tumor population (Nowell, 1976). Depleting cells within a tumor by chemotherapy or other means can restrict clonal phenotypic variation. Poste et al. (1981) demonstrated recently that chemotherapy can restrict phenotypic diversity of B16 melanoma cells *in vivo* to yield a new B16 population; this probably occurred because of the heterogeneity in drug sensitivites between different cells in the polyclonal B16 population (Lotan and Nicolson, 1979; Tsuruo and Fidler, 1981). Once the B16 population was restricted to the cell survivors of chemotherapy, some of which were apparently unstable, a new panel of variant subpopulations was quickly generated returning the tumor to its original heterogeneous phenotypic state (Poste *et al.*, 1981). In order to explain this phenomenon Schirrmacher (1980) has proposed that a preformed genetic program could be activated by environmental signals, and this could lead to widespread changes in genetic expression resulting in phenotypically diverse tumor cell populations.

We have been interested in the cell surface properties of highly malignant cell subpopulations, because of the obvious role of the cell surface in metastasis (Fidler and Nicolson, 1981; Nicolson, 1982). There are a few dramatic differences between RAW117 cells of low and high metastatic potential. First, RAW117 cells can be separated on the basis of their cell surface properties by countercurrent distribution or sequential partitioning in dextran-poly(ethylene) glycol two-phase aqueous buffer systems. Highly malignant RAW117 subpopulations, whether from unselected or selected lymphosarcoma cell populations, always partition to high cavity numbers along the extraction train based on their cell charge and hydrophilic/hydrophobic cell surface properties (Miner *et al.*, 1981). Another difference that is related to metastatic potential is the exposure of cell surface proteins and glycoproteins by surface labeling (Nicolson *et al.*, 1980; Reading *et al.*, 1980a,b), particularly the exposure of a 70,000 molecular weight component. The identity of this component is probably gp70, the major viral envelope glycoprotein found on many types of murine tumor cells. Indeed, when the results of competition radioimmune assays for gp70 were correlated with metastatic potential, a good correlation ($r = 0.93$) was obtained between loss of gp70 and metastasis to liver, suggesting that gp70 is related to the quantitative aspects of RAW117 metastasis. Interestingly, the cells with high gp70 content are recognized and eliminated by the host's immune system. In support of this we have found that while depression of certain host immune mechanisms such as T cell-dependent systems had no effect on the metastatic properties of RAW117 cells *in vivo*, inhibiting macrophage function rendered the low metastatic parental RAW117-P cells highly metastatic (Reading *et al.*, 1982). In addition, unstimulated or poly I:C activated syngeneic macrophages were more effective in killing and suppressing the growth of the high gp70-containing RAW117 sublines than the low gp70-containing sublines *in vitro* (Miner and Nicolson, 1982). Our results are similar to what

Mora *et al.* (1977) found with tumor forming SV40-transformed fibrosarcomas. These authors noted that loss of SV40 cell surface antigens due to immunoselection resulted in tumor cell populations with increased tumorigenic properties.

In terms of metastasis, there are several reports that metastases have antigenic alterations compared to their primary tumors. Sugarbaker and Cohen (1972) examined spontaneous lung metastases of a murine fibrosarcoma, and they found that transplantation antigens were lost or were present in lower amounts in metastases compared to primary tumors. Pimm and Baldwin (1977), Gorelik *et al.* (1979), Fogel *et al.* (1979), and Schirrmacher and Bosslet (1980) have documented that metastases are antigenicly different from primary tumors. Similar to what we have found with RAW117, Shearman and Longenecker (1981) found alterations in antigen expression between avian lymphoma variants of different metastatic properties, and they also correlated the expression of an antigen on lymphoma cells with liver-colonizing potential. Shearman *et al.* (1980) also demonstrated that liver colonization could be inhibited, at least in part, by treating lymphoma cells with antibodies against a specific cell surface antigen. The antigen they studied could be similar to the oncofetal antigen we have found on RAW117 cells, the expression of which is also related to liver metastasis (Nicolson *et al.*, 1982; McGuire *et al.*, 1982).

The relationship between liver colonization of the RAW117 cells and the expression of an oncofetal antigen similar to an embryonic liver antigen is probably not explained by host immune responses. This antigen(s) appears to be similar to the component(s) involved in embryonic liver cell adhesion (Grady *et al.*, 1981). It is expressed on embryonic liver cells but is not expressed on embryonic mouse retinal cells; on adult cells it is expressed, but in low amounts. The expression of this antigen(s) or a cross-reacting species on the RAW117 cells may be related to the embryonic stage when normal fetal lymphoid cells colonize the liver, or it may be present in a rare subpopulation of adult lymphoid stem cells in the monocyte or B cell lineage. Transformation may cause the reexpression on the RAW117 cells of the oncofetal antigen(s) or its permanent expression on a stem cell which may ultimately become the RAW117 tumor cells.

Acknowledgments

These studies were supported by NCI Grant R01-CA29571. I thank C. Reading, P. Belloni, M. Torriani, R. Davis, and M. Hughes for assistance.

References

Brunson, K. W., and Nicolson, G. L. (1978). *J. Natl. Cancer Inst.* **61**, 1499–1503.

Brunson, K. W., and Nicolson, G. L. (1979). *J. Supramol. Struct.* **11**, 517–528.

Brunson, K. W., Beattie, G., and Nicolson, G. L. (1978). *Nature (London)* **272**, 543–545.

Chambers, A. F., Hill, R. P., and Ling, V. (1981). *Cancer Res.* **41**, 1368–1372.

Chow, D. A., and Greenberg, A. H. (1980). *Int. J. Cancer* **25**, 261–265.

Fidler, I. J. (1973). *Nature New Biol.* **242**, 148–149.

Fidler, I. J. (1976). *In* "Fundamental Aspects of Metastasis" (L. Weiss, ed.), pp. 275–289. North-Holland Publ., Amsterdam.

Fidler, I. J., and Kripke, M. L. (1977). *Science (Washington, D.C.)* **197**, 893–895.

Fidler, I. J., and Nicolson, G. L. (1981). *Cancer Biol. Rev.* **2**, 171–234.

Fidler, I. J., Gersten, D. M., and Hart, I. R. (1978). *Adv. Cancer Res.* **28**, 149–250.

Fogel, J., Gorelik, E., Segal, S., and Feldman, M. (1979). *J. Natl. Cancer Inst.* **62**, 585–588.

Foulds, L. (1956a). *J. Natl. Cancer Inst.* **17**, 701–712.

Foulds, L. (1956b). *J. Natl. Cancer Inst.* **17**, 713–754.

Foulds, L. (1956c). *J. Natl. Cancer Inst.* **17**, 755–782.

Foulds, L. (1956d). *J. Natl. Cancer Inst.* **17**, 783–802.

Franks, L. M. (1978). *In* "Chemotherapy of Cancer Dissemination and Metastasis" (S. Garattini and G. Franchi, eds.), pp. 71–78. Raven, New York.

Gorelik, E., Fogel, M., Segal, S., and Feldman, M. (1979). *J. Supramol. Struct.* **12**, 385–402.

Grady, S. R., Graves, P. B., Nielsen, L. D., and McGuire, E. J. (1981). *Dev. Biol.* (in press).

Hart, I. R., Talmadge, J. E., and Fidler, I. J. (1981). *Cancer Res.* **41**, 1281–1287.

Herman, S. H., and Mescher M. F. (1979). *J. Biol. Chem.* **254**, 8713–8716

Kerbel, R. S., Roder, J. C., and Pross, H. F. (1981). *Int. J. Cancer* **27**, 87–94.

Kripke, M. L., Gruys, E., and Fidler, I. J. (1978). *Cancer Res.* **38**, 2962–2967.

Lotan, R., and Nicolson, G. L (1979). *Cancer Res.* **39**, 4767–4771.

Lukes, R. J. and Collins, R. D. (1974). *Cancer* **34**, 1488–1503.

McGuire, E. J., Mascali, J. J., and Nicolson, G. L. (1982), *Proc. Natl. Acad. Sci. U.S.A.* (in press).

Miner, K. M., Walter, H., and Nicolson, G. L. (1981). *Biochemistry* **2**, 6244–6249

Miner, K. M., and Nicolson, G. L. (1982), submitted for publication.

Mollander, D. W., and Pack, G. T. (1964) *In* "Lymphomas and Related Diseases," Vol. IX: Treatment of Cancer and Allied Diseases (G. T. Pack and I. M. Ariel, eds.), pp. 131–167. Harper, New York.

Mora, P. T., Chang, C., Couvillion, L., Kuster, J. M., and McFarland, V. W. (1977). *Nature (London)* **269**, 36–40.

Neri, A., and Nicolson, G. L. (1981). *Int. J. Cancer* **28**, 731–738.

Neri, A., Welch, D., Kawaguchi, T., and Nicolson, G. L. (1982). *J. Natl. Cancer Inst.* **68**, 507–517.

Nicolson, G. L. (1982). *In* "Cancer Invasion and Metastasis" (L. Liotta and I. R. Hart, eds.), Nijhoff, The Hague (in press).

Nicolson, G. L., and Poste, G. (1976). *N. Engl. J. Med.* **295**, 197–203, Part I, 253–258, Part II.

Nicolson, G. L., Brunson, K. W., and Fidler, I. J. (1978). *Cancer Res.* **38**, 4105–4111.

Nicolson, G. L., Reading, C. L., and Brunson, K. W. (1980). *In* "Tumor Progression" (R. G. Crispen, ed.), pp. 31–48. Elsevier North-Holland, Amsterdam.

Nicolson, G. L., Miner, K. M., and Reading, C. L. (1981). *In* "Fundamental Mechanisms in Human Cancer Immunology:" (J. P. Saunders, J. C. Daniels, B. Serrou, C. Rosenfeld and C. B. Cenney, eds.), pp. 31–39, Elsevier North-Holland, New York.

Nicolson, G. L., Mascali, J. J., and McGuire, E. J. (1982). *Oncodev. Biol. Med.* (in press).

Nisonoff, A., Wissler, F. C., Lipman, L. N., and Woernley, B. L. (1960). *Science (Washington D.C.)* **132**, 1770–1771.

Nisonoff, A., Markus, G., and Wissler, F. C. (1961). *Nature (London)* **189**, 293–295.

Nowell, P. C. (1976). *Science (Washington, D.C.)* **194**, 23–28.

Pimm, M. V., and Baldwin, R. W. (1977). *Int. J. Cancer* **20**, 37–43.

Poste, G., and Fidler, I. J. (1980). *Nature (London)* **283**, 139–146.

Poste, G., Doll, J., and Fidler, I. J. (1981). *Proc. Natl. Acad. Sci. U.S.A.* **78**, 6226–6230.

Raschke, W. C., Ralph, P., Watson, J., Sklar, M., and Coon, H. (1975) *J. Natl. Cancer Inst.* **54**, 1249–1253.

Reading, C. L., Belloni, P. N., and Nicolson, G. L. (1980a). *J. Natl. Cancer Inst.* **64**, 1241–1249.

Reading, C. L., Brunson, K. W., Torianni, M., and Nicolson, G. L. (1980b). *Proc. Natl. Acad. Sci. U.S.A.* **77**, 5943–5947.

Reading, C. L., Kraemer, P. M., Miner, K. M., and Nicolson, G. L. (1982), *Clin. Exp. Metastasis* (in press).

Schirrmacher, V. (1980). *Immunobiology* **157**, 89–98.

Schirrmacher, V., and Bosslet, K. (1980). *Int. J. Cancer* **25**, 781–788.

Schirrmacher, V., Bosslet, K., Santz, G., Clauer, K., and Hubsch, D. (1979). *Int. J. Cancer* **23**, 245–252.

Shearman, P. J., Gallatin, W. M. and Longenecker, B. M. (1980). *Nature (London)* **286**, 267

Shearman, P. J., and Longenecker, B. M. (1981). *Int. J. Cancer* **27**, 387–395.

Sugarbaker, E. V. (1979). *Curr. Probl. Cancer* **3**, 3–59.

Sugarbaker, E. V., and Cohen, A. M. (1972). *Surgery* **72**, 155–161.

Suzuki, N., Withers, H. R., and Koehler, M. W. (1978). *Cancer Res.* **38**, 3349–3351.

Talmadge, J. E., Starkey, J. R., Davis, W. C., and Cohen, A. L. 1979). *J. Supramol. Struct.* **12**, 227–243.

Tao, T-W., Matter, A., Vogel, K., and Burger, M. M. (1979). *Int. J. Cancer* **23**,854–857.

Tsuruo, T., and Fidler, I. J. (1981). *Cancer Res.* **41**, 3058–3064.

Yogeeswaran, G., Stein, B. S., and Sebastian, H. (1980). *J. Natl. Cancer Inst.* **64**, 951–957.

7

Mechanisms for and Implications of the Development of Heterogeneity of Androgen Sensitivity in Prostatic Cancer

JOHN ISAACS

I. Overview of the Response of Prostatic Cancer to Hormonal Therapy

One of the fundamental concepts concerning cancer is that malignant tumors characteristically lose their normal responsiveness to growth factors that regulate cellular proliferation. This does not mean, however, that tumors are completely unresponsive and therefore autonomous to all growth factors. On the contrary, it has been known since the pioneering work of Charles Huggins in the 1940s that many types of human tumors do respond to normal growth factors in relation to their proliferation. Indeed, this response is often very similar to that of the normal tissue of origin for the particular tumor type. For tumors of endocrine dependent tissue, these growth factors are often specific tropic hormones. For example, like the normal prostate, which requires a continuous supply of androgen to maintain both cell number and secretory activity, prostatic cancers often retain a similar androgen requirement for stimulation of their growth. This form of cancer is thus often highly responsive to androgen ablation therapy. While approximately 60–70% of all men with metastatic prostatic cancer treated by androgen ablation do respond, indicating that their cancers are initially androgen responsive, essentially all these men eventually relapse to a state unresponsive to further antiandrogen therapy (Menon and Walsh, 1970). What is the mechanism for this relapse phenomenon wherein an initially androgen-sensitive prostatic cancer progresses following androgen ablation to an androgen-insensitive state?

II. Possible Mechanisms for the Relapse of Prostatic Cancer after Androgen Ablation Therapy

One possibility (Fig. 1) is that prostatic cancers are initially composed of tumor cells that are homogeneous at least in regard to their requirement for androgenic stimulation of their growth. Following castration, most of these dependent cells stop proliferating and die, thus producing an initial

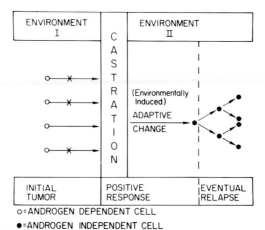

Fig. 1. Environmental adaptation model for the relapse of prostatic cancer to androgen ablation therapy.

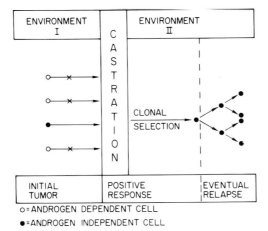

Fig. 2. Environmental selection model for the relapse of prostatic cancer to androgen ablation therapy.

positive response to hormonal therapy. Some of these androgen-dependent cells, however, under environmental pressure, randomly adapt to become androgen-independent. These androgen-independent cells, once formed, proliferate without the requirement for androgenic stimulation, and thus repopulate the tumor producing a relapse after castration. In such an explanation, the changing host environmental conditions following castration are assumed to be critically involved in inducing the adaptive transformation of an initially androgen-dependent to an androgen-independent tumor cell. This process is therefore called the environmental adaptation model. In contrast to this environmental adaptation model where the changing hormonal environment is assumed to play a direct inductive role, an alternative explanation is possible in which the role played by the changing hormonal environment following castration is only indirect (Fig. 2). It is possible that initially prostatic cancers are heterogeneous, at least in regard to their androgen requirements for growth, being composed of preexisting clones of androgen-dependent and -independent tumor cells. Castration, in such a context, would result in the death of only the androgen-dependent cells without affecting the continuous growth of the androgen-independent ones. These independent cells would continue to proliferate following castration. Even if these androgen-independent cells initially represented only a small fraction of the starting tumor, they would eventually not only completely replace any tumor loss due to the death of the androgen-dependent cells, but progressively expand the tumor population producing the relapse phenomenon.

III. Experimental Animal System That Demonstrates the Relapse of Prostatic Cancer after Androgen Ablation: The Dunning R-3327-H Rat Prostatic Tumor

In order to experimentally determine if either the environmental adaptation or selection model is indeed responsible for the relapse of prostatic cancer after androgen ablation therapy, we have utilized the Dunning R-3327-H rat prostatic adenocarcinoma as a test system (Isaacs *et al.*, 1978). This serially transplantable rat prostatic tumor, hereafter called the H tumor, was originally derived by W. F. Dunning in 1961 from a spontaneously occurring primary tumor of the dorsal lobe of a 22-month old male Copenhagen rat (Dunning, 1963). Histological examination of this H tu-

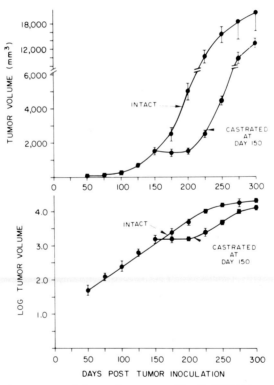

Fig. 3. Growth response of the androgen-sensitive R-3327-H tumor to hormonal therapy. Initially 24 intact male rats were each inoculated with 1.5×10^6 viable H tumor cells. A control group of 12 male rats was allowed to remain intact during the entire tumor growth period while the remaining 12 test rats were castrated after 150 days postinoculation. Upper panel: linear growth plots. Lower panel: semilogarithmic plot of the tumor growth in the control and test animals.

mor reveals a well differentiated prostatic adenocarcinoma composed of distinct well formed acini (Isaacs *et al.*, 1979a). This H tumor has been shown to be an important model for human prostatic cancer since it mimics many of the properties of the human disease (Isaacs and Coffey, 1979b). One of its important similarities is its response to androgen ablation (Isaacs and Coffey, 1981).

When 1.5×10^6 viable H cells are injected subcutaneously into intact adult male rats, H tumors become palpable approximately 40–50 days postinoculation. Once palpable, the growth of these tumors is continuous as revealed by the plot of the tumor volume versus days post tumor inoculation (Fig. 3). This linear growth curve can be replotted as the log of tumor volume versus days post tumor inoculation to demonstrate that between 50 and 180 days the H tumor in intact male rats is growing exponentially with a doubling time of 21 ± 6 days.

At 150 days postinoculation of 1.5×10^6 viable H tumor cells into intact male hosts, the exponentially growing tumors, approximately $1-2$ cm^3 in volume, are histologically uniform, well-differentiated adenocarcinomas with essentially no area of necrosis (Fig. 4A). The tumors are composed of prominent well developed acini, the lumen of which are filled with secretions. In addition, each tumor acinus is surrounded by well-developed stromal elements. If intact rats bearing such exponentially slow growing H tumors are castrated at day 150, the tumor abruptly stops its exponential growth and for approximately 60 days does not increase its volume (Fig. 3). This positive response to androgen ablation demonstrates that the H tumor is highly androgen-sensitive. This sensitivity is revealed not only by the cessation of progressive tumor volume growth, but also by the histological appearance of the tumor during this androgen ablation responsive period (Fig. 4B). One month following castration, not only is there an increase in the proportion of the tumor which is necrotic, but even in areas that appear well preserved grossly, there are now large relatively acellular areas in which very few tumor acini are found. These areas are essentially composed of only the stromal element of the tumor (i.e., collagen and fibroblasts). These areas, depleted of tumor acini, are adjacent to large areas where tumor acini are perfectly maintained with no evidence of acinar involution or cellular death. The acini in these well-maintained areas are fully secretory even during this period of positive response as revealed by the presence of secretions in their lumens. Approximately 2 months following castration, this initial response to androgen ablation is subsequently followed by a renewal of proliferative growth, indicating that the tumor has relapsed to hormonal therapy (Fig. 3). The histological picture of the tumor when it has relapsed to castration, as judged by its renewed exponential growth, is now uniformly well differentiated with very few areas depleted of tumor acini (Fig. 4C).

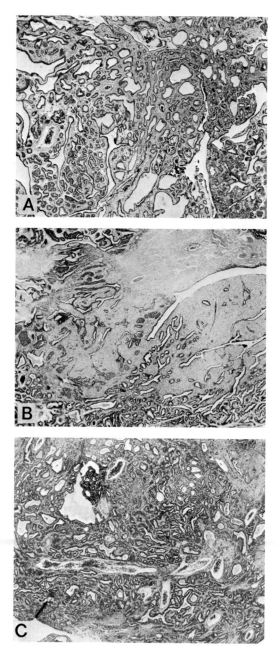

Fig. 4. Histologies of the R-3327-H tumor before, during, and after response to androgen ablation. (A) Tumor growing exponentially in intact male rats before castration. (B) Tumor not growing 1 month following castration. (C) Relapse tumor growing exponentially again 2 months following castration. × 24.

IV. Fluctuation Analysis of the Dunning R-3327-H Tumor: Demonstration of Its Heterogeneous Nature

To determine whether the relapse of the H tumor to hormonal therapy is due to adaptation or clonal selection, fluctuation analysis was performed on the H tumor based on the technique originally developed by Hakansson and Trope (1974) for the demonstration of tumor cell heterogeneity with regard to chemotherapeutic sensitivity (Isaacs and Coffey, 1981). If the H tumor is initially heterogeneous, being composed of substantial areas of androgen-dependent and androgen-independent tumor cells, small trocar pieces of identical size taken at random from the tumor should have the same total number of tumor cells composed, however, of widely fluctuating ratios of androgen-dependent to -independent cells. Therefore, if such trocar pieces are used to individually inoculate rats, each animal will receive a constant number of total tumor cells composed, however, of a highly variable number of androgen-independent cells. If allowed to grow in intact animals, all such trocar inoculums should grow to produce tumors of 1 cm^3 volume with essentially identical times (i.e., small fluctuation in time) since the total number of starting cells in each case is identical and, under such conditions, both androgen-dependent and -independent cells grow equally well. In direct contrast to the consistency in intact rats, the time required for trocar pieces to grow to 1 cm^3 in castrate rats, should require widely fluctuating times if the original H tumor is heterogeneous, since each trocar piece would have varying starting numbers of androgen-independent cells. If the H tumor is not heterogeneous but is instead homogeneously composed of androgen-dependent cells and castration actively induces the random development of androgen-independent cells from the initially dependent tumor cells, then individual trocar pieces of identical cell number inoculated into castrate male rats should each have the same frequency of this induction, and thus, the time required to grow to 1 cm^3 in castrates should be very similar for all trocar pieces. Therefore, the fluctuation in the time required for individual trocar pieces to grow to 1 cm^3 in castrate rats can be used to differentiate between these two different mechanisms for relapse to hormonal therapy. As a control to judge the normal baseline fluctuations in growth response due to technical problems of tumor passage, the entire H tumor remaining after removal of the trocar pieces was enzymatically dissociated into tumor cells. These cells are then carefully mixed so that each cell inoculation will have the same number of starting viable tumor cells as that of the trocar pieces. When these uniform cell suspensions are injected into intact versus castrate rats, the time required for the tumors to grow to 1 cm^3 should be much longer in the castrate hosts since, under this condition, only the androgen-independent cells grow. However, the fluctuation in the time to grow to 1 cm^3 between individual castrate animals inoculated with these uniform cell suspensions should be small since each rat receives an identical number of total viable cells containing the same average number of androgen-independent tumor cells. Therefore, the magnitude of the fluctuation in the time required for these uniform cell suspension inoculations to produce 1 cm^3 tumors in castrate rats can be used to define the upper limit of the random fluctuation expected due simply to technical problems of tumor passage. The data in Fig. 5 demonstrate the actual fluctuation in the time required for tumors to grow to 1 cm^3 in 10 intact and 10 castrate rats individually inoculated with either trocar tumor pieces or uniform cell suspensions (Isaacs and Coffey, 1981). For graphic purposes, each of the tumors was assigned an individual number on the basis of increasing time for the respective tumor to reach 1 cm^3 postinoculation. In this way, the variation in time between tumors number 1 and number 10 graphically illustrates the full range of fluctuation seen for each group. A horizontal line would indicate no fluctuation for all 10 samples. In contrast, an increased slope reflects the degree of fluctuation in the samples. Examination of this figure reveals that the fluctuation for the 10 intact animals inoculated with either trocar pieces or uniform cell suspensions is small and identical. This is expected since under these intact conditions both androgen-dependent and -independent cells grow equally well and thus any variation in the relative proportion of either cell type will not matter, only the total number of cells inoculated, which is identical for all intact animals. In direct contrast, the fluctuation for the 10 castrate rats inoculated with trocar pieces, as compared to castrate rats inoculated with cell suspensions, is not identical. Clearly, the fluctuation in the time required to produce 1 cm^3 tumors in the 10 castrate animals inoculated with trocar pieces is much larger than that seen for the 10 castrate rats inoculated with comparable tumor cell suspensions. The more than three-fold increase in the standard deviation of the mean seen in the castrate group inoculated with trocar pieces ($\pm$ 80) as compared to that of the castrate rats inoculated with cell suspensions ($\pm$ 25) again demonstrates that this large fluctuation is not simply due to technical problems of tumor passage. These results are not compatible with the idea that the H tumor before castration is homogeneously androgen-dependent and that androgen ablation induces the new development postcastration of androgen-independent tumor cells. If this had occurred, the fluctuation in the time required to produce 1 cm^3 tumors should have been very similar between the castrate animals inoculated with trocar pieces as compared to those inoculated with uniform cell suspensions. These results, instead, demonstrate that the H tumor is heterogeneously androgen-sensitive even before androgen ablation therapy is begun.

The relapse of the H tumor to hormonal therapy thus involves a process of clonal selection brought about by androgen ablation therapy of a pre-existing population of androgen-independent tumor cells present within the initially heterogeneous androgen-sensitive H tumor (Fig. 2). The question therefore becomes, how can such tumor cell heterogeneity develop?

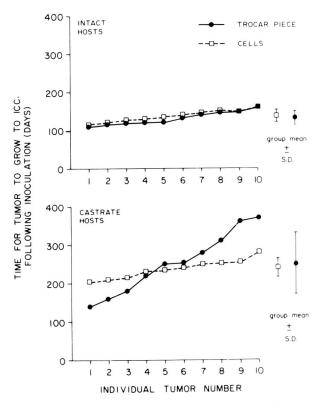

Fig. 5. Fluctuation in the time required for inoculations of solid trocar pieces (10 mg) or cell suspensions (1.5×10^6 viable cells) of the R-3327-H tumor to grow to a size of 1 cm³ in intact versus castrate male rats. Initially, 10 intact and 10 castrate male rats were separately inoculated with tumor cell suspensions and then 10 different intact and 10 different castrate male rats were separately inoculated with solid trocar pieces of tumor. Each tumor was assigned an individual tumor number on the basis of increasing time required for the respective tumor to reach 1 cm³ postinoculation.

V. Mechanisms for the Development of Tumor Cell Heterogeneity in Prostatic Cancer

One possibility is that instead of a monoclonal origin for the original prostatic tumor, the tumor initially arose as a polyclonal mixture of hormonally dependent and independent tumor cells. Indeed, such a possibility has been proposed for human prostatic cancer. This suggestion is based on the observation, obtained by careful pathological step-sectioning of primary human prostatic cancers, that many prostates have anatomically distinct multifocal areas of tumor involvement (Byar and Mostofi, 1972). If some of these distinct tumor areas are hormonally dependent and others independent, then, a heterogeneously sensitive tumor would exist even before hormonal therapy began.

Another possibility is that while a prostatic tumor may initially develop monoclonally from a single androgen-dependent transformed cell, as this parental cell continues to proliferate, eventually an occasional progeny cell becomes genetically unstable. Since this concept of genetic instability in cancer cells will be discussed in detail by Nowell in Chapter 22, I will not develop the general thesis except to say that the development of genetic instability can eventually lead to changes in the tumor genome such that a genetically changed clone of cells with a new phenotype can be added to the original homogeneous tumor. When such an addition occurs, the tumor is no longer homogeneous, but is instead now heterogeneous. Is there any evidence to support the concept of acquired genetic instability as a mechanism for the development of heterogeneity in prostatic cancer? Again, the H tumor can be used to experimentally demonstrate that a genetically stable tumor can develop genetic instability under certain conditions and that this can lead to the addition of new heterogeneous clones of cells to the tumor. The value of using the H tumor for such experimental studies is that this tumor, as will be shown later, has a normal karyotype composed of a diploid number of chromosomes with no markers (Wake et al., 1982). Therefore, any change in this normal karyotype is definitive proof that genetic instability has occurred. The normal genetic stability of the H tumor is demonstrated by the fact that it has been possible to maintain the original characteristics of the H tumor (i.e., diploid chromosomal number, slow growth rate, androgen sensitivity, and well differentiated morphology) for over 20 years in serial passage. At several distinct subpassages during the last 6 years, however, a few random H tumors developed definitive genetic instability (Isaacs et al., 1982). This genetic instability was initially demonstrated by the fact that these H tumors, growing in intact male rats, began growing at rates 8–10 times faster than normal. In these unusual animals, the tumor volume doubling times decreased from approximately 20 to less than 3 days. Histological examination of these unusually fast growing tumors at a time when they are still less than 5 cm^3 revealed heterogeneous tumors composed of distinct areas of well differentiated glandular acini and areas of poorly differentiated anaplastic cells (Fig. 6). When such heterogeneous tumors were passaged, the subsequent tumors uniformly became palpable after only 10 days postinoculation instead of the usual 40–50 day period for normal H tumors. These unusually fast growing tumors doubling in volume in less than 3 days, often grew to the size of the host rat within 60 days. Histological examination of these unusually fast growing tumors revealed uniformly anaplastic tumors with no indication of any areas of well differentiated tumor cells. These fast growing anaplastic tumors are thus termed AT tumors. The spontaneous progression of the slow growing H tumor to fast growing AT tumors has occurred at least three separate times during the last 6 years at Johns Hopkins. Each time such a progression has occurred, we have been able to demonstrate, by flow cytofluorometric techniques, that there has been a substantial increase in DNA content of newly developed AT tumors as compared to the diploid DNA content of the parent H tumor (Isaacs et al., 1982). Fortunately, when the most recent H to AT tumor progression occurred, we were able to demonstrate a concomitant increase in tumor cell ploidy by flow cytometry. In cooperation with Sandberg and Wake of Roswell Park, we documented specific chromosomal changes also (Wake et al., 1982). Wake's chromosomal analysis of the parent H tumor demonstrated a normal diploid karyotype. In contrast to this diploid karyotype, the most recent AT tumor was tetraploid. Karyotype of this tumor demonstrated tetrasomy in almost all chromosomal groups, though deviation from tetrasomy (gain or loss) was observed in a few chromosomes; in addition, there were two unidentified minute chromosomes (Wake et al., 1982). Further chromosomal changes continued to develop with subsequent passage of this AT tumor. For example, five passages later, aneuploidization from tetraploidy (i.e., loss of chromosomes) and the development of structural abnormalities were observed in this AT tumor (Wake et al., 1982).

These results demonstrate that the H to AT tumor progression, each time it has occurred, has consistently involved the development of genetic instability as evidenced by the subsequent development of new anaplastic cell progeny that are genetically distinct from their parental H cell precursors. In addition, these studies have shown that each time an AT tumor has developed, the tumor has been completely androgen-insensitive with relation to its growth; that is, these AT tumors always grow equally well in intact or castrate male rats. This loss of androgen sensitivity occurred even though the tumors always originated in intact male rats. This demon-

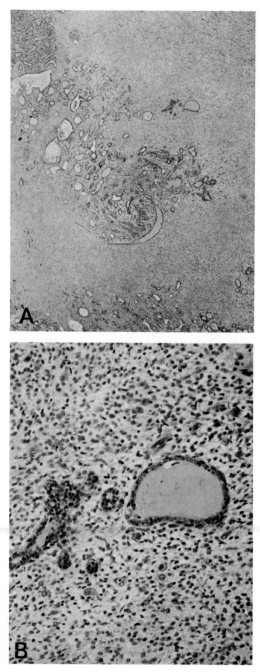

Fig. 6. Histology of the "unusually fast growing" H tumor. (A) × 30 (B) × 210.

strates that changes in the host hormonal environment are not necessarily required for either the acquisition of genetic instability or the subsequent development of new androgen-independent tumor cells.

VI. Conclusions and Therapeutic Implications

In summary, the experimental animal studies that have been presented demonstrate that prostatic cancers can be composed of both androgen-dependent and androgen-independent tumor cells even before hormonal therapy is begun. This heterogeneity can arise via a variety of mechanisms as outlined previously. The therapeutic implication of this preexisting prostatic heterogeneity is that initial therapies based solely on hormonal manipulation will not be able to cure prostatic cancer patients since this therapy affects only a portion of the tumor population. Under these conditions, the use of additional modalities (e.g., radiation therapy and chemotherapy) specifically targeted at the androgen-independent tumor cells, early in the treatment of prostatic cancer, should be combined with androgen ablation therapy.

Acknowledgment

This work was supported by USPHS, National Institutes of Health, Grants Nos. CA 15416 and CA 06973.

REFERENCES

Byar, P., and Mostofi, F. (1972). *Cancer* **30**, 5–13.
Dunning, W. F. (1963). *Natl. Cancer Inst. Monogr.* **12**, 351–369.
Hakansson, L., and Trope, C. (1974). *Acta Pathol. Microbiol. Scand. A.* **82**, 41–47.
Isaacs, J. T., Heston, W . D. W., Weissman, R. M., and Coffey, D. S. (1978). *Cancer Res.* **38**, 4353–4359.
Isaacs, J. T., Isaacs, W. B., and Coffey, D. S. (1979). *Cancer Res.* **39**, 2652–2659.
Isaacs, J. T., and Coffey, D. S. (1979). *Cancer Detect. Prev.* **2**, 587–600.
Isaacs, J. T., and Coffey, D. S. (1981). *Cancer Res.* **41**, 5070–5075.
Isaacs, J. T., Wake, N., Coffey, D. S., and Sandberg, A. A. (1982). *Cancer Res.,* in press.
Menon, M., and Walsh, P. C. (1979). *In* "Prostatic Cancer" (G. P. Murphy, ed.), pp. 175–200. PSP Publishing Co., Littleton, Massachusetts.
Wake, N., Isaacs, J. T., and Sandberg, A. A. (1982). *Cancer Res.,* in press.

PART III

Therapeutic Implications

Drug Resistance and Chemotherapeutic Strategy

JAMES H. GOLDIE

I. Introduction

Drug resistance can be considered to be one of the manifestations of heterogeneity that a tumor cell population will express. Evidence strongly suggests that drug resistance arises as a consequence of spontaneous somatic mutations, with the anticancer drugs functioning as powerful selecting agents. Quantitative analysis yields the conclusion that there will be an increasing likelihood of resistant mutants as the tumor population increases. The risk of resistant cells being present can be minimized by initiating treatment at the earliest time possible (when the tumor size is least) and by utilizing combination chemotherapy. This latter step will be equivalent to dropping the net mutation rate to resistance for the system.

II. Phenotypic Variation and Heterogeneity

A property of most spontaneous malignancies of animals and of man is the great range of phenotypic variation manifested by the constituent cells of these tumors. This marked degree of heterogeneity can be measured by many different techniques. These include identification of morphological variation of the cells themselves and the detection of a wide variety of protein markers present in or elaborated by the tumor cells. Tumors also show a very great range in degrees of sensitivity to many types of antineoplastic agents. In experimental systems this can extend from classes of tumor cells that are susceptible to having their numbers diminished several logs by pharmacologically achievable drug concentrations, to other cell types that are not affected even by the highest drug ranges possible.[1, 2]

Therefore, drug resistance can be seen as one class or subset of phenotypic variation that tumor cell populations can express. In this chapter we will briefly describe some of the mechanisms whereby this range in drug sensitivity and resistance can come about, and how a more quantitative understanding of the process can lead to certain specific conclusions as to how cancer chemotherapy may be directed more effectively.

It is important at the outset to distinguish between two broad classes of phenotypic variation and heterogeneity that may manifest itself in tumor cell populations. The first broad category which we will describe generally as "epigenetic" is based on a significant biological difference that appears to exist between spontaneous tumors and those that have been maintained for protracted periods in laboratory systems, either *in vivo* or *in vitro*. The early studies of Bruce[3] and Bush and Hill,[4] and more recently the large amount of data accumulating from the *in vitro* cloning assays of human tumors,[5] support the hypothesis that spontaneous tumors are characterized by a cellular dynamic organization that is very similar to that of normal cell renewal systems such as the hemopoietic system.

Such a cell renewal system is illustrated schematically in Fig. 1. Present within the cell population is a small subset of cells characterized by the properties of being able to undergo an indefinite process of self-renewal or alternatively to give rise to large numbers of progeny which enter into a differentiation pathway. The stem cell compartment which is labeled A in Fig. 1 is composed of cells that are highly undifferentiated and which upon division may either give rise to two new stem cells or to give rise to progeny which have lost stem cell capacity but which then proceed through a planned program of cellular differentiation. For the integrity of the system to be maintained, the probability of new stem cell formation must always be slightly greater than 0.5 or otherwise the entire cell system will undergo progressive contraction and eventual extinction.[6] The cells that enter the differentiation pathway (labeled B) give rise by a process of clonal expansion to a large number of progeny. As cells progress down this pathway they will increasingly express the morphological and

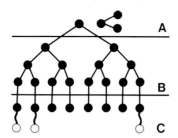

Fig. 1. Schematic representation of a three compartment cell renewal system. (A) Stem cell compartment. These cells can be considered to have a certain probability of dividing to form two new stem cells, or of entering compartment B, where they will undergo a process of clonal expansion, and progressively acquire the properties of differential function. Compartment C represents fully differentiated cells which have lost proliferative capacity and have a finite life-span, during which they undergo senescence and eventual dissolution.

functional characteristics of the terminal differentiated cells that make up compartment C. This latter compartment is composed of fully functional cells which, in the case of the hemopoietic system, have permanently lost the capacity for cell division and which have a finite life expectancy. These cells become effete and are removed from the system and the integrity of the functional compartment C must be maintained by continual input from the proliferative expansion compartment labeled B. In normal cell systems the rate and progression through these compartments is subject to a complex and exquisite system of control such that cell birth is balanced by cell loss so that the total system remains in a steady state. It seems that spontaneous malignancies may be characterized by a cellular organization that is not too dissimilar from that seen in the normal hemopoietic system. Namely, there is a small sub-population of clonogenic or malignant stem cells which is responsible for maintaining the size and progressive expansion of the tumor cell population as a whole. In addition to this small population of stem cells there is a much greater population of morphologically malignant cells which are analogous to the cells present in the normal compartment B. That is, these cells undergo clonal expansion and in the process may acquire, in varying degrees, some of the differentiated properties of the analogous normal cell renewal system from which the tumor line has been evolved. As the tumor cells progress through compartment B they lose proliferative capacity and finally become terminal cells with a variable life expectancy within the end cell compartment. Unlike the normal cell renewal system, however, the balance between cell birth and cell loss is not maintained so that there is progressive expansion of the entire cell population. Likewise, the prog-

eny of the malignant stem lines will not completely express the differentiation programs of the corresponding normal cell lineages. However, in at
least some disorders that are recognized as being fundamentally neoplastic in nature, cells in the proliferating and end cell compartment may express to a very large degree the functional and morphological properties
of their normal counterparts. This is particularly apparent in certain of the
myeloproliferative disorders such as polycythemia vera and chronic
myelogenous leukemia. Such systems are unstable, however, and eventually through a process of clonal evolution display less and less of the normal terminal differentiated cell function and become functionally and
morphologically progressively more undifferentiated.

The reason this process is emphasized in this part of the discussion is
because it is important to distinguish between properties acquired by tumor cells as they pass through scrambled or incomplete differentiation
programs and those properties that are expressed by the tumor stem cells
themselves. As many lines of evidence suggest that in spontaneous tumors the proportion of true stem cells in a neoplastic cell population is
much less than 1% of the recognizable cell forms, then many of the measurements of phenotypic variation and heterogeneity will in fact be measurements of properties of the partially differentiated cells that exist within compartments B and C. These properties may be very important from
the point of view of the effects they have on the host organism, hormone
responsiveness, and response to other homeostatic control mechanisms.
It is apparent, however, that for chemotherapy to be effective in extin-
guishing a neoplastic cell line it must affect the cells of the stem cell compartment. It must be capable of killing these cells outright or at least ren-
dering them sterile in the biological sense.

III. Variation in Drug Sensitivity

In the following discussion we will be concerned with the stem cell
compartment of the tumor. In particular, the question will be addressed as
to what is the basis of variation in drug sensitivity and resistance that is
seen in the cells of this compartment?

The problem is more easily studied if one examines the special case of
neoplastic cell lines that have been propagated continuously in cell culture or by serial transplantation in suitable animal hosts. It can be readily
shown that if at the time of the initial inoculation of malignant cells there
is a variation in the capacity for self-renewal among the stem cells contained in that inoculum, then a process of subculturing or serial passage
will quickly select for those stem cells that have the highest capacity for

self-renewal. Thus, after very few transplant generations one will have a tumor cell population that is largely composed of stem cells which on division give rise to two new stem cells, and where little, if any, differentiation occurs. Such cell systems will be characterized by a considerable degree of morphological and general biological uniformity and a high cloning efficiency when grown in culture or when transplanted from one suitable host to the other.

In recent years much attention has focused on cell kinetic parameters as being a major discriminant in determining drug sensitivity or resistance to particular antineoplastic agents. While cell kinetic phenomena undoubtedly play a role in determining the overall sensitivity of the cell system being considered, there are a number of compelling reasons indicating that this cannot be the sole basis for drug resistance.

It is a commonly observed phenomenon, both in the treatment of experimental neoplasms[7] as well as in the treatment of clinical neoplasia that after an initial regression of a tumor with chemotherapy that the tumor recurs in the face of continued application of the same drugs (and of the same dosage) that were initially effective in inducing a remission. In experimental systems, in virtually every circumstance where this has been examined critically, it is apparent that the cells that recur in the face of continuing therapy are now distinguished by a variety of biochemical alterations which render them resistant to the chemotherapeutic agents that were applied.[7]

In 1943, Luria and Delbruck developed the technique of the fluctuation test to show that the development of resistance in bacterial populations was a consequence of spontaneous mutations arising within those populations and then having a selecting agent remove the sensitive cells, leaving behind a resistant clone.[8] Since their pioneering studies on microbial cells similar types of studies have been carried out on a variety of mammalian tumor cell systems and virtually all of these data are strongly supportive of the hypothesis that resistant tumor cells in experimental systems arise as a consequence of spontaneous mutations.[9, 10] The effect of the chemotherapeutic drugs is to function purely as selective agents eliminating the sensitive cells from the population.

Although the fluctuation test itself does not delineate the mechanism of the origin of the resistant phenotype, it does indicate that the appearance is as a consequence of a spontaneous and random process. It is consistent with what is known about spontaneous genetic mutations resulting in phenotypic variation. More recently, a variety of experimental studies support the conclusion that such resistant phenotypes in fact arise as a consequence of true genetic mutations resulting in hereditable phenotypic changes.[11, 12, 13]

If somatic mutations to resistance are an important factor in conferring overall drug resistance to a population of tumor cells, then this has a number of consequences both with respect to the expected behavior of such a system and as to how one might design therapeutic strategies that will have the maximal likelihood of totally eliminating the neoplastic cell line.

One feature of such cell systems, which are continuously undergoing spontaneous mutations, and which was first noted by Luria and Delbruck, is that both the absolute numbers and proportion of resistant phenotypes increase with the overall increase of the cell population. The process whereby this occurs is illustrated schematically in Fig. 2. Here we postulate a small population of sensitive cells designated S (compartment A) which are undergoing spontaneous conversion to a resistant phenotype at a rate of one in five (this of course is not a realistic value for actual mutation rates but is selected to more readily illustrate the process).

In Fig. 2A one such resistant phenotype has developed at a time when the size of the S population is equal to five. If we now allow the sensitive population to double (Fig. 2A) then there will be on average two more conversions of a sensitive to a resistant phenotype. In addition the initial resistant phenotype developed in Fig. 2A will have also doubled so that there is now a total of four resistant phenotypes in the resistant compartment. Thus, it is readily apparent that not only are the absolute numbers of resistant cells increasing but so is their percentage of the total cell population. This is because resistant phenotypes grow as a consequence of two processes: their own intrinsic growth rate as well as by the added effect of new mutations appearing from the sensitive pool. Even if the back mutation rate to sensitivity is the same as that of to resistance, this will not significantly alter the proportion of resistant phenotypes within the total cell population. This is because in most situations the sensitive cell population will be much larger than that of the resistant one, so that

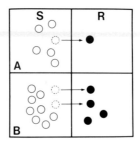

Fig. 2. Schematic representation of the relationship $F = (1\text{-}N\text{-}\alpha)$, to indicate how the resistant subpopulation will come to form a progressively greater percentage of the whole. (A) Initial conditions after one sensitive cell has mutated to a state of resistance. (B) After both populations have undergone one doubling.

even given identical rates there will be a much greater absolute number of entities transitting from sensitivity to resistance than in the reverse direction. Thus, an inherent property of cell systems undergoing spontaneous mutations at a constant rate is that the phenotypic diversity will increase with time. If one imagines more complex scenarios wherein the entities in the resistant compartment undergo further mutational events to double and triple levels of resistance, then one can see that by an acceleration of this effect that, as the cell population expands, its phenotypic diversity and degree of drug resistance will increase disproportionately with time.

This relationship has been developed mathematically by us[14] and can be expressed by the formula F (fraction of resistant cells) $= (1 - N^{-\alpha})$, where N = total tumor size and, α = mutation rate per cell generation.

Thus, one can see that even without invoking other effects associated with expanding tumor mass (related to altered cell kinetics, metabolic and immunological effects on the host organism, and the increasing probability of migration of cells into pharmacologic sanctuaries) that spontaneous mutation will on its own greatly reduce the likelihood of curability of a tumor as it increases in size.

By the appropriate mathematical techniques it is possible to derive a simple equation that estimates the probability of there being zero resistant cells within a cell population of a given size and a given mutation rate.[14] This is given by the formula $P_0 = \exp(-\alpha[N-1])$, where α is the mutation rate per cell generation and N is the size of the cell population of the tumor. If we consider P_0, that is, the probability of there being zero resistant cells present, as the minimum condition required for chemotherapeutic cure to be achieved, then this equation relates the probability of cure to the mutation rate to resistance and the size of the system in cell numbers. It is apparent from this relationship that small tumors will on average be much more likely to have zero resistant cells present within them than tumors that have reached a considerable volume. Thus, the somatic mutation theory provides a readily understandable explanation for the virtually universally observed phenomenon in experimental neoplasms of the inverse relationship between curability and cell burden.[8] Extrapolating this relationship into the treatment of clinical tumors, one would expect that all other things being equal, that neoplasms that are not curable in an advanced stage might be so when treated in the adjuvant situation, when the residual tumor burden is small.

There is another important relationship that can be derived from the equation $P_0 = \exp(-\alpha[N-1])$. If one fixes the value of N to a particular level then plots the probability of zero resistant cells for differing values of the mutation rate, one obtains a curve such as depicted in Fig. 3. This relationship is for a tumor of size 10^6 and we can see the probability of zero resistant cells as it varies with different values for the mutation rate. As might be expected intuitively the lower the mutation rate for the system the greater the probability of there being zero resistant cells present and hence the better likelihood of cure been achieved.

Generally speaking, the only feasible way to drop the net mutation rate for a cell system is by the use of multiple therapeutic agents which are non-cross-resistant in their mode of action. Thus, the probability of any one individual cell within the target population being resistant to several drugs will be substantially less than its probability of being resistant to one. The relationship depicted in Fig. 3 might then be seen to be a rationale for the use of combination chemotherapy. Although many other factors enter into the processes governing the effectiveness of combination chemotherapy, including differential effects at different points in the cell cycle, biochemical synergism between individual agents, and differing pharmacokinetic properties of drugs, again it is apparent that by utilizing combinations of non-cross-resistant agents one greatly enhances the probability of eradicating the cell population. The generally consistent superiority of combination chemotherapy in producing cures in both experimental and in human malignancies has been documented many times. Indeed, most of the progress in clinical cancer chemotherapy over the last decade has come about as a consequence of the recognition of the superiority of combination chemotherapy over even the most effective single agents given in maximum dose.[15]

It is apparent, therefore, that the net mutation rate of a tumor cell system to resistance is in a sense under the control of the therapist. By the

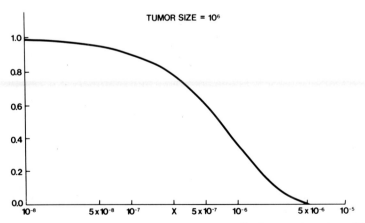

Fig. 3. A plot of the probability of zero resistant cells (i.e., cure) against differing values for the mutation rate for a tumor of size 10^6. $P_0 = \exp(-\alpha[N-1])$. The steepest portions of the curve are where the probability of cure changes from 20 to 60%.

appropriate selection and sequencing of non-cross-resistant agents it should be possible to shift the probability of cure point from a region in the curve where the probability of cure is very low to a point where cure now becomes a realistic possibility for a significant proportion of the patients. It suggests, too, that the most difficult component of this objective may be to move from a point far to the right on the probability of cure curve to a position where at least a small percentage of patients are achieving cure. At this point the probability of cure curve begins to rise in a steep fashion and one might infer from this that the addition of further active non-cross-resistant agents at this juncture may disproportionately push the cure percentages up to a significant degree. It is conceivable that we may have seen something analogous to this process occur during the progressive incremental improvement in the end results of treatment of germ cell tumors of the testes with multiple agent therapy.[16]

The process described above lend themselves to computer simulation,[17] which is important because it becomes difficult conceptually to imagine the effects of a number of interacting and continuously changing variables. Thus, some of the conclusions that such computer simulations yield are at first sight not intuitively obvious. Among the conclusions reached are:

1. The probability of going from a condition of high curability to low curability will occur over a relatively short interval in the tumor's growth history (i.e., to go from a 95% chance of cure to a 5% chance of cure will occur over an increase in size of 1.8 logs). This change could well occur during the subclinical phase of the growth of the tumor and hence emphasizes the importance of the early implimentation of adjuvant chemotherapy.[14]

2. There will be a substantial variability in the number and proportion of resistant cells in histologically identical tumors of equivalent size. This is inherent within the somatic mutation theory and is the basis for the Luria–Delbruck fluctuation test. This will translate into a variable response to chemotherapy by what appear to be tumors of identical type and stage. This variability of response conforms to clinical and experimental observations.[14]

3. It is easy to demonstrate that it is the first one or two courses of therapy that will have the most important impact on subsequent probability of eradication of the tumor. Compromises in treatment strategy during this early phase, both with respect to drug dosage and to the omission of active agents, will result in a diminished probability of cure that cannot easily be compensated for by later changes in the treatment strategy.[17]

4. It can be shown by the appropriate mathematical and computer simulation techniques that if one is dealing with a population of more than one

class of resistant cells that the optimal strategy on average will be to use an approach of alternating equivalent non-cross-resistant treatment arms.[17]

This latter method is already being explored in a number of clinical trials on at least partly empirical grounds but the somatic mutation theory provides a strong theoretical rationale for such strategies.

IV. Conclusion

This brief review has indicated in a general way how the somatic mutation theory contributes to tumor heterogeneity by resulting in an ever-expanding diversity of phenotypic variants as the tumor cell population increases. Such phenotypic diversity operates to defeat the efforts of the therapist attempting to destroy the neoplastic cell population with drugs. Thus, this leads to the conclusion that the strategies that are most likely to be effective in curing tumors are ones applied when the probability of phenotypic diversity is low (i.e., when the tumor population is at its smallest) and ones which incorporate a diversity of therapeutic modalities (i.e., combinations of non-cross-resistant drugs). Many of these approaches have been shown through empirical clinical and experimental testing to be effective in cancer treatment. The somatic mutation model provides a unifying theory wherein it becomes easier to see how various empirically derived strategic options might work, and suggests how these strategies can be refined and improved.

References

1. Skipper, H. E. (1979). On reducing treatment failures due to overgrowth of specifically and permanently drug resistant neoplastic cells. *In* "Cancer Chemotherapy," Vol. 2. Univ. Microfilms Int. Ann Arbor, Michigan.
2. Brockman, R. W. (1975). Circumvention of resistance. *In* "The Pharmacological Basis of Cancer Chemotherapy," pp. 692–710. Williams & Wilkins, Baltimore.
3. Bruce, W. R., and van der Gaag, H. (1963). A quantitative assay for the number of murine lymphoma cells capable of proliferation in vivo. *Nature (London)* **199,** 79–80.
4. Bush, R. S., and Hill, R. P. (1975). Biologic discussion augmenting radiation effects and model systems. *Laryngoscope* **85,** 7, 1119–1133.
5. Salmon, S. E., Hamburger, A. W., Soekalen, V., Durie, V. G. M., Alberts, D. S., and Moon, T. E. (1978). Quantitation of differential sensitivity of human tumor stem cells to anti-cancer drugs. *N. Engl. J. Med.* **298,** 1321.
6. Till, J. E., McCulloch, E. A., and Siminovitch, L. (1964). Stochastic model of stem cell proliferation based on the growth of spleen colony-forming cells. *Proc. Natl. Acad. Sci. U.S.A.* **51,** 29–36.

7. Skipper, H. E. (1978). Reasons for success and failure in treatment of murine leukemias with the drugs now employed in treating human leukemias. *In* "Cancer Chemotherapy," Vol. 1. Univ. Microfilms Int., Ann Arbor, Michigan.

8. Luria, S. E., and Delbruck, M. (1943). Mutations of bacteria from virus sensitivity to virus resistance. *Genetics* **28,** 491.

9. De Mars, R. (1974). Resistance of cultured human fibroblasts and other cells to purine analogs in relation to mutagenesis detection. *Mutat. Res.* **14,** 335.

10. Siminovitch, L. (1976). On the nature of hereditable variation in cultured somatic cells. *Cell,* 1976, **7,** 1.

11. Chan V. L., Whitmore, G. F., and Siminovitch, L. (1972). Mammalian cells with altered forms of RNA polymerase 11. *Proc. Natl. Acad. Sci. U.S.A.* **69,** 3119–3123.

12. Beaudet, A. L., Roufn, D. J., and Caskey, C. T. (1973). Mutations affecting the structure of hypoxanthine: Guanine phosphoribosyl transferase in cultured chinese hamster cells. *Proc. Natl. Acad. Sci. U.S.A.* **70,** 320–324.

13. Cline, M. J., Stang, H., Mercola, K., Morse, L., Ruprecht, R., Browne, J., and Salser, W. (1980). Gene transfer in intact animals. *Nature (London)* **284, 3,** 422–425.

14. Goldie, J. H., and Coldman, A. J. (1979). A mathematic model for relating the drug sensitivity of tumors to their spontaneous mutation rate. *Cancer Treat. Rep.* **63,** 11–12, 1727–1733.

15. De Vita, V. T., Jr., Young, R. C., and Canellos, G. P. (1975). Combination versus single agent chemotherapy: A review of the basis for selection of drug treatment of cancer. *Cancer* **35,** 98.

16. Einhorn, L. H., and Donohue, J. P. (1979). Combination chemotherapy in disseminated testicular cancer: The Indiana University experience. *In* "Seminars in Oncology" (J. W. Yarboro, ed.), Vol. 6, No. 1, p. 87. Grune & Stratton, New York.

17. Goldie, J. H., Coldman, A. J., and Gudauskas, G. A. (1982). A rationale for the use of alternating non-cross-resistant chemotherapy. *Cancer Treat. Rep.* (in press).

The Heterogeneity of Metastatic Properties in Malignant Tumor Cells and Regulation of the Metastatic Phenotype

ISAIAH J. FIDLER AND GEORGE POSTE

I. Introduction

The cellular heterogeneity of neoplasms has been known since the last century when histological studies first identified morphological differences among cells within the same tumor. Since then increasingly sophisticated methods to study tumor cells *in vivo* and *in vitro* have revealed significant heterogeneity in the expression of myriad phenotypic properties by tumor cells in both primary and metastatic lesions in the same host. These include differences in karyotype; antigenicity; immunogenicity; biochemical properties; growth behavior; and cellular susceptibility to chemotherapeutic drugs (see reviews by Poste and Fidler, 1980; Weiss, 1981, for refs.). More recently, studies done in several laboratories using animal tumors of diverse histological origin have revealed significant variation in the metastatic capabilities of subpopulations of cells isolated from the same tumor (Fidler and Kripke, 1977; Dexter *et al.*, 1978; Kripke *et al.*, 1978; Brunson and Nicolson, 1979; Gallimore *et al.*, 1979; Hart, 1979; Tarin and Price, 1979; Brattain *et al.*, 1980; Poste *et al.*, 1980; Suzuki *et al.*, 1980; Chambers *et al.*, 1981; Stackpole, 1981). These findings have attracted considerable attention since they challenge traditional views about the pathogenesis of cancer and pose important questions about the adequacy of current approaches to the therapy of metastasis.

Until the mid-1970s, dogma held that malignant neoplasms were populated by cells with identical metastatic abilities and metastasis was considered to represent a "random" process in so far as any cell from the primary cell was presumed to be capable of generating a metastasis. The demonstration that tumors contain subpopulations with widely differing metastatic capabilities, including subpopulations that are tumorigenic but nonmetastatic, suggests that metastasis is instead a nonrandom process caused by specific subpopulations of cells endowed with the properties needed to successfully complete each step in the metastatic process. As will be discussed later, metastases need not be caused by cells with the highest metastatic potential. The basic tenet of the concept of metastatic heterogeneity is that metastases are caused by cells endowed with the "metastatic phenotype" and that tumor cells lacking this phenotype are unable to generate metastases.

In addition to its importance in improving our understanding of the pathogenesis of cancer metastasis, metastatic heterogeneity has significant implication for the therapy of metastatic disease. The coexistence of nonmetastatic and metastatic cells within the same tumor dictates that any strategy for treating metastases must focus on the therapeutic sensitivities of the metastatic subpopulations. The complexity of this problem must be fully appreciated. The heterogeneous metastatic capabilities of different subpopulations are matched by equivalent heterogeneity in cellular responsiveness to anticancer drugs and other therapies (reviews, Poste and Fidler, 1980; Weiss, 1981). Consequently, successful therapy will be achieved only by modalities that circumvent the extraordinary cellular diversity present not just in the primary tumor but also in different individual metastases. These issues also apply to the design of screening methods for detecting new antimetastatic agents. The majority of current anticancer screening systems merely monitor the response of the primary tumor to therapy. Unfortunately, such assays may not provide any insight into the response of the metastatic cell subpopulations in either the primary lesion or in established metastases.

This chapter provides a brief review of metastatic heterogeneity in tumor cell populations and discusses the factors that may influence the evolution of cellular diversity within tumors and influence expression of the metastatic phenotype.

II. Heterogeneity of Metastatic Properties in Tumor Cells

The possibility that cells with differing metastatic capabilities might coexist within the same tumor was first suggested in 1939 by Koch who isolated a highly metastatic subline from the Ehrlich carcinoma tumor by serially transplanting lymph node metastases. In 1955, Eva Klein demonstrated that gradual conversion of some solid murine neoplasms into ascites variants was due to the selective overgrowth of a small number of cells which differed from the parental population in their ability to proliferate in the peritoneal cavity and metastasize to the lungs. Since the change was stable and heritable, Klein concluded that the gradual conversion of the solid tumor to the ascites form involved mutation/selection and not adaptation. Further evidence of heterogeneity in the metastatic potential of tumor cells has come from more recent experiments in which selective harvesting of cells from metastases during successive passages of tumor cells *in vivo* has yielded cell populations with a greater metastatic potential than cells from the original cell population (Fidler, 1973; Kerbel *et al.*, 1978; Brunson and Nicolson, 1979; Fogel *et al.*, 1979; Hart, 1979; Schirrmacher *et al.*, 1979; Poste *et al.*, 1980).

Definitive evidence that malignant primary tumors contain subpopulations of cells with differing metastatic capabilities was first obtained in 1977 by Fidler and Kripke using the B16 melanoma syngeneic to the C57BL/6 mouse. To investigate whether primary tumors contained cells of differing or uniform metastatic potential, they prepared a cell suspension from a subcutaneous primary tumor and divided it into two aliquots. One part was immediately assayed for its ability to form experimental pulmonary metastases following intravenous injection. From the second part of the original suspension, 17 clones were isolated and their progeny tested for their ability to produce experimental metastases. If the tumor contained cells of uniform metastatic potential, then the cloned sublines should each produce the same number of metastases as the uncloned parental population. This was not the case. The original uncloned parental tumor cell population produced similar numbers of metastases in different animals but the cloned sublines differed markedly in their metastatic potential (Table I). Although the number of metastases produced by any

TABLE I

Heterogeneity of the B16 Melanoma and K-1735 Melanoma Parent Tumors for Experimental Pulmonary Metastasis[a]

B16 melanoma[b]		K-1735 melanoma[c]	
Source of cells	Median no. of pulmonary metastases (range)	Source of cells	Median no. of pulmonary metastases (range)
B16 parent line	40.5 (8–131)	K-1735 parent	33 (0–152)
Clone 16	3.5 (2–15)	Clone 16	0 (0–2)
Clone 15	5 (2–20)	Clone 13	0 (0–2)
Clone 12	6 (0–34)	Clone 11	0 (0–3)
Clone 24	10 (5–29)	Clone 9	0 (0–5)
Clone 19	13 (0–42)	Clone 10	0.5 (0–4)
Clone 7	17 (0–43)	Clone 6	1 (0–1)
Clone 21	18 (1–48)	Clone 23	1 (0–6)
Clone 18	36 (0–91)	Clone 3	1 (0–6)
Clone 5	45.5 (2–171)	Clone 19	1 (0–7)
Clone 6	99 (5–232)	Clone 14	2 (0–10)
Clone 17	150 (104–210)	Clone 8	4 (0–8)
Clone 3	214 (160–450)	Clone 15	7 (0–17)
Clone 1	237 (73–321)	Clone 5	23.5 (4–73)
Clone 2	254.5 (7–450)	Clone 18	55 (11–140)
Clone 13	260 (50–350)	Clone 24	56.5 (23–160)
Clone 14	<500	Clone 17	90 (70–156)
Clone 9	<500	Clone 1	111.5 (44–187)
		Clone 2	123 (41–168)
		Clone 4	156 (101–196)
		Clone 26	209 (48–383)
		Clone 25	257 (15–521)
		Clone 7	320 (82–375)

[a] Data from Fidler and Hart (1982).
[b] Three weeks after the i.v. injection of 50,000 cells.
[c] Five weeks after the i.v. injection of 100,000 cells.

given clone was constant, individual clones showed wide variation in their metastatic potential. Control subcloning experiments demonstrated that the cloning process was not responsible for the variability. These experiments thus demonstrated that the B16 tumor is heterogeneous and that highly metastatic tumor cell variants preexist in the parental tumor cell population.

The B16 melanoma line was established in 1954 and has been maintained by serial passage in either animals or in culture for many times the life-span of its natural host. Metastatic diversity in this tumor might thus be an artifact of its antiquity. However, recent studies have revealed comparable metastatic heterogeneity in clonal subpopulations of another murine melanoma, the K-1735 melanoma, which is of much more recent origin (Fidler and Kripke, 1980; Fidler et al., 1981). This tumor arose in a C3H mouse subjected to ten 1-hour exposures of uv radiation followed by applications of 2.5% croton oil in acetone to the skin of the scapular region for 2 years. The primary tumor was removed and fragments were transplanted into immunodeficient animals to circumvent the possibility of immune selection. Several weeks later, a tissue culture line was established and cells from the fifth passage were used to produce clones whose metastatic properties were assayed. The clones were found to differ dramatically from each other and also from the parent line in their production of lung metastases with regard to their size, number, and pigmentation. Within each injected clone, however, these three characteristics were quite uniform. Thus, lung colonies produced by one clone could be distinguished readily from those produced by another (Table I). Statistical analysis of the results indicated that only 2 of 22 K-1735 clones tested were indistinguishable from the heterogeneous polyclonal parent cell line. The K-1735 melanoma is thus no less heterogeneous than the B16 melanoma.

Clonal variation in metastatic properties is not peculiar to melanomas. Comparable, extensive heterogeneity in metastatic properties has been described in clones isolated from tumors of diverse histological origin from the mouse (Dexter et al., 1978; Kripke et al., 1978; Tarin and Price, 1979; Chambers et al., 1981), rat (Talmadge et al., 1979; Reading et al., 1980), chicken (Shearman and Longenecker, 1980), and hamster (Enders and Diamandopoulos, 1969). In the above studies tumor cell subpopulations with differing metastatic phenotypes were isolated from primary tumors or cultured tumor cell lines. Additional evidence for metastatic heterogeneity is provided by experiments showing that cells isolated from different individual metastases in the same host exhibit significantly different metastatic phenotypes (Eccles et al., 1980; Fidler and Hart, 1982).

Analysis of metastatic heterogeneity in clonal subpopulations isolated from human tumors is only just beginning. Until recently, studies have been hindered by the lack of experimental systems for analyzing the in vivo behavior of human tumor cells. Transplantation into congenitally athymic nude mice has been used widely to assay the tumorigenic potential of human cells. However, a consistent finding has been that in the majority of reported examples the implanted tumors grew but failed to metastasize, including tumor cells isolated originally from metastases. Similar results have been obtained with animal tumors implanted into nude mice. However, it has been found recently that the failure of tumors to metastasize in nude mice is an age-dependent phenomenon. Tumors that are nonmetastatic in nude mice older than 10 weeks of age will metastasize at a high frequency if inoculated into 3-week-old animals (Hanna, 1980).

Recent studies in the laboratory of George Poste have exploited this phenomenon to assay the metastatic properties of a series of clones isolated from a human melanoma. These experiments have revealed extensive heterogeneity in the metastatic properties of the clones (unpublished observations). These data thus indicate that clonal variation in metastatic ability is not a peculiarity of experimental animal tumors. Further studies are in progress to evaluate the clonal heterogeneity of other human melanomas and a series of human squamous cell lines isolated from squamous carcinomas of the head and neck.

The coexistence of clonal subpopulations with differing metastatic properties within the same tumor means that environmental selection pressures may impact differently on individual subpopulations with resulting alteration in the balance between nonmetastatic and metastatic subpopulations and between subpopulations of low and high metastatic potential. By selecting for or against metastatic subpopulations, the metastatic behavior of uncloned tumor cell populations can be increased or reduced. For example, by selective harvesting and propagation of the invasive and metastatic subpopulations present in the B16-F1 melanoma cell line, we have isolated a series of variant B16 melanoma lines with enhanced invasive and metastatic abilities (Fidler, 1973; Hart, 1979; Poste et al., 1980). These lines are heterogeneous, however, and still contain multiple subpopulations with differing metastatic abilities. The selection pressures applied served merely to ''enrich'' the population with subpopulations with high invasive and metastatic abilities.

In addition to selecting for or against tumor cells exhibiting a complex, multifactorial behavioral trait such as metastatic ability, a related strategy is to expose heterogeneous polyclonal tumor populations to selection pressures that select for (or against) cells that exhibit properties considered important for successful metastasis (e.g., production of tissue lytic enzymes; resistance to killing by host defense mechanisms; drug resistance). As in the enrichment method, variants displaying (or lacking) the property of interest are recovered and tested to determine whether their metastatic behavior is altered. This method has been used to examine whether properties as diverse as adhesive characteristics (Briles and Kornfeld, 1978), lectin resistance (Reading et al., 1980), invasive capacity (Poste et al., 1980), resistance to cytotoxic T lymphocytes (Fidler and Bucana, 1977), and resistance to natural killer cells (Hanna and Fidler, 1981) influence the ability of cells to metastasize.

III. Factors Influencing the Evolution of Cellular Diversity in Malignant Tumors

Cellular diversity can arise in tumors by two nonexclusive mechanisms. For tumors of multicellular origin, diversity is present from the outset (Fig. 1). However, even in these tumors, and certainly for tumors of unicellular origin, the available evidence suggests that additional diversity is generated by the emergence of cell variants during progressive tumor growth (Fig. 1). Striking evidence that tumors of unicellular origin can rapidly generate cell variants with differing phenotypes has been obtained by Fidler and Hart (1981a). Individual colonies of BALB/c embryo fibroblasts produced by transformation of single cells by murine sarcoma virus were cultured as cell lines. Subclones were then isolated at intervals and their metastatic properties compared with the original parent lines. Remarkable diversity was detected in the metastatic properties of the subclones within as little as 42 days after transformation of the original parent cell.

Even though the kinetics with which cell variants are generated may

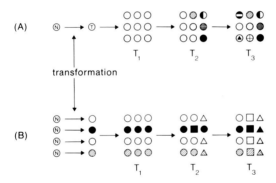

Fig. 1. Schematic representation of possible events in the generation of cellular diversity and metastatic heterogeneity during tumor progression. Following initial transformation of single (scheme A) or multiple (scheme B) normal cells (N), tumor cells are formed and undergo initial proliferation (T_1). In the case of tumors of multicellular origin (scheme B) cellular diversity is present from the outset. With time progressive growth results in the generation of cell variants with different metastatic phenotypes. No time scale is implied for the different time intervals shown (T_1; T_2; T_3). The kinetics of the formation of metastatic variants will probably vary between tumors of different histological origin and between tumors of similar histological origin in different hosts in which tumors will be exposed to a different array of selection pressures imposed by host defense mechanisms and therapy. The formation of new variant subpopulations may not proceed indefinitely and in populations containing multiple subpopulations the rate at which new metastatic variants emerge is lower than in populations containing only a limited number of subpopulations (see Figs. 3 and 4).

vary in tumors of differing histological origin and in tumors of common histological origin in different patients, by the time of initial clinical presentation most tumors will exhibit extensive cellular heterogeneity for a wide range of phenotypes (see Poste and Fidler, 1980, for refs.).

Nowell (1976) has proposed that generation of cell variants is an inevitable and fundamental feature of progressive tumor growth. He proposes that tumor progression occurs via a series of multiple yet independent changes in many different cellular properties, resulting in rapid generation of clonal subpopulations with widely differing phenotypes. At any time during progression, the number of subpopulations present in a tumor, and the extent of their phenotypic diversity, will depend on the selection pressures encountered during the lifetime of the tumor. Selection pressures can be natural (e.g., assault by host defense mechanisms; limiting nutritional conditions) or applied (e.g., therapy).

Nowell's concept of tumor progression also proposes that as successive clonal subpopulations emerge they will display increasing genetic instability. This, coupled with the selection pressures imposed by host defense and/or therapy, will favor relentless emergence of new subpopulations with enhanced metastatic capacities.

The relationship between genetic instability and metastatic ability has been studied recently using clones with low and high metastatic potential isolated from three murine tumors: the UV-2237 fibrosarcoma, the SF-19

TABLE II

Rate of Spontaneous Mutation to Ouabain Resistance of Low or High Metastatic Tumor Cells Isolated from Different Murine Neoplasms [a]

Cell line	Metastatic potential [b]	Rate of mutation [c] ($\times 10^6$ per cell generation)	Increase HMP/LMP
UV-2237 fibrosarcoma LMP-1	Low	0.158	
UV-2237 fibrosarcoma HMP-1	High	0.728	4.61
UV-2237 fibrosarcoma LMP-2	Low	0.0764	
UV-2237 fibrosarcoma HMP-2	High	0.502	6.52
K-1735 melanoma LMP	Low	0.0873	
K-1735 melanoma HMP	High	0.610	6.98
SF-19	Low	0.0178	
SF-19-UV-9	High	0.103	5.78

[a] Data from Cifone and Fidler (1981).

[b] Metastatic potential was determined by the ability of tumor cells to produce spontaneous metastases from a subcutaneously growing tumor or lung metastases after i.v. injection.

[c] The rate of mutation was calculated from the equation originally described by Luria and Delbruck (1943) as adapted in Cifone and Fidler (1981).

fibrosarcoma, and the K-1735 melanoma (Cifone and Fidler, 1981). In all cases the rate of spontaneous cellular mutation to acquire resistance to ouabain or thioguanine was found to be significantly higher in the highly metastatic clones (Table II).

The process of evolution and progression is not limited to the primary tumor but can also occur within metastases. As in the primary tumor, the cellular diversity found in inidividual metastases will be determined both by the properties of the cells responsible for initial formation of the metastasis and by the events that accompany progressive growth of the lesion. For example, if a metastasis arises from the arrest and proliferation of a single tumor cell (Fig. 2A), diversity will be achieved only by generation

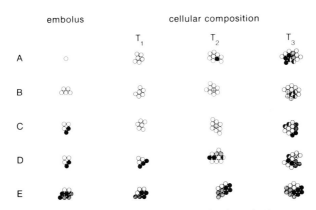

Fig. 2. Schematic representation of possible mechanisms in the generation of cellular diversity within individual metastases. (A) Metastasis formed by the arrest of a single tumor cell which undergoes initial proliferation (T_1). With time (T_2; T_3) new variants are generated. (B) Metastasis produced by arrest of a multicellular embolus composed of cells with identical phenotypes. Irrespective of whether a single cell or several cells survive and proliferate the composition of the initial micrometastasis (T_1) will be similar to that in scheme A. With time new variants will emerge to generate a clonally heterogeneous lesion (T_2; T_3). (C) Metastasis produced by the arrest of a multicellular embolus containing tumor cells with different phenotypes but in which only one cell type survives to generate the intial metastatic lesion (T_1). Subsequent events (T_2; T_3) then follow a similar sequence to schemes A and B. (D) Metastasis produced by arrest of a multicellular embolus containing different cells which survive equally well to establish a micrometastasis that is clonally heterogeneous from the outset (T_1). With progressive growth additional variants are generated to further increase the extent of cellular heterogeneity (T_2; T_3). (E) Metastasis produced by a multicellular embolus containing several different cell types, all of which survive to contribute to the initial micrometastasis (T_1). However, unlike events in scheme D where new variants are quickly generated, in this example the subpopulations interact to limit the rate at which variants are generated in analogous fashion to the events described in Figs. 3 and 4. As a result, progressive growth of the metastasis is accompanied by increases in cell number but subpopulation diversity remains stable (T_2; T_3).

of new cell variants. It is well documented, however, that systemic dissemination of malignant tumors often occurs via clumps or aggregates of tumor cells (see Fidler *et al.*, 1978). The cellular composition of metastases caused by the proliferation of such emboli will then depend on whether the cells in the embolus have similar or dissimilar phenotypes (Fig. 2B–E).

The zonal composition of primary tumors has been recognized on morphological grounds by pathologists for many years. Recently, it has become apparent that these zonal differences are not restricted to morphology alone, but can apply to other biological characteristics of tumor cells (Fidler and Hart, 1981b). We have shown that repeated passage of small, unrepresentative tumor fragments can rapidly impose a uniformity on tumor cell populations that is absent when larger, more representative populations are used (Fidler and Hart, 1981b). It is conceivable that embolic aggregates may arise from a single zone and thus exhibit a degree of uniformity for specific characteristics. Irrespective of whether only one cell or all cells in the embolus survive, the resulting metastatic growth will be analogous to a primary tumor of unicellular origin with regard to the subsequent development of heterogeneity (Fig. 2A and B). The same situation will arise when the embolus is derived from an area of zonal junctions so that the embolus contains populations with varying phenotypes but where selective cell death leads to the survival of only one cell (Fig. 2C). For example, attrition, caused by both specific and nonspecific host defenses, may lead to the death of peripheral cells in the aggregate and the survival of an innermost protected cell. Alternatively many, or all, of the cells forming such a mixed embolus may survive to act as the progenitors of metastatic tumors so that the generation of diversity, as in some primary tumors, is then a consequence of the multicellular origin of the neoplasm (Fig. 2D and E).

Evidence that individual B16 melanoma lung metastases are composed of phenotypically homogeneous cells during the "early" stages of initial metastasis formation but contain phenotypically diverse cells during the later stages of their growth has been obtained in recent studies by Poste *et al.* (1982). These experiments suggest that rapid generation of new cell variants can occur during the lifetime of an individual metastasis, and the data will be described in more detail below when discussing the possible role of interactions between tumor cell subpopulations in regulating the rate at which new variants appear.

Given the role of tumor progression as a mechanism for generating cellular diversity within tumors, and the apparent increasing genetic instability of the new variants generated by this process, how is it that the metastatic properties of uncloned, polyclonal tumor cell lines can remain so constant? For example, the B16 melanoma cell lines, B16-F1 (low metastatic ability) and B16-F10 (high metastatic ability), have maintained their relative metastatic capacities during 8 years of serial passaging *in vitro* and also for long periods of *in vivo* transfer (Poste and Fidler, 1980; Poste *et al.*, 1981). What has prevented these differences from being obliterated by the generation of new variants with different metastatic properties? One reason may be that tumor cells within a polyclonal population do not behave as autonomous units but are affected by the presence of other tumor cells. We have shown recently that different subpopulations of B16 melanoma cells isolated from the B16-F1 and B16-F10 cell lines can affect the behavior of one another and influence the stability of the metastatic phenotype (Poste *et al.*, 1981).

Studies on individual clones isolated from the heterogeneous, polyclonal B16-F1 and B16-F10 lines revealed that their metastatic phenotypes were highly unstable during serial passage *in vitro* and *in vivo* and variant subclones with diverse metastatic phenotypes emerged quickly (Poste *et al.*, 1981). In contrast, the metastatic properties of the uncloned parent cell lines were stable when exposed to the same culture conditions. The "destabilization" of the metastatic phenotype in the individual clones did not occur, however, when several clones were cocultivated together (Fig. 3). The stability of the metastatic phenotype in individual clones during this experiment was verified by using clones bearing stable, drug-resistant markers and by showing that subclones exhibiting resistance to particular drugs had identical metastatic phenotypes to the original clones with the same drug-resistant phenotype.

These experiments suggest that in polyclonal tumors some form of "interaction" is occurring between the constituent clonal subpopulations. Thus, in a polyclonal population containing multiple subpopulations an apparent "equilibrium" exists which, in the absence of any further selection pressure, limits the emergence of new cell variants (or at least variants with altered metastatic properties (Figs. 1 and 3). This type of equilibrium would thus tend to limit the possibility of a few subpopulations or even a single clone dominating the population. This might provide a potent mechanism for the conservation of phenotypic diversity within a tumor and thus increase the likelihood of at least some subpopulations surviving a battery of assaults from the host or from therapy.

Additional studies on the interaction between subpopulations have revealed that imposition of a selection pressure such as drug therapy can alter the "equilibrium" between the subpopulations and restrict subpopulation diversity by eliminating "unfit" subpopulations. If the restriction in subpopulation diversity is substantial, then the "stabilizing" interactions involved in the "equilibrium" state are apparently lost and the surviving subpopulations exhibit marked phenotypic instability and quickly generate a new panel of variants with different metastatic properties (Fig. 3).

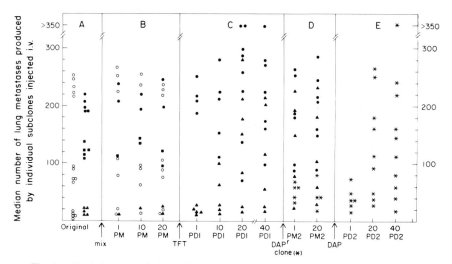

Fig. 3. The influence of clonal diversity on the stability of the metastatic phenotype in B16-F10 melanoma clones. Three wild-type clones (○) and clones resistant to trifluorothymidine (TFT) (▲), ouabain (■) or trifluorothymidine and ouabain (●) with defined metastatic abilities were mixed and cocultivated *in vitro* (Panel A). Subclones were isolated after a further 10 or 20 subcultivations (Panel B) and assayed for their metastatic properties and drug sensitivities. After 20 subcultivations the cultures were treated with TFT. The surviving cells were then passaged (Panel C) and subclones isolated and tested for metastatic properties and for resistance to TFT (▲) or TFT and ouabain (●). After 40 subcultivations a new clone of diaminopurine-resistant (DAP[r]) cells (*) was added. Subclones were isolated from this mixed cell population after 20 subcultivations (Panel D) and their metastatic properties and susceptibility to TFT, ouabain and DAP evaluated. The surviving cells were passaged (Panel E) and subclones isolated at the indicated intervals and tested for their metastatic properties and their ability to grow in HAT medium (DAP[r] variants [*] grow; TFT[r] variants fail to grow). (Reproduced with permission from Poste *et al.*, 1981.)

With time, these variants, in turn, achieve a new equilibrium which persists until a new selection pressure again limits subpopulation diversity and the cycle is repeated (Fig. 3).

This phenomenon is not unique to the B16 melanoma. Similar instability of the metastatic phenotype in clones deprived of interactions with other clonal subpopulations has been reported in two other murine tumors, the UV2237 fibrosarcoma (Cifone and Fidler, 1981) and the RAW117 lymphosarcoma (G. L. Nicolson, personal communication).

The same phenomenon may also occur *in vivo* (Poste *et al.*, 1982). Isolation of multiple clones from individual lung metastases produced by the B16 melanoma has revealed that in "early" metastases excised after 18 days, clones isolated from the same metastasis typically show indistinguishable metastatic properties (i.e., intralesional clonal homogeneity).

This situation was found in approximately 80% of the early metastases tested, though the metastatic phenotypes of clones isolated from different metastases in the same animal do differ significantly (i.e., interlesional clonal heterogeneity). In contrast, in "late" metastases excised after 40 days intralesional clonal homogeneity was found in only 30% of metastases and the remainder yielded two or more clonal subpopulations with differing metastatic properties (i.e., intralesional clonal heterogeneity).

These data suggest that B16 melanoma metastases are populated initially by cells with a uniform metastatic phenotype. This is in agreement with data showing that the majority of experimental metastases result from the arrest and proliferation of a single tumor cell (Poste *et al.*, 1982). This *in vivo* situation is therefore analogous to the *in vitro* experiments described earlier in which individual B16 clones grown in isolation from other clones quickly generated variant subclones with altered metastatic properties. Studies are now in progress using B16 clones bearing drug-resistant markers to study the evolution of clonal heterogeneity within individual metastases *in vivo* in more detail.

IV. Metastatic Heterogeneity in Malignant Tumor Cell Populations: Therapeutic Implications

The problem of cellular heterogeneity in malignant tumors has potentially important implications for experimental efforts to identify new antimetastatic agents and for the treatment of metastatic disease in the clinic.

With the exception of the screening program introduced recently by the Biological Response Modifier Program at the National Cancer Institute, which includes routine evaluation of the antimetastatic activity of candidate compounds, the search for anticancer drugs has relied almost exclusively on assays that screen candidate therapeutic agents for activity against nonmetastatic tumors. Even in assays where metastatic tumors are used, the criterion for activity is often based on the response of the primary tumor rather than metastatic lesions. Although serendipity will allow some agents with antimetastatic activity to be identified in such assays, the probability is equally high that effective antimetastatic agents are being overlooked. The heterogeneity of cellular phenotypes for both metastatic capacity and therapeutic sensitivity is so extensive in most malignant tumor cell populations that evaluation of the response of the primary tumor to therapy may offer little or no insight into the sensitivity of the metastatic cell subpopulations, particularly if these are only a small fraction of the total cell population.

Similarly, heterogeneity among metastatic subpopulations themselves dictates that individual metastases in the same host can show completely different responses to therapy. Consequently, screening assays for anti-metastatic agents must be capable of identifying agents that circumvent this cellular diversity.

The purpose in continuing to use screening methods in which the potential therapeutic agent is administered within hours or a few days of tumor implantation can also be questioned. Although instructive in demonstrating tumoricidal activity, such assays offer no insight into activity against large burdens and established metastases. A much more demanding assay, and one certainly more comparable to the situation encountered by the clinician, is to screen potential agents for their ability to destroy established metastatic lesions.

Metastatic heterogeneity, and the related issue of how the metastatic phenotype is controlled, also merit discussion in the context of current strategies for the clinical therapy of metastatic disease. The finding that tumor cell subpopulations in polyclonal populations influence the behavior of one another and that changes in subpopulation diversity can affect the rate at which new metastatic tumor cell variants emerge have potentially important implications for therapeutic practice. Assuming that similar regulatory interactions between tumor cell subpopulations occur *in vivo* and are common to most, if not all, tumors, then the timing of therapy and its effect on subpopulation diversity may be of crucial importance in determining whether a tumor can be destroyed.

For example, if a particular therapy were to kill the majority, but not all, of the subpopulations in a polyclonal tumor, the surviving subpopulations may be rendered phenotypically unstable because of loss of the regulatory interaction between constituent subpopulations which were previously in "equilibrium." By restricting subpopulation diversity, therapy may perturb this equilibrium and thus provide a stimulus for the rapid generation of new tumor cell variants from the surviving subpopulations (Fig. 4). Generation of variants would then continue until a sufficient level of subpopulation was achieved to again impose a new "equilibrium" via interaction between subpopulations and thus limit the rate at which new variants emerge (Fig. 4). Exposure of the tumor to subsequent treatment regimens would then repeat this cycle (Fig. 4).

If the scheme in Fig. 4 is correct, new therapeutic strategies will need to be devised to frustrate the problem of phenotypic instability in tumor cell subpopulations that survive initial treatment. To achieve this it would be necessary to reduce the time between successive treatment with different therapeutic regimens (Fig. 5). The aim of using a series of different treatment protocols in rapid succession would be to attempt not only to kill

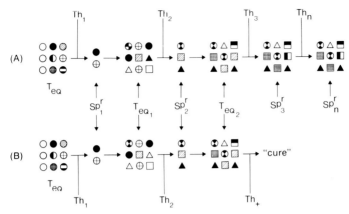

Fig. 4. Schematic illustration of the possible effects of therapy on subpopulation diversity and stability of the metastatic phenotype in neoplastic lesions derived from the experimental data in Fig. 3. By the time of initial clinical detection the lesion contains multiple tumor cell subpopulations. An "equilibrium" state (T_{eq}) exists in which "interaction" between the subpopulations limits the rate at which new metastatic variants are generated as outlined in Fig. 3. On exposure to therapy (Th$_1$), susceptible subpopulations are killed and others survive (SP$_1^r$). As shown in Fig. 3 this restriction of subpopulation diversity may render the surviving subpopulations phenotypically unstable and thus act as a stimulus for the generation of a new panel of tumor cell variants with widely differing metastatic properties. With increasing diversification, a new "equilibrium" state will again be imposed (T_{eq1}). On subsequent exposure to different treatment regimens (Th$_2$; Th$_3$) the cycle of subpopulation restriction and diversification will be repeated until either subpopulations resistant to all therapeutic efforts (SP$_n^r$) kill the patient (scheme A) or a therapeutic modality (Th$_+$) is identified than can kill all subpopulations within the lesion (scheme B).

those subpopulations that survive the previous treatment before they are able to generate large numbers of new variants but also to kill new variant subpopulations as soon as they emerge (Fig. 5). This contrasts with the practice in which subsequent treatment regimens using different agents are often not employed if the first treatment protocol appears successful in eliminating clinically detectable tumor burden. In this situation, additional treatment regimens are implemented only when evidence of a recurrent tumor is detected. By the time such recurrent lesions become detectable, clinically phenotypic diversification of the surviving subpopulations may well have taken place and the lesion is populated by a diverse set of new subpopulations (Fig. 6) which may have widely differing therapeutic sensitivities.

In raising these issues we are mindful of the enormous difficulty that shortening the intervals between successive treatment regimens of the

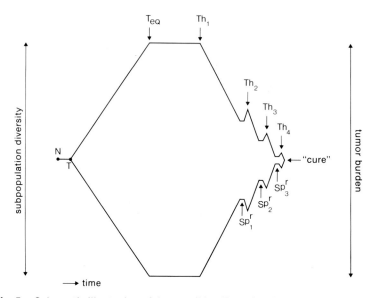

Fig. 5. Schematic illustration of the possible effect of rapid sequential treatment of a neoplastic lesion with a series of different therapeutic regimens. Following initial transformation of a normal cell (N) to establish an initial focus of tumor cells (T), new variants are generated as shown in Fig. 1 to create a heterogeneous lesion populated by diverse subpopulations which eventually establish an "equilibrium" state (T_{eq}) in which the generation of new variants is relatively low. When this population is exposed to therapy (Th_1), the subpopulation diversity and cell mass is reduced by killing susceptible subpopulations. As shown in Figs. 3 and 4, the restriction of subpopulation diversity produced by therapy may provide a stimulus for surviving resistant subpopulations (SP_1^r) to rapidly generate new metastatic variants. However, unlike the example shown in Fig. 6 in which exposure to a second, different treatment regimen is delayed until proliferation of the surviving cells (SP_1^r) creates a clinically detectable lesion, in this example the second treatment regimen (Th_2) is given very shortly after the first treatment protocol even though a residual tumor burden may not be evident clinically. By repeating the process and reducing the interval between successive treatment regimens (Th_1–Th_3), it is hoped that each successive treatment in the series will kill susceptible subpopulations in the tumor fractions (SP_{1-3}^r) that survive the preceding treatment(s) before they are able to generate a large number of new variants which may include variant phenotypes that will prove resistant to all available therapies. By truncating successive treatment regimens into a limited time period, it may be possible to either eradicate tumor cells entirely or reduce the residual tumor burden to a sufficiently low level where host defense mechanisms, perhaps augmented by biological response modifier therapy, can kill any remaining tumor cells.

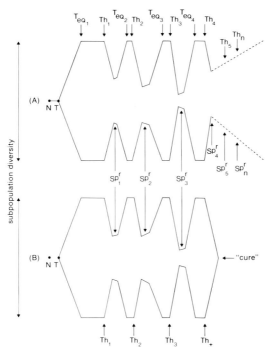

Fig. 6. Schematic illustration of the possible effects of extended staging of successive treatment regimens on subpopulation diversity in neoplastic lesions. Following initial transformation of a normal cell (N) to establish an intial focus of tumor cell (T), extensive phenotypic diversity is generated within the lesion as shown in Fig. 1, creating a heterogeneous lesion populated by diverse subpopulations that interact to establish an "equilibrium" state (T_{eq}) in which emergence of new variant subpopulations is limited. Treatment of such a lesion (Th_1) destroys some, but not all, subpopulations. As described in Figs. 3 and 4, restriction in subpopulation diversity perturbs the preexisting equilibrium and stimulates the surviving subpopulation (SP_1^r) to generate new variants. This diversification process culminates in the establishment of a new "equilibrium" state between the new variants (T_{eq2}). By this time, recurrent tumor growth is detectable clinically and a second, different treatment regimen (Th_2) is initiated and another cycle of subpopulation restriction and diversification ensues. This process will continue until either the patient dies from a tumor burden (SP_3^r) which is refractory to multiple successive treatments (Th_5–Th_n) (scheme A) or a therapy is identified which is able to eradicate the entire remaining tumor burden (scheme B; Th_+). In contrast to the treatment strategy shown in Fig. 5 the extended intervals between successive treatments shown in this figure may allow residual tumor cells to undergo extensive phenotypic diversification between treatments and thus increase the likelihood that new variants refractory to therapy will emerge.

143

kind shown in Fig. 5 would create for both the oncologist and the patient. Given the highly toxic nature of most anticancer agents, legitimate doubt can be expressed as to whether patients could sustain an intensive therapeutic assault of this kind, or would even agree to it!

We do not minimize the dimension of the potential therapeutic problems raised by recent findings on metastatic heterogeneity and the regulation of the metastatic phenotype. Research on these important questions is only just beginning and considerably more work is needed before we would advocate decreasing intervals between successive treatment cycles in clinical practice. Nonetheless, we believe that the potential implications of the research described here are of sufficient importance to merit further study as a matter of some urgency. Similarly, in raising the possibility that therapy may stimulate phenotypic diversification and facilitate emergence of increasingly aggressive tumor cell variants, we are not proposing that current therapies be withheld or abandoned. As emphasized earlier, even if this effect is a consistent feature of therapy the problem may not be insurmountable and can be addressed by changing the timing of therapy.

The more immediate issue is to establish whether the problems discussed here are of limited or general significance in the behavior of malignant tumors. This will require further experiments to determine the effect of different therapeutic modalities and their timing on the phenotypic stability and metastatic behavior of tumor cell subpopulations in neoplasms containing different numbers of identifiable subpopulations. These experiments are conceptually straightforward but the technical resources needed to undertake them may be beyond the capacity of all but the largest research laboratories.

Acknowledgments

Research sponsored by the National Cancer Institute, DHHS, under Contract No. N01-CO-75380 with Litton Bionetics, Inc. (I.J.F.); Grants CA18260 and 30192 from the National Cancer Institute (G.P.). The contents of this publication do not necessarily reflect the views or policies of the Department of Health and Human Services, nor does mention of trade names, commercial products, or organizations imply endorsement by the U.S. Government.

References

Brattain, M. G., Strobel-Stevens, J., Fine, D., Webb, M., and Sarrif, A. M. (1980) *Cancer Res.* **40**, 2142–2146.
Briles, E. B., and Kornfeld, S. (1978). *J. Natl. Cancer Inst. (U.S.)* **60**, 1217–1222.
Brunson, K. W., and Nicolson, G. L. (1979). *J. Supramol. Struct.* **11**, 517–528.
Chambers, A. F., Hill, R. P., and Ling, V. (1981). *Cancer Res.* **41**, 1368–1372.

Cifone, M., and Fidler, I. J. (1981). *Proc. Natl. Acad. Sci. U.S.A.* **78**, 6949–6952.

Dexter, D. L., Kowalski, H. M., Fligiel, Z., Vogel, R., and Heppner, G. (1978). *Cancer Res.* **38**, 3174–3181.

Eccles, S. A., Hackford, S. E., and Alexander, P. (1980). *Br. J. Cancer* **42**, 252–259.

Enders, J. F., and Diamandopoulos, G. T. (1969). *Proc. R. Soc. London, Ser. B* **171**, 431–443.

Fidler, I. J. (1973). *Eur. J. Cancer* **9**, 223–227.

Fidler, I. J., and Bucana, C. (1977). *Cancer Res.* **37**, 3945–3949.

Fidler, I. J., and Hart, I. R. (1981a). *Eur. J. Cancer* **17**, 487–494.

Fidler, I. J., and Hart, I. R. (1981b). *Cancer Res.* **41**, 3266–3267.

Fidler, I. J., and Hart, I. R. (1982). *In* "Genes and Cells" (R. Weber and M. M. Burger, eds.). Alan R. Liss, New York.

Fidler, I. J., and Kripke, M. L. (1977). *Science* **197**, 893–895.

Fidler, I. J., and Kripke, M. L. (1980) *Cancer Immunol. Immunother.* **7**, 201–205.

Fidler, I. J., Gersten, D. M., and Hart, I. R. (1978). *Adv. Cancer Res.* **28**, 149–250.

Fidler, I. J., Gruys, E., Cifone, M. A., Barnes, Z., and Bucana, C. (1981). *J. Natl. Cancer Inst. (U.S.)* **67**, 947–956.

Fogel, M., Gorelik, E., Segal, S., and Feldman, M. (1979). *J. Natl. Cancer Inst. (U.S.)* **62**, 585–588.

Gallimore, P. H., McDougall, J. K., and Chen, L. B. (1979). *Int. J. Cancer* **24**, 477–484.

Hanna, N. (1980). *Int. J. Cancer* **26**, 675–680.

Hanna, N., and Fidler, I. J. (1981). *J. Natl. Cancer Inst. (U.S.)* **66**, 1183–1190.

Hart, I. R. (1979). *Am. J. Pathol.* **97**, 587–600.

Kerbel, R. S., Twiddy, R. R., and Robertson, D. M. (1978). *Int. J. Cancer* **22**, 583–594.

Koch, F. E. (1939). *Krebsforschung* **48**, 495–507.

Kripke, M. L., Gruys, E., and Fidler, I. J. (1978). *Cancer Res.* **38**, 2962–2967.

Luria, E. S., and Delbrük, M. (1943). *Genetics* **28**, 491–511.

Nowell, P. C. (1976). *Science (Washington, D.C.)* **194**, 23–28.

Poste, G., and Fidler, I. J. (1980). *Nature (London)* **283**, 139–146.

Poste, G., Doll, J., Hart I. R., and Fidler, I. J. (1980). *Cancer Res.* **40**, 1636–1644.

Poste, G., Doll, J., and Fidler, I. J. (1981). *Proc. Natl. Acad. Sci. U.S.A.* **78**, 6226–6230.

Poste, G., Doll, J., Brown, A. E., Tzeng, J., and Zeidman, I. (1982). *Cancer Res.* (in press).

Reading, D. L., Belloni, P. N., and Nicolson, G. L. (1980). *J. Natl. Cancer Inst. (U.S.)* **64**, 1241–1248.

Schirrmacher, V., Bosslet, K., Shantz, G., Claver, K., and Hubsch, D. (1979). *Int. J. Cancer* **23**, 245–252.

Shearman, P. J., and Longenecker, B. M. (1980). *Int. J. Cancer* **25**, 363–369.

Stackpole, C. W. (1981). *Nature (London)* **289**, 798–800.

Suzuki, N., Williams, M., Hunter, N. M., and Withers, H. R. (1980). *Br. J. Cancer* **42**, 765–771.

Talmadge, J. E., Starkey, J. R., Davis, W. C., and Cohen, A. L. (1979). *J. Supramol. Struct.* **12**, 227–243.

Tarin, D., and Price, J. E. (1979). *Br. J. Cancer* **39**, 740–754.

Weiss, L. (1981). *Pathobiol. Annu.* (in press).

10

Different Susceptibilities of Tumor Cell Subpopulations to Cytotoxic Agents and Therapeutic Consequences

CLAES TROPÉ

I. Introduction

As the number of drugs with demonstratable cytostatic activity increases exponentially year by year, so the job of selecting appropriate drugs for a given tumor becomes increasingly difficult. Not only will the response to new agents vary between different types of tumor, but individual tumors may vary within one histological type and class. Added to this is the difficulty of monitoring a response and the vast increase in complexity resulting from triple and quadruple combinations. Drug sensitivity of cultures derived from the tumor have often been used to predict the response of individual tumors (for review see Kaufmann, 1980).

TUMOR CELL HETEROGENEITY

Extrapolation of *in vitro* drug testing results to the *in vivo* situation is difficult, as the effect of the cytostatic drug therapy on malignant disease depends on many factors that cannot be studied *in vitro* (e.g., factors such as drug excretion and metabolism, tumor–host interaction, drug distribution, and vascularization of the tumor). Furthermore, there is a risk that the parts of the tumor tested *in vitro* are not representative of the whole tumor.

When organ cell cultures are used, only a fraction of all explanted tumors will grow *in vitro* (on average 60%). When this occurs, the result can be a selection of tumor cells which create a cell population with a sensitivity to cytostatic drugs differing from that of the original tumor. In order to reduce the risk of cell selection during the *in vitro* test, studies were made on short-term effects of drugs on tumor cell metabolism.

In our laboratory we have used such a method to study the effect of hormones on human endometrial tissue, normal and malignant, and human breast cancer. It was also used for studies of the effect of cytostatic drugs on normal cells. In these studies, cellular response to drugs was measured as changes in DNA synthesis, evaluated by incorporation of labeled thymidine.

In a series of studies, we further explored the possibility of using this method for investigating the effect of cytostatic drugs on tumor cells. For this purpose, we choose to work with experimental animal tumors in order to get a controlled system where the significance of the effects studies *in vitro* could be evaluated. The main studies were made on mouse subcutaneous sarcomas induced with methylcholanthrene. Thereby, a large number of different tumors could easily and rapidly be obtained. By using an inbred mouse strain, C57B1/6J, it was also possible to study such tumors after serial subcutaneous transplantation.

II. Technical Aspects of the *in Vitro* Short-Term Incubation Method

The method used in the present study consists of the following steps (Fig. 1): A suspension of tumor tissue is prepared in a culture medium, and the suspension is incubated with or without added drug for 3 hours at 37°C. Then tritiated thymidine or uridine is added and incubation is continued for a further hour. The amount of incorporated thymidine and uridine is measured by liquid scintillation counting and the cpm are normalized for the number of tumor cells (estimated as amount of DNA). Thymidine incorporation is expressed in a logarithmic form (so-called *a*

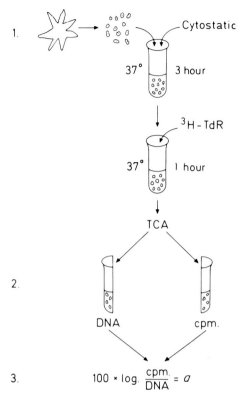

Fig. 1. Technical aspects of the *in vitro* short-term incubation method. For further explanation see the text.

values), partly to ensure a near-normal distribution of variates, and partly to make statistical calculations easier. The drug effect is expressed as the difference between the thymidine incorporation before and after the drug was added. The difference thus really expresses a multiplicative factor. The use of *a values* has made it possible to analyze the findings with various statistical methods, especially variance analysis. The composite nature of many of the experiments made it necessary to use this type of analysis in order to ensure that the recorded differences could not have arisen by random variations.

In some experiments, effect values were used instead. The effect value of a tumor is the difference between the *a value* recorded in control tubes and the *a value* recorded in the drug-treated tubes.

Thymidine and uridine uptake might not mirror activity in DNA synthe-

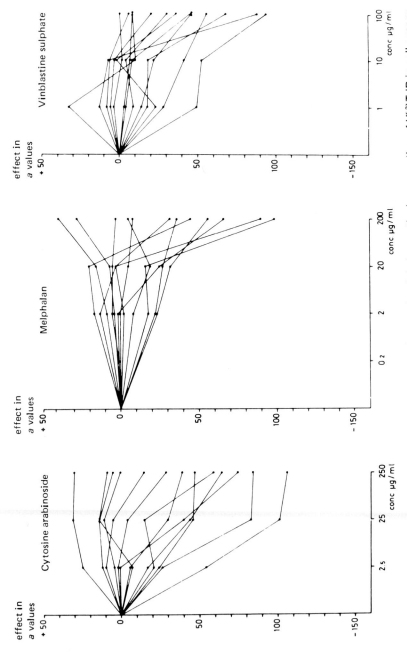

Fig. 2. Effect of cytosine arabinoside, vinblastine sulfate, and melphalan on the incorporation of H[³]TdR in cell suspensions from primary methylcholanthrene induced mouse sarcomas.

sis. The size of the nucleotide pools might change, or salvage enzymes be inhibited or even stimulated by the drug. Such changes can appear as alterations in DNA synthesis. O. D. Håkansson, my collaborator, discussed these questions at some length and found that the reduced incorporation of radiolabeled thymidine and uridine is probably not due to changes in pool size, but mirrors decreased DNA synthesis.

In our experimental series of investigations, three drugs were used: cytosine arabinoside (250 μ/ml), melphalan (200 μ/ml), and vinblastine sulfate (100 μ/ml). The concentrations of cytostatic drugs used in the *in vitro* tests in the present investigations were chosen from the results obtained on normal mouse thymocytes and on methylcholanthrene induced sarcoma cells. Each tumor should be tested at many different concentrations in order to reach a maximum discriminative effect, but technical limitations made such a project impossible. We therefore chose concentrations that gave marked effects on normal tissue and discriminated well between a number of sarcomas (Fig. 2). It is quite possible, however, that tumors that respond vigorously in the *in vitro* test do react *in vivo* to the drug in question. Undoubtedly, the concentrations used in the present study are high, and the question of unspecific toxicity springs to mind; therefore the correlation between *in vitro* results and *in vivo* effects can *a priori* be seriously questioned.

III. Heterogeneity in Tumors with Respect to Drug Sensitivity

Many tumors are composed of more than one cell type. The mosaic composition of some experimental and human malignant tumors has been demonstrated by, for instance, karyological and cytochemical methods. Karyological analyses of mammalian tumors have shown that most cancers are mosaics of different somatic karyotypes within the same tumor cell populations (Bishun *et al.*, 1973; Mitelman, 1971).

As stressed above, the *in vitro* method could demonstrate differences in reactivity between different primary methylcholanthrene induced mouse sarcomas (Fig. 3). Further studies also showed that different parts in a tumor could show different reactivity. In one study, a number of tumors were divided into quarters, each quarter being used to prepare a cell suspension which was tested *in vitro* (Fig. 4). The degree of heterogeneity varied markedly between individual tumors. When the primary tumors were compared with a group of serially transplanted tumors, the latter were not significantly less heterogeneous. This experiment showed that

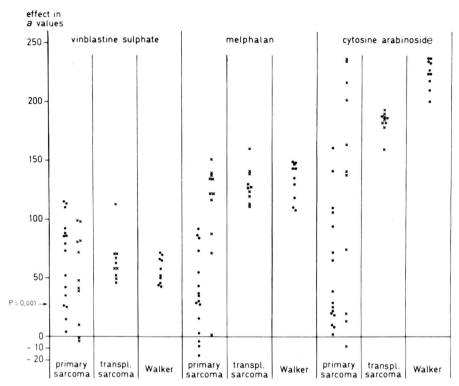

Fig. 3. Diagram showing effect values, i.e., differences in a-values for control tubes and tubes containing the drug to be tested. Three groups of tumors: primary methylcholanthrene induced sarcomas in the mouse, serially transplanted sarcomas, rat Walker 256 adenocarcinomas. Ten of the primary sarcomas were tested parallel to the one serially transplanted; they are marked with x and are to the right of the other primary sarcomas.

the degree of heterogeneity varied considerably in different primary sarcomas: Some appeared nearly homogeneous, others showed a marked degree of heterogeneity. This is to be expected if large regions with different properties exist in a tumor cut arbitrarily into four pieces. This great initial heterogeneity in the tumors made it impossible to demonstrate an effect of serial transplantation on the degree of heterogeneity. In another study (Fig. 5), tumors developing after grafting small tumor fragments were compared with tumors developing after injection of a cell suspension. This study showed that a difference does exist between primary tumors and serially transplanted ones, the primary being more heterogeneous with respect to cell composition.

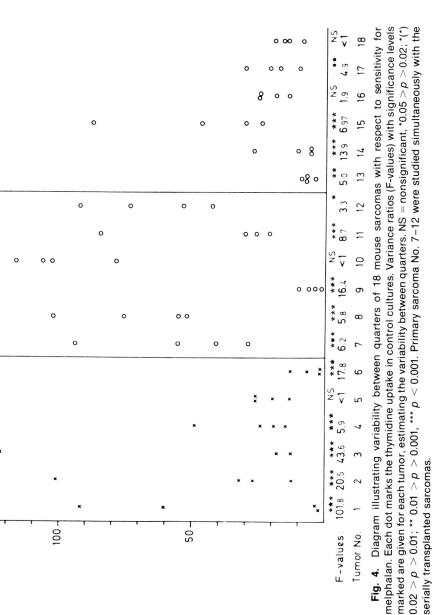

Fig. 4. Diagram illustrating variability between quarters of 18 mouse sarcomas with respect to sensitivity for melphalan. Each dot marks the thymidine uptake in control cultures. Variance ratios (F-values) with significance levels marked are given for each tumor, estimating the variability between quarters. NS = nonsignificant, *0.05 > p > 0.02; (*) 0.02 > p > 0.01; ** 0.01 > p > 0.001, *** p < 0.001. Primary sarcoma No. 7–12 were studied simultaneously with the serially transplanted sarcomas.

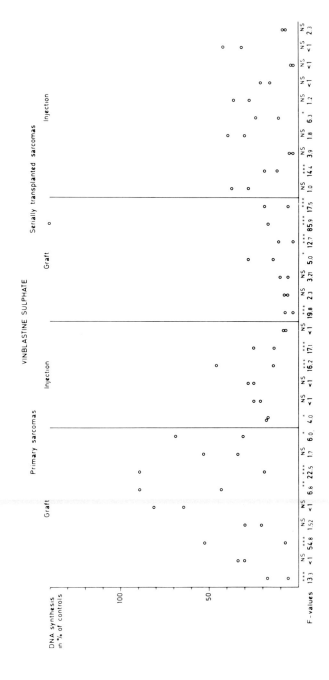

Fig. 5. Diagram illustrating variability between daughter tumors with respect to sensitivity for vinblastine sulfate (A), melphalan (B), and cytosine arabinosine (C). Each circle marks the thymidine uptake per DNA units in the presence of the drug expressed in percent of uptake in control tubes. Variance ratios (F-values) obtained for each animal is given at the bottom of the figure. NS, nonsignificant; *0.05 > p > 0.02; **0.01 > p > 0.001; ***p < 0.001 (see pp. 155 and 156).

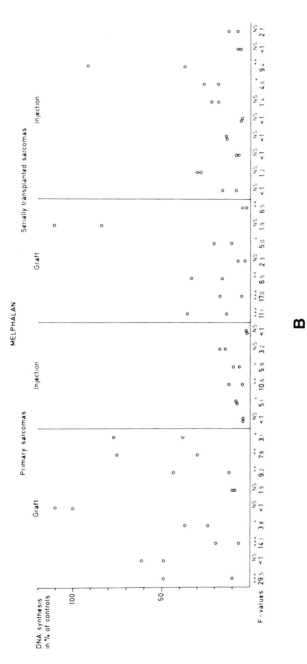

MELPHALAN

Primary sarcomas | Serially transplanted sarcomas

Graft — Injection | Graft — Injection

DNA synthesis
in % of controls

Fig. 5 (*Continued*)

B

155

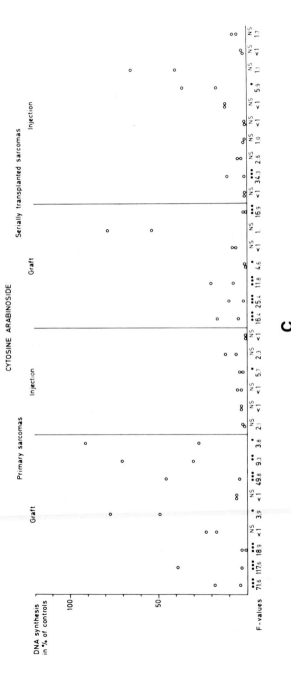

Fig. 5 (Continued)

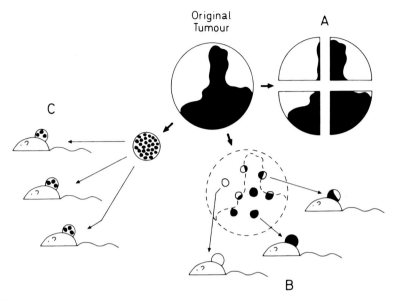

Fig. 6. Principles in experiments on heterogeneity. Original tumor built up by two clones, marked black and white, respectively. A, division of tumors into quarters followed by *in vitro* testing of each quarter. B, transplantation of small grafts selected at random and *in vitro* testing of tumors that develop. C, transplantation of homogeneous cell suspension and testing *in vitro* of tumors that develop.

Figure 6 illustrates schematically the principles of these methods. For simplicity, only two clones with different sensitivity to cytostatic drugs are shown. In the first method the tumors were divided into quarters and tested separately *in vitro*. Some tumors were found to be heterogeneous; others were not. Considered from this point of view, primary and serially transplanted tumors did not differ. This might indicate that the tumors were still markedly heterogeneous even after serial transplantation for ten generations in the absence of evolutionary pressure; the tumors were permitted to grow without any drug treatment of the animals. But it is also possible that the tumors had developed toward less heterogeneity during the serial transplantation, although this could not be demonstrated with the method used. Differences in heterogeneity between different kinds of tumors can be obscured, e.g., the quartering of the tumor can be done in many different ways with quite variable results, even if only two unevenly distributed clones are present in the tumor. Thus, the intertumor variation with respect to the degree of heterogeneity will be highly influenced by the way a tumor is quartered.

The present method was developed to analyze the heterogeneity of tu-

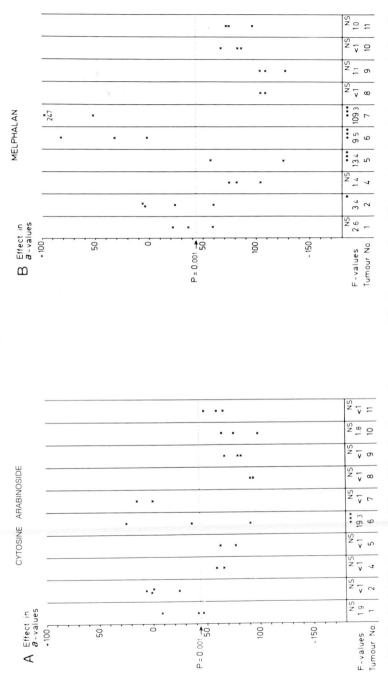

Fig. 7. Variability between different biopsies from colon cancers. Effect expressed as difference in values between controls and treated cells (see pp. 159 and 160).

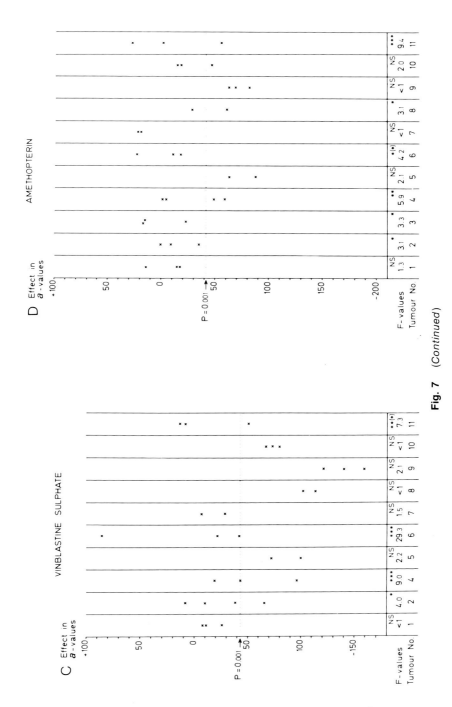

Fig. 7 (*Continued*)

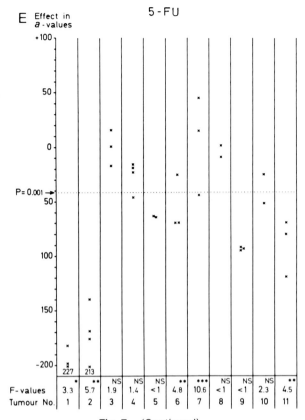

Fig. 7 *(Continued)*

mors further. Small pieces of an original tumor were grafted to a number of animals. The tumors that developed from the grafts were then tested for their sensitivity to cytostatic drugs *in vitro*. If the original tumor is built up by the different clones that are not intermingled, the small pieces of the tumor ought to be different in their clonal makeup; consequently, tumors developing from such pieces ought to be different. On the other hand, heterogeneity can develop during the further growth of the graft in the recipient mouse. Selection processes and mutations might be operative; furthermore, local factors such as nutritional effects could cause an apparent heterogeneity. To evaluate the importance of such processes, parallel experiments were made with tumors obtained from injections of cell suspensions. These suspensions should give a representative average of the cell composition of the tumor, and all transplanted tumors should develop from similarly composed samples. If there is a heterogeneity, this

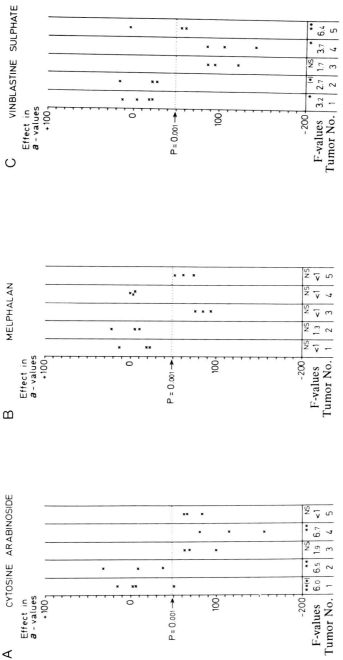

Fig. 8. Variability between different biopsies from stomach cancers (see p. 162).

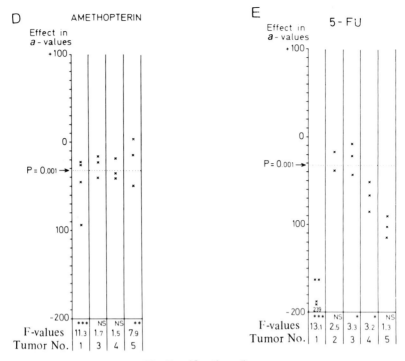

Fig. 8   (Continued)

could reasonably develop during tumor growth and not be due to variations in tumor cell inocula. When tumors obtained from a primary sarcoma were investigated in this way, those obtained by graft transplantation
showed a marked degree of heterogeneity, significantly greater than that
obtained with tumors obtained by injection transplantation. However, a
heterogeneity was present also among the latter; this is reasonably explained by factors of the type discussed above.

When tumors obtained from a serially transplanted sarcoma (10 generations) were used, no difference in heterogeneity could be shown among
tumors developed from grafts and those from injected cell suspensions. In
both groups, a heterogeneity exists, but they are of the same size. Again,
this is reasonable due to the processes commented on above. The picture
suggested by these data is: In primary induced sarcoma there exist at least
two, and perhaps many, different clones of cells differing in sensitivity
in vitro to cytostatic drugs. The clones are not completely intermingled,
but form spatially separate tumor regions. They have developed either
from separate foci of carcinogenetically transformed cells, or during the
further evolution of the sarcoma. During serial transplantation the

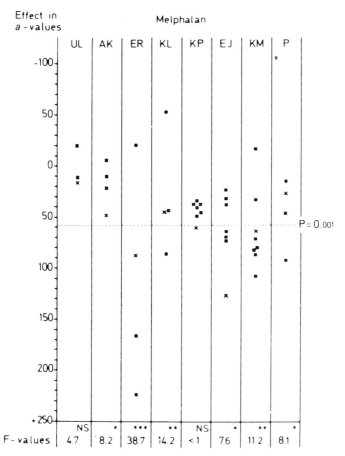

Fig. 9. Effect of melphalan on [³H]TdR incorporation *in vitro* into primary tumors and solid metastases (solid squares) and into ascitic cells (crosses) from nine patients with ovarian cancer. Effect values, i.e., difference between control tubes and melphalan treated tubes, are given in the graph. The 0.1% significance level is marked as a horizontal dashed line. Variance ratios (F-values) and their significance levels, estimating the variance between effects in primary tumor, solid metastases and ascitic cells from a patient, are given at the bottom. NS, not significant, $*p < 0.05$; $**p < 0.01$; $***$ $p < 0.001$.

tumor becomes more homogeneous, i.e., it is built up by fewer clones or the existing clones become strongly intermingled. This will increase the chance for the transplanted pieces of the original tumor to become rather identical; thus the difference due to transplantation technique will be reduced.

A similar heterogeneity pattern for cytostatic drugs, as in methylchol-

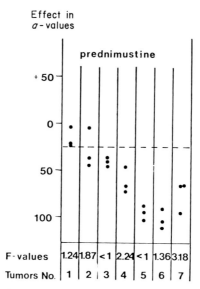

Fig. 10. Differences in sensitivity to cytostatic treatment *in vitro* between different biopsies from lymphomas. Effect expressed as difference in a-values between controls and drug-treated cells.

anthrene-induced sarcomas, has been found in human adenocarcinomas of the stomach and colon, in advanced ovarian carcinoma and in non-Hodgkin's lymphoma *in vitro* (Figs. 7, 8, 9, and 10).

IV. Predictive Value of *in Vitro* Testing for Sensitivity to Cytostatic Drugs

As mentioned in the Introduction, several attempts were made to develop *in vitro* tests that could predict the sensitivity of malignant tumors to cytostatic drugs. So far, no system has been described with an adequate *in vivo–in vitro* correlation. Many reports on *in vitro* tests for cytostatic sensitivity deal with human tumors; this renders the evaluation of the *in vivo* results very difficult. The correlation described in these reports is therefore often uncertain. The situation is somewhat better when human leukemic cells are tested *in vitro*. A relatively good correlation between *in vitro* and *in vivo* cytotoxic effects has been found, but the predictive value of the *in vitro* tests for obtaining hematological remission was low. For ovarian carcinoma we have found a 70% correlation between *in vitro* and *in vivo*. We have used our *in vitro* test model to mea-

MELPHALAN	In vitro	
	Sensitive	Resistant
In vivo		
OR	10	2
SD	2	2
PD	4	4
	16	8	24

MELPHALAN ADRIAMYCIN	In vitro	
	Sensitive	Resistant
In vivo		
OR	10	2
SD	0	0
PD	0	4
	10	6	16

Fig. 11. Correlation between *in vitro* results and response *in vivo*.

sure sensitivity of human ovarian cancer cells to melphalan and melphalan combined with adriamycin. With this model we studied the possible correlation between the *in vitro* results and the response to these cytostatic drugs *in vivo*. Cancer cells from 40 patients with advanced ovarian cancer were tested. The *in vitro* effects of the drugs were measured as differences in incorporation of labelled [^{3}H]thymidine in drug-containing tubes and in control tubes (Fig. 11). The effects of the drugs on the different cancer cells varied greatly from strong sensitivity to resistance. *In vitro* and *in vivo* results were compared 1 year after start of patient treatment. The overall agreement was 28/40, 70%. The *in vitro* method thus estimated a tumor cell characterstic which has a biological meaning also for *in vivo* conditions.

Cell suspensions from nine of 24 human ovarian primary cancers, their metastases, and ascitic cells were treated *in vitro* with melphalan. The results show that there are differences in the response to melphalan treatment *in vitro* between tumor biopsies from one patient with metastasizing ovarian cancer which thus contain cell lines with varying sensitivity toward that drug. The present work indicates that various clones may exist in human ovarian cancers which explains why the correlation between *in vitro* and *in vivo* was not better than 70%. In contrast to these solid tumors, lymphomas of non-Hodgkin's type are not heterogeneous toward cytostatic drugs *in vitro*. In seven patients there was a correlation between the therapeutic effect of prednimustine and its effect in the *in vitro* test model (Table I).

In our laboratory we also use an *in vivo* method for predicting chemosensitivity, namely, the nude mouse model. Tumor take rate for ovarian cancers and head and neck cancers is about 40%. There was a correlation between *in vivo* results in nude mice and the *in vivo* results in patients in 20 successful cases. In 16/20 cases there was a good correlation (Table II).

TABLE I

Presentation of the Histologic Type of the Lymphomas and the Effect of Prednimustine Treatment *in Vivo* and *in Vitro*

Patient No.	Histologic type (Rappaport)	Stage (Ann Arbor)	Prednimustine treatment		Effect *in vitro*[a]
			Therapy dose	Effect *in vivo*	
1	Undifferentiated lymphoblastic	II	60 mg daily	Progressive disease	16.53
2	Diffuse histiocytic	III	120 mg daily for 5 days	Progressive disease	29.45
3	Diffuse histiocytic	III	60 mg daily	Complete remission of short duration	41.18
4	Diffuse lymphocytic, poorly differentiated	IV	60 mg daily	Complete remission more than 2 years	62.34
5	Diffused mixed	III	—	—	95.52
6	Nodular lymphocytic, poorly differentiated	III	200 mg daily for 5 days every other week	Complete remission more than 2 years	102.36
7	Nodular lymphocytic, poorly differentiated	III	60 mg daily	Complete remission more than 2 years	75.79

[a] Mean of the effect values of the three biopsies from each lymph node.

TABLE II

Correlation between *in Vivo* Results in Nude Mice and Patient Response *in Vivo*

		in Vivo nude mice	
		OR	PD
	Melphalan		
In vivo patient			
Objective response		8	—
Static disease		1	1
Progressive disease		—	3
	Adriamycin–Melphalan		
In vivo patient			
Objective response		3	—
Static disease		1	1
Progressive disease		—	2

V. Discussion

The best correlation has been with leukemias and non-Hodgkin's lymphomas, probably because of the monoclonal character of these tumors. For solid adenocarcinomas, however, no system has been devised which gives adequate correlation *in vitro* or *in vivo*. A likely explanation of this fact is the demonstrated heterogeneity. This heterogeneity is a drawback for predictive tests, i.e. cells tested *in vitro* are not necessarily representative of the tumor as a whole, and a tumor of clinically significant size probably contains several subpopulations of cells with special characteristics of chemosensitivity. To overcome this problem one has to take several biopsies from the primary tumor, from different metastatic locales, and test all the biopsies *in vitro*. Then, the various subpopulations of malignant cells in a primary tumor and their metastases can be defined better and a median sensitivity pattern for all subpopulations be determined.

VI. Conclusion

While there are many limitations in the use of tissue culture predictive testing, there are good reasons to suppose that its potential has not been exploited fully. Assays designed with due regard to cell kinetics and cell population heterogeneity must be employed for screening for initial chemotherapy. Also, careful analysis of clonal variation, both preexisting and induced by drug exposure, may enable the design of follow-up regimens aimed at small resistant fractions. This phase is probably the most critical and should be considered an integral part of any predictive screening program (Biörklund *et al.*, 1980).

References

Biörklund, A., Hakansson, L., Stenstam, B., Trope, C., and Akerman, M. (1980). On heterogeneity of non-Hodgkin's lymphomas as regards sensitivity to cytostatic drugs. *Eur. J. Cancer* **16**, 647-654.

Bishun, N. P., Mills, J., Lloyd, N., and Williams, D. C. (1973). Chromosomal examination of various cell clones in (*in vitro*) derived from a DMBA induced male rat breast tumor. *Eur. J. Cancer* **9**, 865.

Kaufmann, M. (1980). Clinical applications of *in vitro* chemosensitivity testing. *In* "Advances in the Biosciences" (Newman *et al*, eds.), Vol. 26. Pergamon, Oxford.

Mitelman, F. (1971).The chromosomes of fifty Rous rat sarcomas. *Hereditas* **69**, 155.

11

Gene Amplification in Human Tumor Systems

BRUCE J. DOLNICK AND JOSEPH R. BERTINO

I. Introduction

Development of resistance to methotrexate (MTX) in tissue culture systems has been known for approximately 20 years (for a review see Bertino *et al.*, 1981). In recent years, gene amplification leading to elevation of dihydrofolate reductase (DHFR) in some MTX-resistant tumor cell lines has been demonstrated to be the underlying mechanism for the development of drug resistance (Alt *et al.*, 1978). Although other mechanisms have been documented whereby tumor cells become resistant to MTX, (i.e., decreased uptake and altered DHFR), the most common mechanism of resistance to MTX documented in experimental tumors is an increase in DHFR (Bertino *et al.*, 1981). The cell culture systems developed have proved useful for both the study of drug resistance as well as gene structure and gene expression. The status of knowledge about these gene amplified systems is reviewed in this chapter with the emphasis being on the heterogeneity observed intraspecifically in gene amplified systems and the comparison of mouse to human gene amplified systems.

II. A Brief Review of Gene Amplification in Methotrexate-Resistant Cells

It is still not clear as to what the molecular mechanism of gene amplification is. The location of DHFR genes in MTX-resistant gene amplified cells is variable dependent on whether the cells are stably or unstably resistant (Dolnick *et al.*, 1979; Haber and Schimke, 1981; Kaufman *et al.*, 1979; Nunberg *et al.*, 1978). In stably resistant cells, most or all of the DHFR genes appear to be located in homogeneously staining regions (HSRs) (Dolnick *et al.*, 1979; Nunberg *et al.*, 1978). However, Schimke's laboratory has determined that in unstably resistant cells (i.e., cells that lose most of their amplified genes upon removal to medium lacking MTX) the DHFR genes are localized in double minute chromosomes (Haber and Schimke, 1981; Kaufman *et al.*, 1979). When unstably resistant cells become stably resistant, the double minutes are lost. Presumedly, there is a relationship between the double minutes and the HSRs but this relationship is not clearly established. The answer to the question of why some cells develop double minutes and are unstably resistant as opposed to why some cells develop HSRs and are stably resistant may provide an answer to the mechanism of gene amplification.

Perhaps one of the most interesting observations to date is the discovery that some known tumor promoters can facilitate gene amplification (Varshavsky, 1981). Although isolation of DHFR gene amplified cells with MTX is required to observe the newly amplified cells, the presence of the tumor promoter (12-O-tetradecanoyl-phorbal-13-acetate, TPA) is required only during the selection of MTX-resistant cells indicating the TPA effect is permanent and does not involve a lowering of the effective MTX concentration intracellularly (and, therefore, does not act as a metabolic modulator). It is reported that insulin causes a similar phenomenon (Varshavsky, 1981). Determination of the DHFR gene dosages in the newly developed MTX-resistant cells indicated they were indeed amplified. Further investigation of gene amplification in this system may lead to an understanding of why some tumor cells in tissue culture are more disposed to become gene amplified than others and whether there is one or more mechanism of gene amplification.

III. Organization of the Dihydrofolate Reductase Gene, Human versus Mouse

The organization of the DHFR gene in MTX-resistant murine cells has been elucidated by Schimke and colleagues. They have shown that the DHFR gene is approximately 40 kilobase pairs (kbp) in length, about 70 times as large as the coding portion of the mature mRNAs for DHFR (Nunberg *et al.*, 1980). In addition, the mouse DHFR gene contains five intervening sequences. One intervening sequence resides within the 5' untranslated region and the others lie within the structural region of the gene. The restriction map is also consistent among a number of murine gene amplified and nonamplified cell lines as well as DNA from normal mouse tissue, indicating that no substantial gene reorganization has taken place during the amplification and that the gene mapped represents the normal DHFR gene (Nunberg *et al.*, 1980; Table I). Thus, the DHFR gene appears to be conserved in the murine cell population.

The study of recently developed DHFR gene amplified human cell lines is presenting a picture of significant divergence from the murine DHFR gene. The *Eco*RI pattern obtained with the MTX-resistant cell line K562C, an undifferentiated leukemia with erythroid features, is shown in Fig. 1. This pattern is identical to that obtained with another gene amplified cell line KB, a human epidermoid carcinoma cell line developed by

TABLE I

Comparison of Restriction Enzyme Fragments in Mouse and Human DNA

Species	Cell line	Restriction enzyme fragments (kb)	
		*Eco*RI	*Pst*I
Mouse	L5178YR[a]	16, 6.2, 5.8, 3.5	3.9, 2.8, 2, 1.6, 1.6
	L1210R	16, 6.2, 5.8, 3.5	3.9, 2.8, 2, 1.6, 1.6
	S-180/AT 3000	16, 6.2, 5.8, 3.5	3.9, 2.8, 2, 1.6, 1.6
	3T6	16, 6.2, 5.8, 3.5	3.9, 2.8, 2, 1.6, 1.6
Human	KBR	6, 4, 1.7, 1.5	8.5, 7.5, 4
	K562CR	6, 4, 1.7, 1.5	ND[b]
	HL60	6, 4	ND
	Colon	6, 4, 1.7, 1.5	ND
	Colon tumor	6, 4, 4[c], 1.7, 1.5	ND

[a] R denotes an MTX-resistant gene amplified cell line.
[b] ND not determined.
[c] 4 kbp doublet appears in some colon tumor preparation which has pBR322 homology.

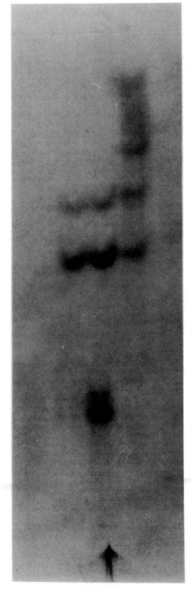

Fig. I. Southern blot of *Eco* RI digested K562CR high molecular weight DNA. 5 or 10 μg DNA were digested with an excess of *Eco* RI and electrophoresed in a 0.8% agarose gel to assure completeness of digestion. The DNA was transferred to diazotized paper and hybridized with nick-translated [³²P]pDHRF26 (Chang *et al.*, 1978; Wahl *et al.*, 1979).

Cheng's laboratory in Chapel Hill. This pattern has now been observed for over five cell types, both methotrexate resistant and sensitive in tissue culture cells and clinical tissue (Table I). The mouse gene and the human gene each contain four bands upon restriction with $EcoRI$ (Table I) but the molecular weights of these bands clearly differs from the mouse restriction pattern. Thus, while the mouse DHFR gene contains a 16 kbp band, the largest band displayed in the human DHFR gene is only 6 kbp. This species specific difference in gene structure is further emphasized by a comparison of the $PstI$ pattern of the human versus mouse gene (Table I). Whether these differences result from sequence divergence of the structural or intervening sequence portions of the DHFR gene between the two species is not resolved and awaits characterization of the human gene with a cDNA probe derived from a human mRNA and DNA sequence analysis. Table I also demonstrates possible polymorphism in the human DHFR gene. While most cell lines and clinical DNA samples display two low molecular weight bands of 1.7 and 1.5 kbp after restriction of their DNA with $EcoRI$, at least one cell line (i.e., HL60) does not. This is true for both the MTX-sensitive and MTX-resistant sublines of this promelocytic leukemia. This cell line is somewhat unusual in that it can be induced to differentiate to a high degree upon the administration of a number of agents (Breitman et al., 1980; Gallagher et al., 1979). The two gene amplified human cell lines (i.e., KB and K562C) both contain HSRs (Medina and Bertino, Cheng et al., unpublished results) and should provide interesting systems for mapping the DHFR gene from human cells and localizing the chromosomal position of the DHFR gene(s) in man.

IV. Expression of the Dihydrofolate Reductase Gene, Multiple Messenger RNAs

The gene amplified MTX-resistant cell lines lend themselves to analysis of gene expression by Northern blotting of their RNA gene products (Alwine et al., 1977, Wahl et al., 1979). The analysis of the RNAs with DHFR coding sequences has been carried out by several laboratories with similar results in two different species (Dolnick and Bertino, 1981; Lewis et al., 1981; Setzer et al., 1980). Thus, it appears that in both murine and chinese hamster cell lines with amplified DHFR genes there are multiple mRNAs coding for DHFR. This is demonstrated in Figs. 2 and 3 for the gene amplified subclone of L5178R, L5178YC$_3$. As Fig. 2 indicates, there are approximately six species of RNA in the cytoplasm of L5178YC$_3$ which are easily detectable and contain DHFR coding sequences (Dolnick and Bertino, 1981). The six predominant species have molecular weights

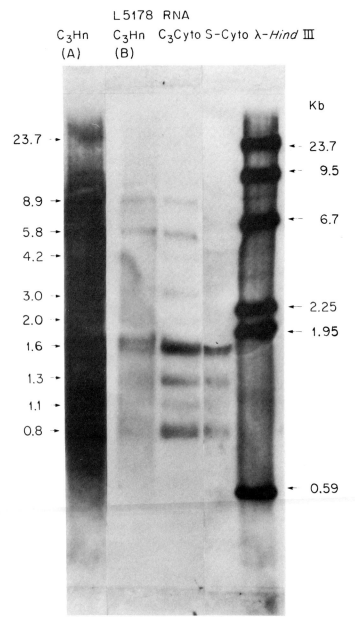

Fig. 2. Northern blot of DHFR cytoplasmic RNA from L5178Y MTX-sensitive and -resistant cells, nuclear RNA (C₃Hn) from MTX-resistant cells. Conditions as described previously (Dolnick and Bertino, 1981).

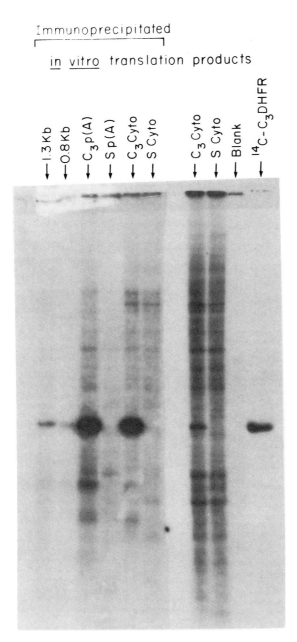

Fig. 3. Immunoprecipitation and identification of DHFR mRNA species translated *in vitro* in a 15% polyacrylamide gel (Dolnick and Bertino, 1981).

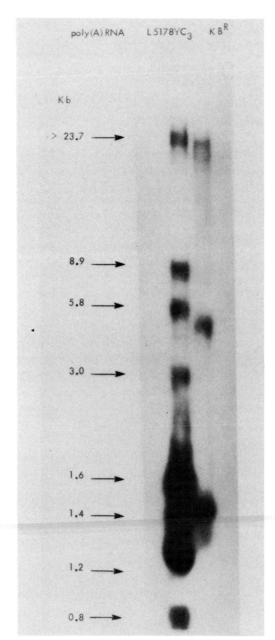

Fig. 4. Northern blot of DHFR-poly(A) RNA from human (KBR) or mouse (L5178YC$_3$) DHFR-gene amplified cell lines. Poly(A) RNA was electrophoresed in a 1.4% agarose gel containing 10 m*M* methyl mercury hydroxide. Transfer and hybridization conditions were as described in legend to Fig. 1.

of 8.9, 5.8, 1.9, 1.6, 1.2, and 0.8 kb. Only three of these appear to predominate in the nucleus (i.e., the 8.9, 5.8, and 1.6 kb species). Of the major cytoplasmic species, three of these have been shown to translate to DHFR *in vitro*. This is demonstrated for the 1.2 and 0.8 kb species in Fig. 3. The difference between the 0.8 kb and other DHFR coding sequence bearing RNAs is in the 3' nontranslated region (Dolnick and Bertino, 1981; Setzer *et al.*, 1980), but some of the other species may represent processing intermediates observed in the gene amplified cells due to the extremely high levels of amplification (300- to 400-fold). Similar patterns have been obtained with gene amplified L1210 and Sarcoma-180 cells (Setzer *et al.*, 1980). The parental cell lines also display multiple mRNAs for DHFR, the species being observed are identical in molecular weight to four of the major species observed in the gene amplified cells, but there may be differences as the 8.9 and 5.8 kb species are not observed in the MTX-sensitive parental cells, though present in comparably high levels to the other major bands in the amplified cells (Fig. 2). Thus there may be some differences in gene expression in gene amplified versus nonamplified cells in some cases. In some gene amplified cell lines from the same species, four of the major DHFR RNA species are found but not all of those from the L5178YC$_3$ clone are displayed in some other cell lines, notably the gene amplified Sarcoma-180 cell line (Setzer *et al.*, 1980). Though amplification of the DHFR gene appears to be a uniform phenomenon of cultured tumor cells in response to MTX, it is clear that expression of the DHFR gene is dependent on the species in question. Thus, if one compares the DHFR RNA patterns from human versus mouse gene amplified cells on a Northern blot a very different picture emerges (see Fig. 4). As Fig. 4 illustrates, there are qualitatively fewer RNA species with DHFR specific sequences in human as compared to mouse poly(A) RNA. This emphasizes the difficulty in extrapolating biochemical data interspecifically and indicates a basic difference in organization of the mouse and human DHFR gene systems.

V. Discussion

Increased enzyme activity of a target enzyme for a drug as a mechanism of resistance has now been documented for several drugs (Table II). In at least three of these circumstances, in which gene copy numbers have been quantitated, gene amplification has occurred. Thus, the phenomenon of gene amplification as a mechanism of drug resistance appears not to be limited to MTX. The findings of double minute chromosomes in several tumor cell types not previously exposed to drugs, the correlation

TABLE II

Examples of Enzyme Elevation in Response to Drug Treatment

Drug	Enzyme increased	Gene amplification
MTX	Dihydrofolate reductase	Yes
PALA	CAD protein	Yes
Cd^{2+}	Metallothionein	Yes
Hydroxyurea	Ribonucleotide reductase	ND[a]
FudR	Thymidylate synthetase	ND
Asparagenase	Asparagine synthetase	ND

[a] ND, not determined.

with an increase in the number of these structures as resistance develops, and a decrease in their number as resistance decreases in a population indicate that some neoplastic cells have the ability to rapidly adapt to selective pressures imposed by drug therapy. In some cell lines, double minutes are not seen as resistance develops, but rather the emergence of a HSR when the cell line becomes markedly resistant. In general, when HSR regions are present in a resistant line, the resistant cell lines do not lose resistance or the HSR when propagated out of MTX for many generations (Dolnick *et al.*, 1979; Kaufman *et al.*, 1979). In the two human neoplastic sublines developed that are markedly resistant to MTX with 200–400 increases in DHFR, both have HSRs and the KBR cells are stably resistant (Y. C. Cheng, personal communication). Obviously, additional human lines will have to be examined to determine if human lines do not amplify via double minute amplification. In this regard, it would be of interest to develop a MTX-resistant line from a human cell line that contains double minute chromosomes (e.g., neuroblastoma).

The availability of human amplified lines should allow a determination of the sequence of the human enzyme, as well as an understanding of gene organization and regulation. It will be of great interest to determine if heterogeneity exists in the enzyme sequence. If sufficient DHFR specific cDNA from a normal human tissue, in particular marrow or gastrointestinal tissue, can be obtained and sequenced, it can be determined whether sequence differences exist between normal and neoplastic tissue. This may be exploitable with appropriately designed drugs. In addition, the availability of a human cDNA probe will allow quantitation of gene copies from tumor cells of patients treated with MTX who have become resistant to this drug. From a basic science view, a human cDNA probe will allow a finer picture of the organization and expression of the human DHFR gene to be developed.

References

Alt, F. W., Kellems, R. E., and Schimke, R. T. (1978). *J. Biol. Chem.* **251**, 3063–3074.

Alwine, J. C., Kemp, D. J., and Stark, G. R. (1977). *Proc. Natl. Acad. Sci. U.S.A.* **74**, 5350–5354.

Bertino, J. R., Dolnick, B. J., Berenson, R. J., Scheer, D. I., and Kamen, B. A. (1981). *In* "Molecular Actions and Targets for Cancer Chemotherapeutic Agents," pp. 385–397. Academic Press, New York.

Breitman, T. R., Sclonick, S. E., and Collins, S. J. (1980). *Proc. Natl. Acad. Sci. U.S.A.* **77**, 2936–2940.

Chang, A. C. Y., Nunberg, J. H., Kaufman, R. J., Erlich, H. A., Schimke, R. T., and Cohen, S. N. (1978). *Nature (London)* **275**, 617–624.

Dolnick, B. J., and Bertino, J. R. (1981). *Arch. Biochem. Biophys.* **210**, 691–697.

Dolnick, B. J., Berenson, R. J., Bertino, J. R., Kaufman, R. J., Nunberg, J. H., and Schimke, R. T. (1979). *J. Cell Biol.* **83**, 394–402.

Gallagher, R., Collins, S., Trujillo, J., McCredie, K., Ahearn, M., Tsai, S., Metzgar, R., Aulakh, G., Ting, R., Ruscetti, F., and Gallo, R. (1979). *Blood,* **54**, 713–733.

Haber, D. A., and Schimke, R. T. (1981). *Cell* **26**, 355–362.

Kaufman, R. J., Brown, P. C., Schimke, R. T. (1979). *Proc. Natl. Acad. Sci. U.S.A.* **76**, 5669–5673.

Lewis, J. A., Kurtz, D. T., and Melera, P. W. (1981). *Nucleic Acids Res.* **9**, 1311–1322.

Nunberg, J. H., Kaufman, R. J., Schimke, R. T., Urlaub, G., and Chasin, L. A. (1978). *Proc. Natl. Acad. Sci. U.S.A.* **75**, 5553–5556.

Nunberg, J. H., Kaufman, R. J., Chang, A. C. Y., Cohen, S. N., and Schimke, R. T. (1980). *Cell* **19**, 355–364.

Schimke, R. T., Kaufman, R. J., Alt, F. W., and Kellems, R. F. (1978). *Science (Washington D.C.)* **202**, 1051–1055.

Setzer, D. R., McGrogan, M., Nunberg, J. H., and Schimke, R. T. (1980). *Cell* **22**, 361–370.

Varshavsky, A. (1981). *Cell,* **25**, 561–572.

Wahl, G. M., Stern, M., and Stark, G. R. (1979). *Proc. Natl. Acad. Sci. U.S.A.* **76**, 3683–3687.

12

Clinical Implications of Cancer Cell Heterogeneity

PAUL CALABRESI AND DANIEL L. DEXTER

I. Introduction

Some of the most recent important developments in cancer biology have evolved in the area of tumor cell heterogeneity. The documentation of intratumor heterogeneity, the isolation and characterization of subpopulations of cancer cells from an individual tumor, and studies of the implications of intraneoplastic diversity for treatment of cancer have provided us with information vital to our understanding of the behavior of tumors and to the development of more effective treatment protocols for neoplastic diseases. Many laboratories have demonstrated heterogeneity in animal tumors (Fidler and Kripke, 1977; Gray and Pierce, 1964; Mitelman *et al.*, 1972; Haschka and Levan, 1958; Henderson and Rous, 1962; Klein and Klein, 1956; Pimm and Baldwin, 1977; Prehn, 1970; Sluyser and Von Nie, 1974; Becker *et al.*, 1973; Dexter *et al.*, 1978; Hakansson and Trope, 1974a). Although less work has been reported on human tumor heterogeneity, a number of relevant studies have been conducted on human neoplasms. This report reviews some of the research performed on human intraneoplastic diversity, and attempts to place the phenomenon in an appropriate clinical perspective. The clinical implications of tumor cell heterogeneity are crucial to the individual afflicted with cancer, and our success in treating neoplastic disorders will depend, to a large extent, on how well we understand and exploit the phenomenon of intraneoplastic diversity.

II. Evidence for Intraneoplastic Diversity in Human Tumors

For many years, experimental and clinical oncologists have considered cancer a monotonous and homogeneous disease characterized by propagating daughter cells identical in most respects to their progenitors (Calabresi *et al.*, 1979). Tumors were thought to be monoclonal in nature, without obvious variation or diversification. Accordingly, experimental models were developed in cancer research that were representative of this relatively limited and oversimplified notion. Some of these models, such as the murine leukemia L1210, have been extremely helpful in screening for agents that have brought about a large percentage of cures in such diseases as acute lymphoblastic leukemia and Burkitt's lymphoma. These neoplasms, however, are largely comprised of cells that are morphologically and probably biologically homogeneous.

By contrast, the clinical observations of some oncologists and pathologists have provided a totally different picture of neoplasia. A number of clinical examples can be cited to illustrate the intraneoplastic diversity of human cancers. Germinal tumors have been recognized to contain various neoplastic cell types, such as seminomas, embryonal carcinomas, and gonadoblastomas within the same tumor. Mixed testicular tumors may give rise to distinct metastatic foci, each containing a tumor of a different cell type. Malignant melanomas can manifest the same phenomenon and give rise to melanotic and amelanotic metastases. Tumor cell heterogeneity has been recently reported in carcinomas of the breast by using fluorescein-labeled estradiol to detect the presence or absence of estrogen receptors (Lee, 1979). It is not uncommon for pathologists to observe histological heterogeneity in carcinomas of the colon, pancreas, stomach, lung, head, and neck, as well as in ovarian, bladder, and brain tumors.

Recent studies have shown that many human solid tumors are heterogeneous at the time of surgical removal. Petersen *et al.* (1979) have reported that five of six colorectal carcinomas they studied contained hyperploid subpopulations that were karyotypically distinct from a diploid majority subpopulation. They concluded that these subpopulations with an abnormal chromosome content might also differ in other properties as well. Siracky (1979) has elegantly documented the phenomenon of human tumor heterogeneity in studies with three distinct types of human carcinomas. First, sequential sampling of tumor cells from ascitic fluids of 12 patients undergoing chemotherapy treatment for inoperable ovarian cancer revealed a number of changes in chromosome distribution with time for a given patient. Second, cell suspensions were prepared from different regions of primary and secondary ovarian and colon cancers. Antineoplastic drugs were added to the suspensions, which were then exposed to [^{3}H]TdR. Differential labeling was observed both between distinct parts of the same tumor and between a primary tumor and its metastases. Third, a series of 20 human endometrial cancers was analyzed for secretory conversion following progesterone treatment. Results showed that not all the cells within a given human endometrial carcinoma underwent this conversion. These data provided evidence that these human carcinomas contained subpopulations of cancer cells and were heterogeneous neoplasms.

Vindelov et al. (1980) using flow-cytometric DNA analysis demonstrated considerable heterogeneity in human small cell carcinoma of the lung. Results were obtained with samples from needle biopsies of metastases from small cell carcinoma in 29 patients. In each of six patients, two different subpopulations were present either in the same metastasis or in different metastases. The authors further concluded that their method would underestimate the extent of intraneoplastic diversity in small cell cancer, and that many of these carcinomas are heterogeneous. Convincing biochemical and morphological evidence for heterogeneity in small cell carcinoma of the lung has also been reported by Abeloff and co-workers (1979).

Other laboratories have reported isolating distinct subpopulations from human solid tumors or from cell lines established from human neoplasms. Quinn et al. (1979) have established two karyotypically distinct human cancer cell lines from a heterogeneous carcinoma of the sigmoid colon. Kimball and Brattain (1980) exposed human colon carcinoma HT29 cells to fluorouracil and isolated a drug-resistant subpopulation. Shapiro and co-workers (1981) examined human gliomas for evidence of intraneoplastic diversity and eight tumors were shown to be karyotypically heterogeneous. Bronson et al. (1980) have established a cell line from a metastasis of a human testicular cancer that contained four histological types of neoplastic cells.

III. Differential Sensitivities of Subpopulation of Human Cancer Cells to Therapeutic Modalities

The human colon cancer cell line DLD-1 was established from a biopsy obtained from a patient with a carcinoma of the sigmoid colon (Dexter *et al.*, 1979; Dexter *et al.*, 1981). On histological examination, this tumor appeared morphologically heterogeneous, varying from moderately to poorly differentiated (Fig. 1). Chromosome analysis of DLD-1 cells that had been growing only 1 month after transfer of the primary cell culture revealed the presence of two karyotypically distinct populations. Most of the cells were diploid, but 5–10% of the cells were hyperploid (Table I). When DLD-1 cells were seeded in agar, two morphologically distinct colony types were observed. Clones of each type were isolated, and these gave rise to the A and D subpopulations. Clone A cells produce poorly differentiated adenocarcinomas, and clone D cells produce moderately differentiated adenocarcinomas in nude mice. Parent DLD-1 cells produce moderately to poorly differentiated adenocarcinomas in these mice; this histology is quite similar to that of the original human tumor. The histological variation observed in the original human neoplasm and the morphological and karyotypic heterogeneity detected in early passage cultures of the DLD-1 cell line indicate that the patient's adenocarcinoma and the parent cell line were both heterogeneous. The morphologies, karyotypes, and tumor histologies of clones A and D indicate that they are representative of the two subpopulations that are responsible for the variation observed in this system. The biological properties of the DLD-1 cell line and its derivative A and D clones are shown in Table I. All the variation in the parent line can be accounted for by the properties and characteristics of the two subpopulations.

The sensitivities of clones A and D to several anticancer drugs *in vitro* were determined in the following manner. On day 1, replicate tissue culture dishes were inoculated with 5×10^4 cells. Cells were harvested by trypsin treatment from two of the dishes on day 2 and counted with a hemacytometer in order to determine the number of cells per dish at the time of drug addition. Drugs were added in varying concentrations to other cultures on day 2. Drug treated and control cultures were harvested by trypsin treatment on day 5, and the number of cells was determined. The number of doublings for nontreated cells was calculated from the cell number in control dishes on days 2 and 5. The drug concentration required to inhibit the number of doublings in the 72-hour period by 50% was then calculated from the dose–response curve in which cell numbers were plotted against molar drug concentrations on logarithmic paper (Calabresi *et al.*, 1979).

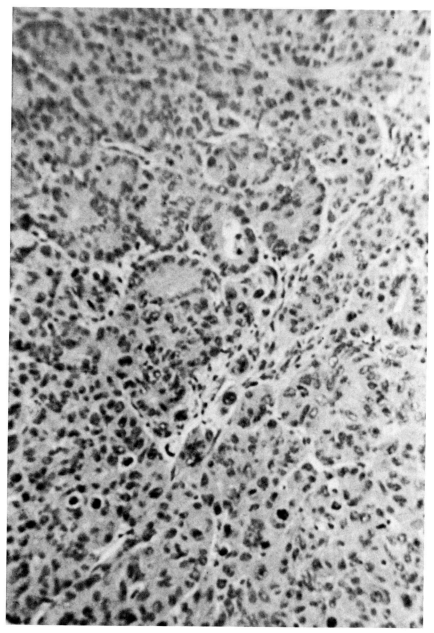

Fig. 1. DLD-1 tumor in the nude mouse. Section shows histological heterogeneity, with solid areas and some areas containing small glands. Hematoxylin and eosin stain ×100.

TABLE I

Properties of the DLD-1 Human Colon Cancer Cell Line and Its Derivative Clone A and Clone D Subpopulations[a]

Cell line	Cloning efficiency (%)	Saturation density (cells/cm²)	Chromosome number	Tumor histology[b]
DLD-1	42	8.9×10^5	Mostly diploid, 45–46; a few with 70–90	Moderately to poorly differentiated
Clone A	77	2.8×10^5	Hyperploid, mostly 70–90	Poorly differentiated
Clone D	24	6.8×10^5	Diploid, 45–46	Moderately differentiated

[a] Adapted from Dexter et al. (1979).

[b] Tumors were produced by s.c. inoculation of nude mice with 1×10^6 cells, and tumor tissue was analyzed for histology. Nude mice used in this study bear the nu/nu gene on an outbred Swiss background, and are bred and maintained in the Roger Williams General Hospital Animal Care Facility.

The growth inhibitory effects of six commonly used chemotherapeutic drugs were determined for the parent cell line (DLD-1) and for each of its two clones (A and D). The results are shown in Table II. Actinomycin D produced the most potent growth inhibitory effect, whereas methyl CCNU had the least effect on these cell lines. Significant (greater than 300%) differences in sensitivity to a given drug were observed among the three lines for three agents. With actinomycin D, parent DLD-1 cells were the most sensitive; DLD-1 cells were 460 and 440% more sensitive to the

TABLE II

Sensitivities to Chemotherapeutic Drugs of Subpopulations Isolated from the Heterogeneous DLD-1 Human Colon Carcinoma Cell Line[a]

Drug	DLD-1 (M)	Clone A (M)	Clone D (M)
Methyl CCNU	2.7×10^{-5}	3.0×10^{-5}	5.7×10^{-5}
5-FU	4.5×10^{-6}	1.5×10^{-6}	3.6×10^{-6}
Actinomycin D	1.6×10^{-9}	7.4×10^{-9}	7.0×10^{-9}
Vincristine	4.3×10^{-7}	5.0×10^{-7}	4.9×10^{-7}
Mitomycin-C	6.1×10^{-8}	1.2×10^{-9}	3.8×10^{-8}
Ara C	1.4×10^{-6}	7.3×10^{-7}	9.0×10^{-7}

[a] Adapted from Dexter et al., 1981 (in press). Clone A or clone D cultures were exposed to drugs for 72 hours, and then the cells were counted. The numbers of cells in treated cultures were compared to those determined for control cultures, and ID_{50} values were calculated. The ID_{50} is defined as the molar concentration of drug required to inhibit the number of doublings by 50%.

drug than were clone D and clone A cells, respectively. In contrast, clone A was the line most sensitive to 5-FU and mitomycin-C. Clone A cells were 5000% more sensitive to mitomycin-C than were parent DLD-1 cells, and they were about 3000% more sensitive to the drug than were clone D cells. Thus, differential sensitivities among the parent line and its clones were observed with three agents, but the ranking of the responses of the lines differed depending on the drug. The mitomycin-C data are striking, and indicate that differential drug sensitivities among subpopulations of a heterogeneous human cancer may be quite marked (Dexter *et al.*, in press).

The carcinoma of the lung LX-1 cell line was established by M. Chu at our Cancer Center from a human neoplasm transplanted in a nude mouse (Giovanella *et al.*, 1978). Using the soft agar cloning technique, four clones were isolated by Chu and were designated LX-1 sub 1, LX-1 sub 2, LX-1 sub 3, and LX-1 sub 9 (Chu *et al.*, 1979; Chu *et al.*, submitted for publication). These lines differ morphologically, and were tested for their sensitivities *in vivo* to three anticancer drugs, selected because of demonstrated activity against the parent tumor. Antithymocyte serum-immunosuppressed $B_6D_2F_1$ mice were inoculated s.c. with tumor cells on day 0, and then received i.p. injections of anguidine, procarbazine, or mitomycin-C on days 1 and 2. Animals were sacrificed on day 10, and the tumors were removed and weighed.

The results clearly demonstrated heterogeneity of the parent LX-1 cell line with respect to sensitivity to chemotherapeutic drugs (Figs. 2–4). Subline 9 was completely unresponsive to doses of anguidine (8 mg/kg/day) or mitomycin-C (0.4 mg/kg/day) that inhibited parent LX-1 tumor growth by 51 and 72%, respectively. Subline 1 tumor growth was not affected by procarbazine (25 mg/kg/day), whereas this dose of drug inhibited parent LX-1 tumor growth by 88%. The other sublines also responded differentially to each of the three drugs. It is evident that LX-1 contains subpopulations, which are quite resistant to drugs that are effective in inhibiting the growth of the heterogeneous parent tumor. Furthermore, the degree of sensitivity appears to be subline dependent (Chu *et al.*, 1979; Chu *et al.*, submitted for publication). Certainly our data suggest that a combination of drugs would be required to treat this particular cancer successfully, particularly if individual subpopulations had metastasized in the patient.

Other laboratories have also demonstrated differential sensitivities of tumor cell subpopulations from a single neoplasm to anticancer drugs. A number of studies have been reported on both animal (Hakannson and Trope, 1974a; Barranco *et al.*, 1978; Hakannson and Trope, 1974b; Hepner *et al.*, 1978; Lotan and Nicolson, 1979; Schable, 1975; Schable *et al.*, 1979) and human neoplasms (Barranco *et al.*, 1972; Biorklund *et al.*, 1980;

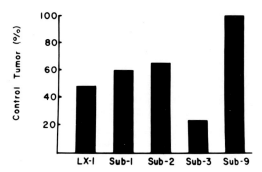

Fig. 2. Activity of anguidine against human carcinoma of the lung, LX-1, and its clones *in vivo*. Note differences in sensitivity among the various clones.

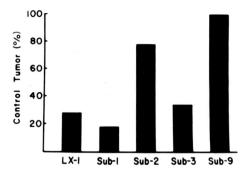

Fig. 3. Activity of mitomycin-C against human carcinoma of the lung, LX-1, and its clones *in vivo*. Note differences in sensitivity among the various clones.

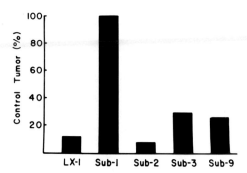

Fig. 4. Activity of procarbazine against human carcinoma of the lung, LX-1, and its clones *in vivo*. Note differences in sensitivity among the various clones.

Trope, 1975; Trope et al., 1979; Trope et al., 1975; Barranco et al., 1973). Differences in chemosensitivities between cells from a primary tumor and cells obtained from a metastasis of that tumor have also been documented (Fugmann et al., 1977; Schable, 1975; Schable et al., 1979; Trope, 1975).

Our lung and colon cancer cell lines have also been tested for their sensitivities in vitro to X-irradiation. This work was done in collaboration with our colleagues (John Leith et al., 1980). As was the case with chemotherapeutic agents, there were significant differences in radiosensitivity among the lines for each neoplasm (Table III). Among the colon lines, parent DLD-1 cells are the most resistant to X-rays. By contrast, the LX-1 sub 1 clone of the lung carcinoma lines is the most resistant in that system. The difference between the D_q values of 0.19 Gy and 0.00 Gy for LX-1 parent and LX-1 sub 9 compared to a D_q of 2.06 Gy for LX-1 sub 1 cells is marked. Thus, subpopulations from a human carcinoma can show significant differences in their responses to ionizing radiation as well as to drugs. These results also show that cells from either a cloned or a parent line can be more radioresistant, depending on the tumor (Leith et al., 1980, 1982, in press). Our findings again underscore the importance of multimodality treatment of heterogeneous human cancers.

Hyperthermia studies were also performed in the DLD-1 system in collaboration with Glicksman and Leith (Table IV). As might be expected, the colon cancer lines showed differential sensitivities to heat (Leith

TABLE III

Sensitivities to X-Irradiation of Cultured Human Colon and Lung Carcinoma Subpopulations [a]

Cell line	Subline	Extrapolation no.	Quasithreshold dose (D_q, Gy)	Mean lethal dose (D_o, Gy)
Colon carcinoma	Parent (DLD-1)	11.7	2.34	0.95
	Clone A	8.20	2.23	1.06
	Clone D	5.80	1.89	1.08
Lung carcinoma	Parent (LX1)	1.20	0.19	1.14
	LX1-1	8.54	2.06	0.96
	LX1-2	2.48	0.88	0.96
	LX1-3	20.3	2.05	2.68
	LX1-9	1.00	0.00	1.12

[a] Data adapted from Leith et al. (1980, submitted for publication). Cells were plated in replicate flasks, and exponentially growing cultures were treated with X-irradiation at graded doses. The cells were removed from the flasks, and were plated at appropriate inocula in culture dishes. After 8 days, dishes were stained with crystal violet, and colonies of more than 50 cells were scored. Parameters were determined from survival curves generated from colony counts.

TABLE IV

Sensitivities to Heat of Cultured Human Colon Carcinoma Cells[a]

Cell line	Extrapolation no.	Quasi-threshold time (T_o, min)	Inactivation rate (T_o, min)
Parent (DLD-1)	3.9	33.0	24.2
Clone A	1.4	30.8	55.5
Clone D	2.3	41.6	49.3

[a] Adapted from Leith *et al.* (in press). Cells were plated in replicate flasks, and exponentially growing cultures (wrapped in parafilm) were immersed in a 43°C water bath with bath temperature maintained to within 0.01°C. Flasks were heated for varying periods of time, then the cells were removed from the flasks and were replated at appropriate inocula in culture dishes. After 8 days, dishes were stained with crystal violet, and colonies of more than 50 cells were scored. Parameters were determined from survival curves generated from colony counts.

et al., in press). The parent DLD-1 cells, however, were the most sensitive to this modality [see inactivation rates (T_0), Table IV], in contrast to the results with X-rays, which showed that DLD-1 cells were the most resistant to ionizing radiation. Both clones were significantly more resistant to hyperthermia. This provides further evidence that the relative sensitivity of parent and subpopulations of cancer cells from the same tumor mass vary for different therapeutic modalities.

The question of whether cancer cells that survive one treatment modality are more resistant to a second type of therapy was addressed in our laboratory using the DLD-1 system. DLD-1, clone A, or clone D cells were injected s.c. into nude mice. The resulting tumors were X-irradiated at graded doses, the tumors were immediately excised, prepared as single cell suspensions, and cultures were reestablished from the irradiated (IR) tumors as well as from unirradiated control (CON) xenografts. Distinct morphological differences were seen between IR and CON cultures for each of the three lines. Karyotypic analysis showed that 65% of DLD-1 CON cells were pseudodiploid (like clone D). DLD-1 IR cells (from a tumor that received 10.71 Gy) had a modal number of 76 chromosomes, and 95% of the cells were hyperploid (like clone A). An intermediate shift in karyotype was observed with 3.50 Gy; 80% of the DLD-1 cells were hyperploid (see Figs. 5–7). This significant and dose-dependent shift in karyotype following irradiation suggested selection of a subpopulation with a different inherent sensitivity to certain drugs. Karyotypic patterns were also somewhat different between IR and CON cultures for clone A or D. IR or CON cell cultures were treated with anticancer drugs, and their chemosensitivities were compared (Table V). DLD-1 IR cells were about threefold more sensitive to mitomycin-C ($ID_{50}=2.7 \times 10^{-8} M$) than were cells cultured from the CON tumor ($ID_{50}=6.8 \times 10^{-8} M$). The DLD-1 IR

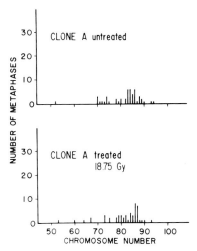

Fig. 5. Chromosome ranges of clone A cells from X-irradiated or unirradiated human colon cancer xenografts. Nude mice were inoculated with clone A cells, and animals were divided among the various control and treatment groups when tumors reached a size of 5 × 5 mm. Tumors were subjected to X-irradiation followed by immediate excision. Graded doses of X-rays from 2.0 Gy to 18.75 Gy were used on 10 xenografted tumors; control tumors were not irradiated prior to excision. Single cell suspensions were prepared with standard mechanical and enzymatic dissociation methods. Cells were plated in tissue culture flasks, and cultures obtained from unirradiated and irradiated tumors were designated CON and IR cultures, respectively. The karyotypes were determined on early passage IR and CON cultures.

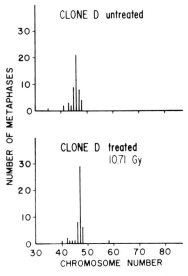

Fig. 6. Chromosome ranges of clone D cells from X-irradiated or control human colon cancer xenografts. See legend to Fig. 5.

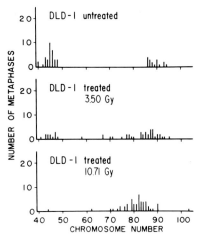

Fig. 7. Chromosome ranges of parent DLD-1 cells from X-irradiated or control human colon cancer xenografts. See legend to Fig. 5.

cells were also 250% more sensitive to 5-fluorouracil ($ID_{50} = 3.9 \times 10^{-6}$ M) than were DLD-1 CON cells ($ID_{50} = 1.0 \times 10^{-5}$ M). In contrast, clone D IR cells were at least fourfold more resistant to methyl CCNU (ID_{50} greater than 10^{-4}; limits of sensitivity of our assay) than were clone D CON cells ($ID_{50} = 2.4 \times 10^{-5}$ M). These results suggest that differential sensitivities to other drugs or modalities may exist between IR and CON cultures, and provide a further rationale for combination therapy of cancer (Dexter *et al.*, submitted for publication).

It is important to extend the experimental approaches outlined in the preceding paragraphs to aggressive subpopulations in human cancers. We have recently begun to use the chicken chorioallantoic membrane (CAM) to select highly invasive or metastatic tumor cell subpopulations from the murine melanoma B16-BL6 and the rat glioma C6 cell lines. Tumor cells were deposited on the CAM of eggs 10 days postfertilization. Upon hatching, chickens were autopsied, and organs were removed, minced, and implanted s.c. in C57BL/6 mice (for melanoma) or nude mice (for glioma). A glioma growing s.c. from a chicken lung implant metastasized to the liver of the recipient nude mouse, and a melanoma growing s.c. from a chicken liver implant metastasized to the lung of its murine host. The s.c. melanoma contained distinct black and gray areas. Cell lines were established from the s.c. glioma (C6-V) and from the "black" and "gray" regions of the melanoma (Fig. 8). Marked differences in lung colonization were seen 14 days after 1×10^5 parent BL6, "gray," or "black" cultured cells were injected into the tail vein of C57BL mice. Mean numbers

TABLE V

Drug Sensitivities of Human Colon Cancer Cells from Control and X-Irradiated Xenograft Tumors[a]

Cell line (radiation dose)[a]	ID_{50} values for antineoplastic drugs (M)			
	5-FU	Mitomycin-C	Methyl CCNU	8-Azaadenosine
DLD-1	$1.0 \pm 0.3 \times 10^{-5}$	$6.8 \pm 1.2 \times 10^{-8}$	$2.2 \pm 0.6 \times 10^{-5}$	$1.7 \pm 0.1 \times 10^{-6}$
DLD-1 X-ray (10.71 Gy)	$3.9 \pm 1.3 \times 10^{-6b}$	$2.7 \pm 0.1 \times 10^{-8b}$	$2.5 \pm 0.7 \times 10^{-5}$	$1.3 \pm 0.04 \times 10^{-6}$
Clone A	$6.7 \pm 0.9 \times 10^{-6}$	$2.1 \pm 0.2 \times 10^{-8}$	$3.4 \pm 0.8 \times 10^{-5}$	$2.4 \pm 0.4 \times 10^{-6}$
Clone A X-ray (18.75 Gy)	$6.4 \pm 0.4 \times 10^{-6}$	$2.7 \pm 0.7 \times 10^{-8}$	$2.6 \pm 0.4 \times 10^{-5}$	$1.7 \pm 0.1 \times 10^{-6}$
Clone D	$3.3 \pm 0.9 \times 10^{-5}$	$2.9 \pm 1.2 \times 10^{-8}$	$2.4 \pm 0.2 \times 10^{-5}$	$2.0 \pm 0.1 \times 10^{-6}$
Clone D X-ray (10.71 Gy)	$4.6 \pm 1.4 \times 10^{-5}$	$2.8 \pm 0.5 \times 10^{-8}$	1×10^{-4b}	$1.4 \pm 0.3 \times 10^{-6}$

[a] Adapted from Dexter et al. (submitted for publication). Drug sensitivities were determined as described in the text. Methyl CCNU, 5-FU, and azaadenosine were tested against cultures of all lines in their second to fifth passages from primary cultures. Mitomycin-C was tested against the various cell lines in their tenth or eleventh passage.

[b] Statistically significant difference ($\pm$SEM).

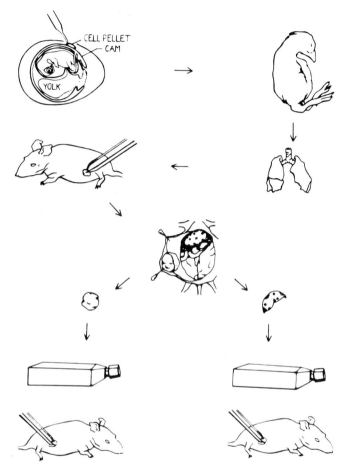

Fig. 8. Schematic illustration of method for selecting aggressive neoplastic sub-populations using the CAM. See text for details.

($\pm$SEM) of pulmonary metastases for BL6, "gray," and "black" cells were 7 ± 2, 96 ± 6, and 493 ± 12 foci/mouse. Tumor volume doubling times for "black" and "gray" tumors trocared s.c. into mice were 6.1 and 4.4 days, respectively. C6-V cells are morphologically distinct from C6 cells. The two lines also differ in their plating efficiencies on plastic (67% for C6 vs. 48% for C6-V), and C6-V cells do not adhere to glass surfaces whereas C6 cells do. These results from our preliminary investigations indicate that it may be possible to select cancer cells with metastatic potential from heterogeneous human tumors with this technique. We are currently testing this hypothesis with cells from human colon and pancreatic carcinomas and melanomas.

IV. Clinical Implications of Intraneoplastic Diversity

A number of interesting and important clinical implications of cancer cell heterogeneity must be considered and incorporated into our approach to patients with neoplastic disorders. These include the fundamental consequences of this concept for the problem of metastases, the reliablity of tumor markers, the interpretation of data obtained using the stem cell (clonogenic) assay, and most important, our rationale toward therapy.

When considering the problem of metastases, it is essential to realize that metastases are a relatively unusual phenomenon in the pathogenesis of most neoplasms. Since there are approximately one billion cancer cells present in a small tumor 1 cm in diameter, it is evident that not all cancer cells are capable of metastasizing successfully; otherwise we would expect to see hundreds or thousands of metastases, a rare event even in a patient with an advanced neoplasm. Accordingly, only a few cancer cells from a select population may have all the necessary properties to complete the metastatic process. These might include exfoliation, invasiveness, survival in the circulation, immunity to host defenses, ability to produce entrapment (possibly by platelet aggregation), and perhaps the capability of secreting tumor angiogenesis factor. Although a convenient model for a metastatic system using human cancer cells is not available, Fidler and co-workers (Fidler and Kripke, 1977; Post et al., 1980; Hart and Fidler, 1981) have successfully used the B16 murine melanoma to demonstrate the presence of subpopulations of tumor cells with high metastatic or invasive potential. It is apparent that similar studies with human cancer cells could be most informative and, as we discussed earlier in this review, these investigations are currently being pursued in our laboratories with the CAM model. We are also interested in preliminary evidence that suggests a variability in the capacity of human neoplastic cells from the same tumor to evoke platelet aggregation in vitro. We are currently studying the various clones from our heterogeneous human tumors for differences in collagenase and elastase activity. Liotta et al. (1980) have reported that the invasive variant BL6 isolated from the murine melanoma line B16-F10 produces high levels of type IV collagenase compared to the parent line.

Tumor markers are proteins or related substances that are secreted by a cancer into the circulation or other body fluids and serve as indirect indicators of neoplastic proliferation. Increasing elevations in titers of a marker, such as carcinoembryonic antigen (CEA) in patients with carcinoma of the colon, may be extremely helpful in detecting early recurrence or progression of disease. Conversely, a reduction in titer should indicate a favorable response to therapy. Production of CEA, however, appears to be correlated to the degree of cellular differentiation, with higher titers measurable in patients with well-differentiated carcinomas of the colon, as compared to those with the more anaplastic variety. Our studies with the DLD-1 tumor indicate that clone D, which is better differentiated than clone A, produces more CEA than its anaplastic counterpart, clone A (Hager *et al.*, 1980). While this is in accord with accepted clinical experience (Denk *et al.*, 1972, 1974; Von Kleist and Burtin, 1969), it raises serious questions about the reliability of tumor markers in heterogeneous neoplasms. With the DLD-1 tumor, for instance, recurrence or metastatic progression would be detected only if clone D cells were involved, since they are primarily responsible for the elaboration of CEA. Because a particular clone may be preferentially eradicated by therapy, a recurrence or metastatic progression by another clone incapable of producing the specific marker would escape early detection (Fig. 9). Accordingly, tumor markers are reliable indicators of total tumor growth only if they are produced by all the subpopulations of cancer cells within a given neoplasm.

There has been a great deal of interest in recent years in the development of clonogenic (stem cell) assay to predict the sensitivity of individual patients' tumor cells to chemotherapeutic drugs. Reports have been made of correlations between *in vitro* sensitivity in a soft agar cloning system and patient response, with ovarian cancer and myeloma (Salmon *et al.*, 1978). The usefulness and general applicability of the clonogenic assay for treatment of patients with carcinomas of the breast, colon, lung, and pancreas remain to be determined. Certainly such an approach should be examined in the context of what is currently known regarding human intraneoplastic diversity. We, as well as others, have shown that human carcinomas do not always clone well in soft agar (Crabtree *et al.*, 1981; Stiles *et al.*, 1976). Failure to clone out all the subpopulations present in a tumor would result in misleading data from a clonogenic assay if the cells

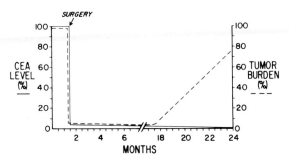

Fig. 9. Diagram showing recurrence of a cancer due to growth of a subpopulation that does not produce CEA; the marker would be unreliable for diagnosis in this situation.

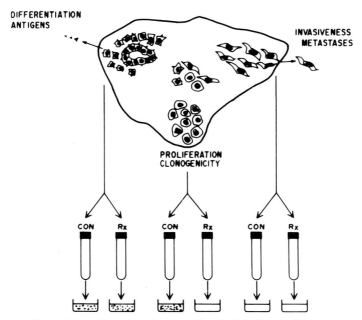

Fig. 10. Illustration of the effect intraneoplastic diversity could have on the interpretation of data from a clonogenic drug sensitivity assay. If an aggressive subpopulation does not clone in agar, the test cannot predict for the tumor cells that will be responsible for the demise of the patient.

that invaded or metastasized in the patient failed to grow in agar culture (Fig. 10). The problem is further complicated by the fact that many human carcinomas simply do not grow at even the low cloning efficiencies (0.05%) often set as the lower limit required to perform the assay on cells from a given patient's tumor. Other investigators have also discussed these limitations to the stem cell assay (Smith *et al.*, 1981; Tsuruo and Fidler, 1981; Shrivastav *et al.*, 1980).

Another approach would be to perform the clonogenic assay on cells from secondary neoplasms. If these cells grow in agar, then drugs might be selected that are effective against the metastatic cancer usually responsible for the demise of the patient. Alternatively, cells with metastatic or invasive potential could be isolated from a patient's tumor via the CAM or other selection methods. These aggressive variants could be tested for their sensitivity to drugs, and the patient undergoing adjuvant chemotherapy could be treated with the most appropriate regimen. Chemotherapy in the adjuvant setting is often administered for several years. Thus, even if several months were required to obtain the results with aggressive variants, there would be time to modify or change therapy. Tumor heterogeneity must be considered in analyzing the limitations of the clonogenic assay and in designing *in vitro* sensitivity tests that predict for responsiveness of those cells most likely to result in the death of the patient.

The most important clinical implications of cancer cell heterogeneity concern our approach to antineoplastic therapy. An increasing number of disseminated and regional neoplasms have been successfully cured during the past 20 years (Calabresi and Parks, 1980). In most of these, a key factor has been the use of combination chemotherapy and treatment with combined modalities, such as surgery, irradiation, and drugs (Calabresi, 1979). It is evident from our investigations and those of others that cancer cells within a particular neoplasm differ markedly in sensitivity to different drugs as well as to doses of irradiation and hyperthermia; they are also variable with respect to immunological determinants and surface receptors for hormones. Accordingly, it is not surprising that treatment with one drug or one therapeutic modality may have a far lower chance of eradicating all the subpopulations of cancer cells than administration of combination chemotherapy or the use of multiple modalities. An important challenge for the future is the rational selection of the most appropriate sequences and schedules of administration for multiple agents. For example, drugs used in combination chemotherapy are most often given concomitantly, with the rationale that they hit different targets in the same cell. This may be true for some cancer cells, and some agents may even potentiate each other when used in combination. It may be wiser, however, to administer the same drugs in sequential rotation (Fig. 11), in an effort to eliminate more effectively each differentially sensitive subpopulation of cancer cells in a heterogeneous tumor with acceptable tox-

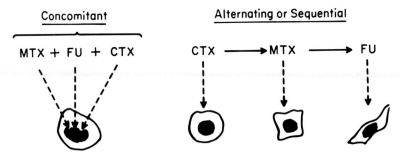

Fig. 11. Diagrammatic representation of different sequences and schedules of drug administration in combination chemotherapy. The rationale for concomitant versus sequential, rotational, or cyclical administration of agents is discussed in the text from the standpoint of cancer cell heterogeneity. CTX (cytoxan), MTX (methotrexate), and FU (fluorouracil), are three drugs used in the popular CMF regimen for carcinoma of the breast.

icity for the patient. This strategy would allow the use of considerably higher doses of each agent than would be possible if the drugs were used together and had similar toxic manifestations. Furthermore, rotational or alternating schedules could be developed that would allow individual drugs or combinations of agents to be administered safely and effectively on a cyclical basis. A recent report suggests that much better therapeutic results may be obtained by repeatedly alternating two different, non-cross-resistant drug combinations, MOPP (mustargen, oncovin, procarbazine, and prednisone) and ABVD (adriamycin, bleomycin, vinblastine, and dacarbazine), in Stage IV Hodgkin's disease than by using one combination alone (Santoro et al., 1980).

Essential to any therapeutic approach is a clearer insight into the cellular basis for resistance. Experiments are in progress at our Clinical Cancer Research Center to determine whether recurrence of a tumor and resistance to therapy are the result of selection and emergence of a preexisting resistant subpopulation after successful eradication of other more sensitive cancer cells in the same neoplasm. Our results with DLD-1 CON and IR cells indicate that this may well be the case. It is also important to define whether different therapeutic modalities, including chemotherapy, radiotherapy, immunotherapy, hormones, hyperthermia, and biological modifiers, exert unique and non-cross-resistant antineoplastic activity on the individual subpopulations of human cancers. The efforts of investigators studying these aspects of tumor cell heterogeneity should produce more effective regimens for treatment of neoplastic diseases.

In conclusion, intratumor heterogeneity not only provides an explanation for many of the clinical problems that medical oncologists have experienced, but it also suggests the approaches necessary for more efficacious treatment protocols. Although a formidable biological and clinical obstacle, intraneoplastic diversity may provide the essential clue that is required to design and implement effective therapy.

References

Abeloff, M. D., Eggleston, J. C., Mendelsohn, G., Ettinger, D. S., and Baylin, S. B. (1979). *Am. J. Med* **66,** 757–764.

Barranco, S. C., Ho, D., Drewinko, B., Romsdahl, M. M., and Humphrey, R. M. (1972). *Cancer Res.* **32,** 2733–2736.

Barranco, S. C., Drewinko, B., and Humphrey, R. M. (1973). *Mutat. Res.* **19,** 277–280.

Barranco, S. C., Haenelt, B. R., and Gee, E. L. (1978). *Cancer Res.* **38,** 656–660.

Becker, F. F., Klein, K. M., Wolman, S. R., Asofsky, R., and Sell, S. (1973). *Cancer Res.* **33,** 3330–3338.

Biorklund, A., Hakansson, L., Stenstam, B., Trope, C., and Akerman, M. (1980). *Eur. J. Cancer* **16,** 647–654.

Bronson, D. L., Andrews, P. W., Solter, D., Cervenka, J., Lange, P. H., and Fraley, E. E. (1980). *Cancer Res.* **49,** 2500–2506.

Calabresi, P. (1979). *In* "Cecil Textbook of Medicine" (P. B. Beeson, W. McDermott, and J. B. Wyngaarden, eds.), pp. 1922–1941. Saunders, Philadelphia.

Calabresi, P., and Parks, R. E., Jr. (1980). *In* "The Pharmacological Basis of Therapeutics" (A. G. Gilman, L. S. Goodman, and A. Gilman, eds.), pp. 1249–1313. MacMillan, New York.

Calabresi, P., Dexter, D. L., and Heppner, G. H. (1979). *Biochem. Pharmacol.* **28,** 1933–1941.

Chu, M. Y., Takeuchi, T., Yeskey, K. S., Bogaars, H., and Calabresi, P. (1979). *Proc. Am. Assoc. Cancer Res.* **20,** 151.

Chu, M. Y., Takeuchi, T., Yeskey, K. S., Bogaars, H., and Calabresi, P. (1982). *Cancer Res.* (submitted).

Crabtree, G. W., Dexter, D. L., Stoeckler, J. D., Savarese, T. M., Ghoda, L. Y., Rogler-Brown, T. L., Calabresi, P., and Parks, R. E. Jr. (1981). *Biochem. Pharmacol.* **30,** 793–798.

Denk, H., Tappeiner, G., Eckerstorfer, R., and Holzner, J. H. (1972). *Int. J. Cancer* **10,** 262–272.

Denk, H., Tappeiner, G., Davidovits, A., Eckerstorfer, R., and Holzner, J. H. (1974). *J. Natl. Cancer Inst.* **53,** 933–942.

Dexter, D. L., Kowalski, H. M., Blazer, B. A., Fligiel, Z., Vogel, R., and Heppner, G. L. (1978). *Cancer Res.* **38,** 3174–3181.

Dexter, D. L., Barbosa, J. A., and Calabresi, P. (1979). *Cancer Res.* **39,** 1020–1025.

Dexter, D. L., Spremulli, E. N., Fligiel, Z., Barbosa, J. A., Vogel, R., VanVoorhees, A., and Calabresi, P. (1981). *Am. J. Med.* **71,** 949–956.

Dexter, D. L., McCarthy, K., Leith, J. T., Glicksman, A. S., and Calabresi, P. (1982). *Cancer Res.* (submitted).

Fidler, I. J., and Kripke, M. L. (1977). *Science (Washington, D.C.)* **197,** 893–895.

Fugmann, R. A., Anderson, J. C., Stolfi, R. L., and Martin, D. S. (1977). *Cancer Res.* **37,** 496–500.

Giovanella, B. C., Stehlin, J. S., Jr., Williams, L. J., Lee, S. -S., and Shepard, R. C. (1978). *Cancer* **42,** 2269–2281.

Gray, J. M., and Pierce, G. B. (1964). *J. Natl. Cancer Inst.* **32,** 1201–1211.

Hager, J. C., Gold, D. V., Barbosa, J. A., Fligiel, A., Miller, F., and Dexter, D. L. (1980). *J. Natl. Cancer Inst.* **64,** 439–446.

Hakansson, L., and Trope, C. (1974a). *Acta. Pathol. Microbiol. Scand. Sect. A.* **82,** 35–40.

Hakansson, L., and Trope, C. (1974b). *Acta. Pathol. Microbiol. Scand. Sect. A.* **82,** 41–47.

Hart, I. R., and Fidler, I. J. (1981). *Biochem. Biophys. Acta.* **651,** 37–50.

Hauschka, T. S., and Levan, A. (1958). *J. Natl. Cancer Inst.* **21,** 77–135.

Henderson, J. S., and Rous, P. (1962). *J. Exp. Med.* **115,** 1211–1229.

Heppner, G. H., Dexter, D. S., DeNucci, T., Miller, F. R., and Calabresi, P. (1978). *Cancer Res.* **38,** 3758–3763.

Kimball, P. M., and Brattain, M. G., (1980). *Cancer Res.* **40,** 1574–1579.

Klein, G., and Klein, E. (1956). *Ann. N.Y. Acad. Sci.* **63,** 640–661.

Lee, S. H. (1979). *Cancer* **44,** 1–12.

Leith, J., Zeman, E., Dexter, D., Calabresi, P., and Glickman, A. (1980). *Proc. Am. Assoc. Cancer Res.* **21,** 274.

Leith, J. T., DeWyngaert, J. K., Dexter, D. L., Calabresi, P., and Glicksman, A. S. (1982). *J. Natl. Cancer Inst.* (in press).

Leith, J. T., Dexter, D. L., DeWyngaert, J. K., Zeman, E. M., Chu, M. Y., Calabresi, P., and Glicksman, A. S. (1982). *Cancer Res.* (in press).

Liotta, L. A., Tryggrason, K., Garbisa, S., Hart, I., and Folts, C. M. (1980). *Nature (London)* **284**, 67–68.

Lotan, R., and Nicolson, G. L. (1979). *Cancer Res.* **39**, 4767–4771.

Mitelman, F., Mark, J., Levan, G., and Levan, A. (1972). *Science (Washington, D.C.)* **176**, 1340–1341.

Petersen, S. E., Bichel, P., and Lorentzen, M. (1979). *Eur. J. Cancer* **15**, 383–386.

Pimm, M. V., and Baldwin, R. W. (1977). *Int. J. Cancer* **20**, 37–43.

Post, G., Doll, J., Hart, I. R., and Fidler, I. J. (1980). *Cancer Res.* **40**, 1636–1644.

Prehn, R. T. (1970). *J. Natl. Cancer Inst.* **45**, 1039–1045.

Quinn, L. A., Moore, G. E., Morgan, R. T., and Woods, L. K. (1979). *Cancer Res.* **39**, 4919–4924.

Salmon, S. E., Hamburger, A. W., Soehnlen, B., Durie, B. G. M., Alberts, D. S., and Moon, T. E. (1978). *N. Engl. J. Med.* **298**, 1321–1327.

Santoro, A., Bonadonna, G., Bonfante, V., and Valagussa, P. (1980). *Proc. Am. Soc. Clin. Oncol.* **21**, 470.

Schable, F. M., Jr. (1975). *Cancer (Philadelphia)* **35**, 15–24.

Schable, F. M., Jr., Griswold, D. P., Jr., Corbett, R. H., Laster, W. R., Jr., Mayo, J. G., and Lloyd, H. H. (1979). *Methods Cancer Res.* **17**, 3–40.

Shapiro, J. R., Yung, W. -K. A., and Shapiro, W. R. (1981). *Cancer Res.* **41**, 2349–2359.

Shrivastav, S., Bonar, R. A., Stone, K. R., and Paulson, D. F. (1980). *Cancer Res.* **40**, 4438–4442.

Siracky, J. (1979). *Br. J. Cancer* **39**, 570–577.

Sluyser, M., and Von Nie, R. (1974). *Cancer Res.* **34**, 3253–3257.

Smith, H. S., Lan, S., Ceriani, R., Hackett, A. J., and Stampfer, M. R. (1981). *Cancer Res.* **41**, 4637–4643.

Stiles, C. D., Desmond, W., Chuman, L. M., Sato, G., Saier, M. H., Jr. (1976). *Cancer Res.* **36**, 3300–3305.

Trope, C. (1975). *Neoplasma (Bratisl.)* **22**, 171–180.

Trope, C., Hakansson, L., and Dencker, H. (1975). *Neoplasma* **22**, 423–430.

Trope, C., Aspergren, K., Kullander, S., and Astedt, B. (1979). *Acta Obstet. Gynecol. Scand.* **58**, 543–546.

Tsuruo, T., and Fidler, I. J. (1981). *Cancer Res.* **41**, 3058–3064.

Vindelov, L. L., Hansen, H. H., Christensen, I. J., Spang-Thomsen, M., Hirsch, F. R., Hansen, M., and Nissen, N. I. (1980). *Cancer Res.* **40**, 4295–4300.

Von Kleist, S., and Burtin, P. (1969). *Int. J. Cancer* **4**, 874–879.

PART IV

Epigenetic Mechanisms

13

Transforming Growth Factors Produced by Tumor Cells

GEORGE J. TODARO,
HANS MARQUARDT,
DANIEL R. TWARDZIK,
PATRICIA A. JOHNSON,
CHARLOTTE M. FRYLING, AND
JOSEPH E. DE LARCO

I. Introduction

Tumor cells differ from one another in many different ways. One way, which first came to our attention several years ago, involved the number of growth factor receptors that could be found unoccupied on their surface membranes. When compared to their normal counterparts, it was found that certain tumor cells had lost their ability to bind labeled epidermal growth factor (EGF) while other tumor cells no longer could bind the insulin-like growth factors (IGFs). It was suggested, then, that the reason for their inability to bind externally provided ligand was because they had (re)acquired the ability to make specific growth factors. Subsequent experiments have shown that some tumor cells, especially those that have no apparent EGF membrane receptors, produce potent growth factors called transforming growth factors (TGFs) that are related in some ways to EGF.

The TGFs that will be discussed in this chapter are polypeptides that are functionally related to EGF, but, unlike EGF, confer the transformed phenotype on normal fibroblasts *in vitro*. The production of TGF appears to be a common property of tumor cells of different origins and is also characteristic of RNA tumor virus-transformed cell cultures. Several polypeptides with the properties of TGF have been partially purified from the conditioned medium of Moloney murine sarcoma virus-transformed mouse 3T3 cells, designated sarcoma growth factor (SGF) (De Larco and Todaro, 1978), from RNA tumor virus-transformed rat fibroblasts (Ozanne *et al.*, 1980) and from various human tumor cells (Todaro *et al.*, 1980). An intracellular form(s) of TGF has been detected also in tumor cells and transformed cells growing both in culture and in the animal (Roberts *et al.*, 1980); some of these do not interact with the EGF receptor.

The TGFs produced by the virus-transformed cells and by certain human tumor cells interact with EGF-specific receptors. Certain human sarcoma and carcinoma cells (Todaro and De Larco, 1978) and most melanomas (Fabricant *et al.*, 1977) lack EGF receptors (Table I): Some of these have been shown to produce TGFs (Todaro *et al.*, 1980). EGF-related TGF was not detectable in fluids from cultures of cells, including tumor cells, with high numbers of free EGF membrane receptors or from normal human fibroblasts. In addition, Abelson virus (AbLV)-transformed rat

TABLE I

EGF-Specific Receptors in Human Tumor Cells

Cells	[^{125}I]EGF bound/10^6 cells
Diploid human (avg. 12)	8,700
Rhabdomyosarcoma (A204)	11,400
Rhabdomyosarcoma (A673)	<200
Epidermoid carcinoma (A431)	146,000
Pancreatic carcinoma (A549)	23,400
Bronchogenic carcinoma (9812)	<200
Glioblastoma (A172)	17,600
Other carcinomas (avg. 4)	21,900
Other sarcomas (avg. 6)	7,900

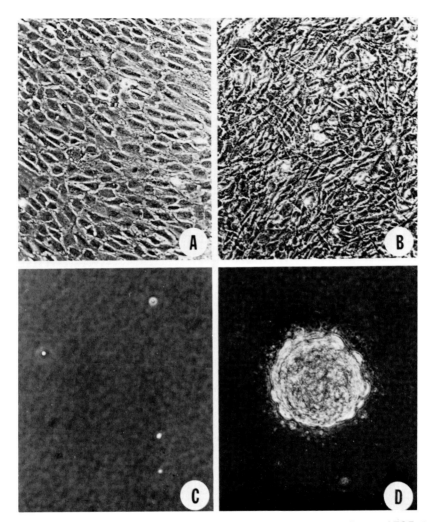

Fig. 1. Normal rat kidney cells. (A) Untreated; (B) treated with an aliquot of TGF at 10 μg/ml and photographed 6 days later. The cells have grown to considerable higher cell density and display a morphology similar to that of viral transformed cells. × 125. (C and D) Normal rat kidney cells were plated in 0.3% soft agar. (C) Untreated; (D) treated with an aliquot of TGF at 10 μg/ml and photographed 2 weeks after treatment. The untreated cultures show primarily single cells with two or three cell colonies, but none of larger size. In the treated cultures many colonies contained well over 500 cells. × 250.

cells produce TGF while the same cells transformed by a transformation-defective (td) mutant of AbLV produced no detectable TGF (Twardzik *et al.*, 1982b).

TGF is acid and heat stable, produces profound morphological changes in rat and human fibroblasts, and enables normal anchorage-dependent cells to grow in soft agar (see Fig. 1). Removal of the transforming protein results in a reversion of cell phenotype back toward the normal. When soft agar colonies formed by untransformed fibroblasts, under the stimulation of TGF, are selected and plated as monolayer cultures in the absence of TGF, they grow as normal contact-inhibited, growth-arrested fibroblasts. They will not form soft agar colonies when plated in the absence of TGF; however, if TGF is added as an overlay, even 1 week after these cells are plated in soft agar, they will form three or four cell colonies within 3 days and eventually give rise to colonies containing greater than 100 cells.

II. Isolation and Characterization of TGF from Human Melanoma Cells

A small molecular weight human TGF (hTGF$_S$) was isolated from serum-free conditioned medium of the highly transformed human metastatic melanoma cell line A2058 (Marquardt and Todaro, 1982). The quantitation of hTGF$_S$ was based on two of its properties: the capacity to induce anchorage-independent growth of normal rat kidney fibroblasts in soft agar, and the ability to compete with [^{125}I] EGF for the EGF receptor sites on A431 human carcinoma cells. A summary of the steps leading to the isolation of hTGF$_S$ and its recovery is presented in Table II.

To remove serum proteins, A2058 cells were washed extensively with Waymouth's medium prior to their culture in serum-free medium. The supernatant fluids were collected every other day for a 2-week period. Culture conditions were such that at the end of the period more than 90% of the cells were still viable and attached as monolayers. The initial clarified A2058-conditioned medium of 136 liters, containing 1.02 gm of total protein and 4525 units of EGF-competing activity, was concentrated to about 900 ml using a hollow fiber concentrator with cartridges of 5000 molecular weight cutoff. The total EGF-competing activity was retained and a recovery above 95% was obtained.

Dialysis of the concentrated A2058-conditioned medium against acetic acid and subsequent centrifugation resulted in 95% recovery of the initial total EGF-competing activity. The acid-soluble, partially purified hTGF

TABLE II

Purification of hTGF$_s$ from Conditioned Medium of Human Melanoma Cells, A2058

Purification step	Protein[a] recovered (mg)	EGF-competing activity recovered (units)[b]	Relative specific activity (units/mg)	Degree of purification (-fold)	Recovery (%)
1. A2058-conditioned medium	1,020	4,525	4.4	1	100
2. Acid-soluble supernatant	837	4,299	5.1	1	95
3. Bio-Gel P-10					
pool P-10-A	29.7	2,077	70	16	45.9
pool P-10-B	14.5	2,033	140	32	44.9
4. μBondapak C$_{18}$ (acetonitrile)	0.202	1,628	8,059	1,823	36.0
5. μBondapak C$_{18}$ (1-propanol)	0.0015	1,476	984,000	223,636	32.6

[a] Total protein was determined using bovine serum albumin as a standard. The quantitation of step 5 hTGF$_s$ was based on amino acid analysis. The absolute specific activity of a companion aliquot was found to be 1–1.5 × 10 units/mg (see text).

[b] One EGF-competing activity unit is defined as the amount of protein that inhibits the binding of [^{125}I]EGF to its receptor by 50%.

was subjected to gel permeation chromatography on Bio-Gel P-10. The column was eluted with 1 *M* acetic acid. A representative chromatogram is illustrated in Fig. 2. The bulk of the contaminating protein was eluted in the exclusion volume of the column and was well separated from the EGF-competing activity and growth-stimulating activity. Two peaks of activity were found to be well resolved from each other. Fractions with both EGF-competing and growth-stimulating activity (P-10-A and P-10-B) had apparent molecular weights of 10,500 and 6800, respectively. Fractions having only one of the two activities were not observed. hTGF-containing fractions were pooled as indicated, lyophilized, and further purified. The larger molecular weight TGF (hTGF$_L$) eluted from the column in a broad peak (P-10-A) and appeared to be associated

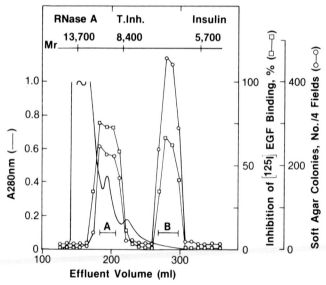

Fig. 2. Gel permeation chromatography of A2058-conditioned medium on Bio-Gel P-10 (420-ml bed volume). Elution pattern of 69.7 mg of protein (acid-soluble protein from 9.2 liters of A2058-conditioned medium). The elution was performed with 1*M* acetic acid at 22°C at a flow rate of 12 ml/hour. 4.8-ml fractions were collected. Aliquots of the indicated fractions were lyophilized and assayed for (1) EGF-competing activity with 100-µl aliquots (□); (2) soft agar growth with 200-µl aliquots (○). The solid line gives the protein absorbance at 280 nm. The following proteins and peptides were used to construct standard plots of log molecular weight versus elution volume: bovine pancreatic ribonuclease A, RNase A, molecular weight 13,700; lima bean trypsin inhibitor, T.Inh., molecular weight 8400; bovine pancreatic insulin, Insulin, molecular weight 5700. The elution volumes of the standard peptides are indicated.

with polypeptides of different sizes. The small molecular weight TGF ($hTGF_S$) eluted from the column in a sharp peak (P-10-B) and represented 45% of the initial total EGF-competing activity. The cumulative yield of total input EGF-competing activity from step 1 through the gel permeation chromatography step was 91% (Table II). hTGF was eluted as these two distinct major peaks that varied quantitatively from one preparation to another. In some preparations of A2058-conditioned medium essentially all the growth-promoting activity was in the $hTGF_S$ region.

Pool P-10-B ($hTGF_S$) was reconstituted in 0.05% trifluoroacetic acid in water, and then further purified using reverse phase high pressure liquid chromatography (rpHPLC) on a μBondapak C_{18} column. $hTGF_S$ was well separated from the bulk of contaminating protein which eluted at higher concentrations of organic solvent. The fractions with the maximal activity were pooled, lyophilized, and rechromatographed. A 57-fold purification of $hTGF_S$ after gel permeation chromatography was obtained. Eighty percent of the initial EGF-competing activity in pool P-10-B was recovered. Rechromatography of the $hTGF_S$-containing fractions on μBondapak C_{18} support was chosen for the final purification step since only relatively small losses of EGF-competing activity were observed on these columns. In order to obtain a distinct separation of $hTGF_S$ from impurities, it was necessary to use a shallow linear 1-propanol gradient in 0.035% trifluoroacetic acid. EGF-competing and growth-stimulating activities copurified with a distinct absorbance peak at 13% 1-propanol. The purification of $hTGF_S$ was approximately 7000-fold after gel permeation chromatography with a yield of 33% of the initial total EGF-competing activity. The overall recovery of $hTGF_S$ from step 3 through the final rpHPLC step was 73%, and the recovery range per step was 80–100% (Table II).

The receptor reactivity of $hTGF_S$ was compared with EGF in the radioreceptor assay. The quantitation of $hTGF_S$ was based on amino acid analysis of a companion aliquot. Both $hTGF_S$ and EGF competed with [^{125}I] EGF for the EGF receptor sites on A431 human carcinoma cells as shown in Fig. 3. The specific EGF-competing activity of $hTGF_S$ was found to be $1-1.5 \times 10^6$ units/mg; 1.1 ng of $hTGF_S$ or EGF were required to inhibit EGF binding by 50%.

$hTGF_S$ enabled normal anchorage-dependent rat kidney cells, clone 49F, to grow in soft agar. The half-maximal response of $hTGF_S$ in soft agar was reached with 1 EGF-competing unit, or 1.1 ng of $hTGF_S$, whereas EGF does not stimulate growth of these cells in soft agar even when tested with up to 10 μg (Fig. 3B). The specificity of the radioreceptor assay was further exemplified by the close correlation between $hTGF_S$

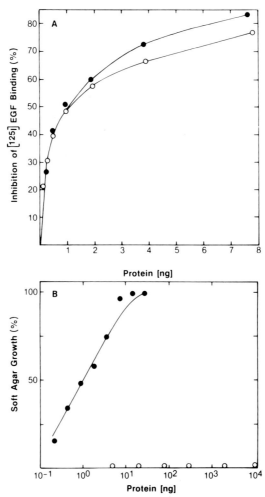

Fig. 3. Dose–response curves of EGF and hTGF$_s$. (A) Inhibition of [^{125}I]EGF binding to the EGF receptor of formalin-fixed A431 human carcinoma cells by EGF (○) and by hTGF (●). Cells, 8×10^3/dish, were incubated with [^{125}I] EGF (0.4 ng/dish; 74 μCi/μg) and unlabeled peptides at the indicated concentrations. The [^{125}I] EGF bound was determined, and nonspecific binding (binding in the presence of 2 μg of EGF) was 2.9% and has been subtracted. One hundred percent specific binding corresponds to 15.1% of the input radioactivity. (B) Soft agar growth assay as a function of protein concentration. Normal rat kidney fibroblasts, clone 49F, 1×10^4 cells/dish were incubated with increasing amounts of hTGF$_s$ (●) and EGF (○) in 2.3 ml of 0.3% agar in Dulbecco's modified Eagle's medium, supplemented with 10% calf serum, on a 2-ml base layer of 0.5% (w/v) agar in the same medium. The number of colonies ($>$10 cells) were scored at 2 weeks and are presented as percent maximum effect. One hundred percent maximum response corresponds to 440 colonies/4 fields. No colonies, in the absence of hTGF$_s$, have been seen on control plates.

levels determined by the radioreceptor assay and the soft agar growth assay (Fig. 3). The purity of the final hTGF$_s$ preparation was determined by analytical SDS-polyacrylamide gel electrophoresis as shown in Fig. 4. The gel was stained with silver. One major polypeptide band, with an apparent molecular weight of 7400, was observed. The same pattern was obtained when samples were electrophoresed under nonreducing conditions.

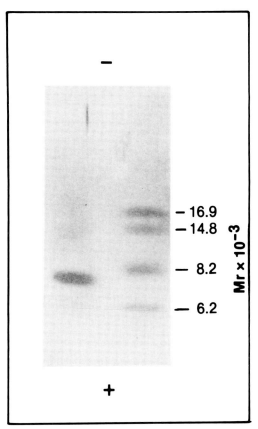

Fig. 4. SDS-polyacrylamide gel electrophoresis of hTGF$_s$ on a 15–30% acrylamide gradient slab (Laemmli, 1970). The sample (100 ng) was dissolved in 10 μl of sample buffer containing 1% SDS and 1% β-mercaptoethanol and incubated at 100°C for 2 minutes. After electrophoresis, gels were fixed in 50% methanol, 10% acetic acid for 2 hours, washed in 5% methanol, 7% acetic acid overnight, and stained with silver (Oakley *et al.*, 1980). The positions of marker polypeptides used to construct standard plots of log molecular weights versus mobility are indicated: horse-heart myoglobin, 16,900 MW, and its cyanogen bromide peptides, 14,400, 8200, 6200, and 2500 MW (BHD Chemicals Ltd.) (Dautrevaux *et al.*, 1969). The 2500 MW cyanogen bromide peptide was detected only with sufficient loading.

The amino acid composition of human melanoma cell-derived hTGF$_S$ is shown in Table III. The closest approximation to integral values for all residues was obtained by assuming that hTGF$_S$ has a molecular weight of 7400. A molecular weight of 7350 was calculated for the peptide chain of hTGF$_S$ on the basis of its amino acid composition. The contribution of tryptophan and proline to the size of the peptide chain was not taken into account. No free sulfhydryl groups could be found by S-amidomethylation with iodo[1-^{14}C]acetamide in 6 M guanidine-HCl without prior reduction. A comparison of the amino acid compositions of hTGF$_S$ with that of human EGF does not suggest any similarities (Table III).

TABLE III

Amino Acid Compositions of Human TGF$_S$ and Human EGF

Amino acid	Residues/mole[a]	
	hTGF$_S$[b]	hEGF[c]
Aspartic acid	5.1 (5)[d]	7
Threonine[e]	2.9 (3)	0
Serine[e]	5.8 (6)	3
Glutamic acid	9.8 (10)	5
Proline	ND[f]	1
Glycine	7.1 (7)	4
Alanine	5.2 (5)	2
Half-cystine[a]	5.8 (6)	6
Valine	6.0 (6)	3
Methionine	0 (0)	1
Isoleucine	0.9 (1)	2
Leucine	3.8 (4)	5
Tyrosine	0 (0)	5
Phenylalanine	2.8 (3)	0
Histidine	4.1 (4)	2
Lysine	3.9 (4)	2
Arginine	3.9 (4)	3
Tryptophan	ND[f]	2

[a] Residues per peptide.
[b] Values are based on two aliquots (350 ng each) hydrolyzed for 24 hours and calculated by assuming a 7400 MW.
[c] Residues per peptide, determined by amino acid sequence analysis.
[d] Nearest integer.
[e] Corrected for hydrolytic losses.
[f] ND, not determined.
[g] Determined as cysteic acid after performic acid oxidation. The sample was hydrolyzed for 24 hours.

III. TGF from Abelson Murine Leukemia Virus-Transformed Rat Cells

Abelson murine leukemia virus (AbLV) is a prototype replication-defective mammalian transforming virus initially generated as a result of genetic recombination between the Moloney strain of murine leukemia virus (MuLV) and transformation-specific sequences of mouse cell origin (Scolnick et al., 1975; Witte et al., 1978; F. H. Reynolds et al., 1978a; R. K. Reynolds et al., 1978b). In the presence of an appropriate type C helper virus, AbLV transforms embryo fibroblasts in cell culture (Scher and Siegler, 1975) and induces a rapid B cell lymphoid leukemia in vivo (Abelson and Rabstein, 1970; Rosenberg and Baltimore, 1976). A characteristic property of AbLV-transformed embryo fibroblasts is a marked reduction in available binding sites for EGF (Blomberg et al., 1980).

Culture fluids from AbLV nonproductively transformed rat embryo fibroblasts were harvested, concentrated, acid ethanol extracted, and subjected to molecular size analysis by gel filtration chromatography (Fig. 5). Individual column fractions were assayed for competition with ^{125}I-labeled EGF for binding A431 cell membrane receptors and for transformation of normal rat kidney (NRK) cells as measured by ability to form progressively growing colonies in soft agar. As shown in Fig. 5, two peaks of EGF-competing activity were identified; these eluted with apparent molecular weights of approximately 10,000 (fractions 75–85) and 20,000 (fractions 45–55) respectively. Activities in both peaks morphologically transform cells in monolayer culture and support anchorage independent growth of NRK cells in soft agar. EGF, in contrast, did not promote soft agar growth in this assay. Thus, the activities produced and released into the culture fluids by AbLV-transformed rat cells demonstrate many of the characteristics described for growth factors produced by Moloney murine sarcoma virus (MSV)-transformed mouse fibroblasts (De Larco and Todaro, 1978; De Larco et al., 1980) and human melanoma cells (Todaro et al., 1980).

AbLV TGF activities are distinguished from EGF on the basis of several immunological and biochemical criteria. For instance, neither molecular weight form of AbLV TGF exhibited detectable reactivity in a competition radioimmunoassay for mouse EGF. AbLV TGF is further distinguished from EGF by its differential solvent elution profile in rp-HPLC. Whereas mouse EGF elutes at 28.7% acetonitrile in 0.05% trichloroacetic acid from a μBondapak C_{18} column, the 10,000 MW AbLV TGF elutes at 19.5% acetonitrile concentration.

The low molecular weight growth factor released by AbLV-transformed cells closely resembles the sarcoma growth factor (De Larco et

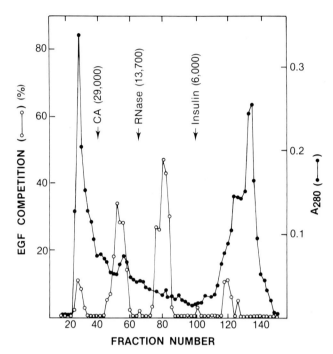

Fig. 5. AbLV nonproductively transformed Fisher rat embryo cell monolayers were washed twice with serum-free medium; culture fluids were collected at three sequential 12-hour intervals, clarified by low speed centrifugation, concentrated using a hollow fiber concentrator DC2 (Amicon, Scientific Systems, Inc.), dialyzed against 1% acetic acid, and lyophilized. The lyophilizate from 6.0 liters of culture fluid was extracted using a modification of the previously described acid ethanol procedure (Twardzik *et al.*, 1982a; Roberts *et al.*, 1980) and applied to a 2.5 x 100 cm Bio-Gel P-100 column in 1*M* acetic acid. Individual fractions (3.5 ml) were collected and aliquots were tested for competition with ^{125}I-labeled EGF for binding to membrane receptors of A431 cells (De Larco and Todaro, 1978; De Larco *et al.*, 1980).

al., 1980) from culture fluids of Moloney MSV-transformed mouse cells. Growth factors associated with transformation by each of these viruses morphologically transform cells *in vitro* (De Larco and Todaro, 1978), compete with EGF for binding to homologous cell surface receptors (De Larco *et al.*, 1980), and induce tyrosine phosphorylation of EGF membrane receptors (Blomberg *et al.*, 1980). The similarities in growth factors produced by cells transformed by retroviruses containing genetically distinct acquired cellular sequences favor the conclusion that TGFs represent cellular rather than direct viral gene products.

The mechanism by which cells convert to the transformed phenotype as a result of exogenous exposure to TGFs is, as yet, unclear. Since tyrosine phosphorylation of EGF receptors is induced by both EGF and TGF, this event, in itself, does not appear sufficient for transformation. Indeed, in certain situations EGF receptor phosphorylation can be distinguished from growth stimulation (Schreiber *et al.*, 1981; Gill and Lazar, 1981). The present findings indicate that TGF production may be a relatively common feature of retrovirus-transformed cells, including those transformed by AbLV, and that such factors may be induced either directly or indirectly by phosphorylation of one or more cellular tyrosine acceptor sites. The demonstration of tyrosine phosphorylation of the EGF receptor by TGFs produced by human tumor cells (Reynolds *et al.*, 1981) argues that identification of cellular pathways involved in the expression of the transformed phenotype will have significance for the understanding of cancer causation.

IV. Relationship between TGF and EGF

As described above the family of peptides (TGF) produced by the EGF receptor-negative lines (RNA virus-transformed rodent cells and certain human tumor cells) produce a rapid, readily detectable morphological transformation of various indicator cells; they also specifically bind to EGF membrane receptors. Table IV summarizes the similarities and differences between TGF and EGF. Both are heat stable (100°C for 5 min-

TABLE IV

Comparison of Properties of EGF and TGF

Similarities
1. Heat-stable, acid-stable peptides sensitive to reducing agents and to proteases
2. Specificially interact with and produce their biologic effects through membrane EGF receptor
3. Stimulate cell proliferation of fibroblasts and epithelial cells with nanogram quantities

Differences
1. Molecular weight (TGF: 7.4K; EGF: 6.0K)
2. Isoelectric point (TGF: pI 6.8; EGF: pI 4.5)
3. Amino acid composition (TGF: no Tyr, no Met, 3 Phe, 3 Thr; EGF: 5 Tyr, 1 Met, no Phe, no Thr)
4. Elution from rpHPLC (TGF: 21%; EGF: 29%)
5. TGF induces anchorage independent growth; EGF does not
6. Antibodies to EGF do not recognize TGF
7. Binding protein for EGF does not bind TGF
8. Tumor cells produce TGFs, not EGF

utes), acid stable (stored in 1 M acetic acid for months with no diminution of activity) polypeptides that are very sensitive to reducing agents; disulfide bonds are crucial for their activity. Both bind to specific EGF receptors at neutral pH and can be eluted from the membranes of formalin-fixed, receptor-rich A431 human carcinoma cells (Fabricant *et al.*, 1977; Haigler *et al.*, 1978) by treatment with weak acid. This procedure has been useful in the purification of mouse SGF (De Larco *et al.*, 1980). In addition, both polypeptides are active in inducing cell division in growth-arrested cultures of epithelial cells as well as fibroblasts.

Antibodies to EGF do not detect TGF in either radioimmunoassays or immunoprecipitation tests. The binding protein from mouse serum that complexes to EGF does not bind to any detectable level to TGF. Nevertheless, both EGF and TGF bind to the 160,000 molecular weight EGF membrane receptor protein, and both bring about the specific phosphorylation of tyrosine residues in the receptor as a result of this binding.

The most striking difference between these growth factors, however, is in their effects on susceptible cells. TGF produces a profound phenotypic alteration in cultured cells and confers on them the ability to behave as transformed cells. As the result of a single exposure to TGF, single cells seeded in agar give rise to progressively growing colonies that contain hundreds, even thousands, of cells. The cells are not permanently transformed, however, for when they are reseeded in agar in the absence of SGF they are unable to proliferate. EGF, in contrast, has only a slight effect on monolayer cultures and does not produce large, progressively growing colonies in soft agar. While TGFs are produced by the RNA tumor virus-transformed cells, we have never detected EGF production by the transformed cells. We conclude that mouse salivary gland EGF, or a close relative of it, is not the substance activated by the virus transformation. Instead, a different and much more biologically active family of peptides are produced, TGF. When this family is fully characterized it may turn out to have a relationship to EGF similar to that found when the somatomedins or insulin-like growth factors (IGFs) are compared to insulin itself (Blundell and Humbel, 1980). We have suggested that TGF may be normally produced during the course of embryonic development and have a role in the expansion and/or migration of different populations of fetal cells. Support for this comes from recent experiments where acid–ethanol extracts of 10- to 11-day-old mouse embryos were found to contain measurable levels of a 9000–10,000 MW TGF that could be readily separated from the 6000 MW EGF which was also present (Twardzik *et al.*, 1982a). Nexo *et al.*, (1980) have also shown that in early mouse embryos a radioreceptor assay detects considerably more EGF-like activity than does the more specific radioimmunoassay for EGF.

V. Presence of TGF-Like Activities in Human Urine

TGF-like activities can also be detected in the urine of pregnant and tumor-bearing humans. A 10,000 MW TGF-like activity is found in the urine of mid- to late-term pregnant females and untreated patients with small cell carcinoma of the lung (SCCL). These activities have not been detected in urine pools derived from normal males and nonpregnant females. In addition to the 10,000 MW activity, the urine of pregnant females contains a 17,000–20,000 MW component. The exact source of TGF-like activity in urine from pregnant females has yet to be established, but experiments with mice have identified TGF activity at 10,000 and 17,000–20,000 MW in 10- to 11-day-old embryos (Twardzik *et al.*, 1982a) suggesting that the human fetus may also be capable of producing such factors. All urine specimens examined also contained a common 8000 MW soft agar growth-stimulating activity eluting slightly ahead of human EGF. This factor(s), present in urine of normal individuals as well as tumor patients, is not sufficiently characterized and, thus, its relationship to TGF and EGF is still unclear.

Figure 6 shows a comparison of the Bio-Gel P-100 column profiles comparing the urine from a patient with soft tissue sarcoma and a normal control. Both show the lower molecular weight activity but the urine from the tumor patient also contains a distinct peak of EGF-competing activity and growth-stimulating activity in the 30,000–35,000 MW range.

The activity of the TGF-like 10,000 MW component from the urine of pregnant donors and from a small cell carcinoma of the lung patient was susceptible to treatment with trypsin or dithiothreitol (Table V), as reported previously for sarcoma growth factor (De Larco and Todaro, 1978) and TGFs from human tumor cells (Roberts *et al.*, 1980; Twardzik *et al.*, 1982a). In addition, the activity was also heat stable in 1 M acetic acid solutions and recoverable after repeated lyophilization. The EGF-competing and soft agar growth-stimulating activity for the urine-derived 30,000 MW TGF-like activity also exhibits typical dose response curves (data now shown) and, as with the TGFs isolated from cell culture fluids, have both transforming growth activity and EGF-competing activity. These data indicate a functional similarity between TGF-like activities found in urine from tumor-bearing humans and those identified in conditioned media from tumor cell cultures. We have not yet succeeded in purifying any of the urine TGFs to homogeneity and do not know what relationship they have to the smaller factors seen in the urine or to the factors purified from cell culture fluids; to the extent that they have been purified, however, the transforming activity and EGF receptor binding coelute.

In addition to having the 10,000 MW factor, urine derived from previ-

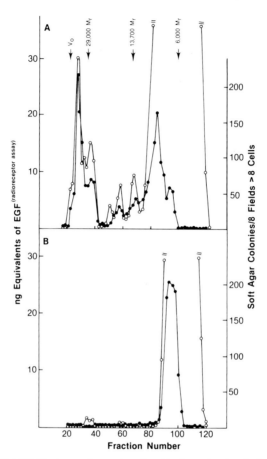

Fig. 6. Bio-Gel P-100 chromatography of acid-ethanol extracted urine from a patient with alveolar cell soft tissue sarcoma (A) and a normal control (B). The number of NRK colonies consisting of >6 cells in four random low power fields (○) and EGF-competing activity calculated as nanogram equivalents from a standard curve (●) are plotted against column fraction. Column markers included carbonic anhydrase (29,000 MW), RNase (13,900), and insulin (6000). The column void is designated by V_o.

ously untreated cancer patients (18 of 22) with a variety of carcinomas, including lung, breast, and colon, also contain this major TGF-like activity with an apparent molecular weight of 30,000–35,000 (Sherwin *et al.,* in preparation). This activity has not been detected in the urine from an equal number of age and sex matched controls. Since small cell carcinoma of the lung cells *in vitro* have been shown to produce soft agar growth stimulating factors (Sherwin *et al.,* 1981) it can also be postulated that the unusually large TGF-like activity in the urine of the patient with small cell

TABLE V

Stability of the 10,000 MW TGF-Like Activity from the Urine of a Previously Untreated Small Cell Carcinoma of the Lung Patient

Treatments[a]	Soft agar colonies/8 fields > 10 cells
Trypsin control	220
Trypsin	<1
Dithiothreitol control	203
Dithiothreitol	<5
Acetic acid control	188
Acetic acid 4°C, 24 hours	200
22°C, 24 hours	210
37°C, 24 hours	205
Relyophilization (2X)	182

[a] The Bio-Gel P-100 10,000 MW TGF-like activity (fractions 72–78 from urine from a SCCl patient) was pooled and equivalent aliquots were lyophilized and redissolved in 0.1 M NH_4HCO_3, pH 7.8. A control solution and one containing trypsin at 50 gm/ml was incubated at 37°C for 2 hours after which soybean trypsin inhibitor was added to give 100 μg/ml. For dithiothreitol treatment, a control solution and one containing 0.075 M DTT were incubated at 22°C for 2 hours followed by extensive dialysis against 0.2 M acetic acid. Each sample was then made 1 M in acetic acid and lyophilized. Acid stability studies were conducted in samples made 1 M in acetic acid prior to lyophilization. All samples were redissolved in binding buffer and assayed for soft agar growth promoting activity as previously described (De Larco and Todaro, 1978; Todaro et al., 1980).

lung cancer is derived from the tumor cells. Since TGF is secreted into tumor cell culture fluids, we propose that these tumor cells products (TGFs) are released from tumor cells *in vivo* and subsequently cleared into the urine. We must however also entertain the possibility that this tumor "associated" activity may be a host response to the tumor burden. The detection of peptides with diverse biological effects in the urine is not a novel observation as, for example, peptides which stimulate capillary–endothelial cell migration have been found in the urine of patients with bladder tumors (Chodak et al., 1981). What is interesting, nevertheless, is that this family of growth-stimulating peptides found in the urine of tumor patients is biologically active, changing nontransformed cells to the transformed phenotype, and it may prove to be a useful biological marker in certain types of cancers.

A large number and variety of tumor cells produce "ectopic" hormones such as corticotropin (ACTH), and calcitonin. If, among all the polypeptide hormones that tumor cells produce there is one, such as TGF, that the tumor cell can use to facilitate its own growth, then the ability to produce these peptide hormones would be of great selective advantage to the tumor cell. Even if the tumor cells produced a variety of hormones it could not use, if *any* one facilitated growth then the ability to "turn on" the whole system would be advantageous to the tumor cell population, although not to the host.

The pituitary hormones corticotropin (ACTH) and β-lipotropin are among several potent hormones formed from a large common precursor (Nakanishi *et al.*, 1979); this precursor and its cleavage products are also expressed in small cell carcinomas and other tumors (Tsukada *et al.*, 1981). From the DNA sequence of pro-opiomelanocortin, a cysteine-rich peptide, function unknown, is seen at the amino-terminal end in both the bovine and human forms (Chang *et al.*, 1980). TGF, which in the urine is found on a 30,000–35,000 MW polyprotein, may be produced by the selective processing of one of these master polyhormone precursors, perhaps even promelanocortin itself. More complete sequence analysis of the purified TGFs will be needed to test this hypothesis.

While we have proposed, for simplicity, a model of a continually expanding population of tumor cells, each producing and responding to potent growth stimulators that the tumor cells, themselves, are able to produce, we are aware that the actual situation may be considerably more complex, given what is known about the extent of tumor cell heterogeneity. For example, we could imagine a tumor cell population that requires a critical level of three different peptide hormones, each interacting with its receptor system. In that population, an individual tumor cell might produce enough of only one factor itself and would be dependent on receiving enough hormone from other cells in the population to continue cell division. No one tumor cell would be completely autonomous, yet the tumor population as a whole could be. Those rare tumor cells that are able to break away from the mass and to colonize distant sites might be relatively more autonomous, perhaps producing more different growth factors or higher levels of some critical rate-limiting hormones.

VI. Growth Inhibitory Factors

While we have concentrated so far on modulators of cell growth that increase proliferative capacity of cells we have also become aware of potent tumor cell growth inhibitory factors (TIFs) produced by normal cells and certain tumor cells. The biological and biochemical properties of TIFs are summarized in Table VI. These factors, some of which are also acid-stable peptides in the 5000–20,000 MW range, inhibit the growth of tumor cells in agar and inhibit the TGF-dependent growth of normal cells in suspension culture. They do not compete directly with either EGF or

TABLE VI

Properties of Tumor Cell Growth Inhibitory Factors (TIFs)

Biological
1. Released into supernatant fluid by normal cells and by certain tumor cells
2. Has no detectable antiviral (interferon-like) activity, no apparent species specificity
3. Blocks tumor cell growth in agar and also TGF-dependent growth of normal cells
4. Does not block TGF or EGF binding to receptors but does block the induction of tyrosine phosphorylation

Biochemical
1. Heat-stable, acid-stable peptides sensitive to reducing agents and to proteases
2. Major activity has apparent MW of 20,000, smaller forms also seen
3. Much more "sticky" than the TGFs
4. Elute later from rpHPLC than does TGF or EGF

TGF at the level of the initial receptor interaction but block their growth-stimulating effects on cells. Unlike the interferons they have no detectable antiviral activity and little or no species specificity. Our laboratory has tested a variety of sources (buffy coats, normal brain, amniotic fluid, supernatant fluids from normal and certain tumor cell cultures), the most common TIF has an apparent MW of 20,000, but others in the 5000 MW range also have been partially purified. Holley *et al.,* (1980) have described an inhibitory factor in the supernatant fluid of monkey kidney cells, BSC-1, that act on BSC-1 cells; their peak has an approximate MW of 15,000 and may be similar to one of the TIFs we are studying.

The TIFs have several properties that are similar to growth factors. They are acid-stable peptides with the major activity from Bio-Gel P-60 having apparent MWs from 5000 to 20,000. On HPLC they elute close to the growth factors. Further studies will be needed to determine how many different families of inhibitory factors there are and whether they, like the growth factors, interact with specific membrane receptors.

References

Abelson, H. T., and Rabstein, L. S. (1970). *Cancer Res.* **30,** 2213–2222.

Blomberg, J., Reynolds, F. H. Jr., Van de Ven, W. J. M., and Stephenson, J. R. (1980). *Nature (London)* **286,** 504–507.

Blundell, T. L., and Humbel, R. E. (1980). *Nature (London)* **287,** 781–787.

Chang, A. C. Y., Cochet, M., and Cohen, S. N. (1980). *Proc. Natl. Acad. Sci. U.S.A.* **77,** 4890–4894.

Chodak, G. W., Scheiner, C. J., and Zetter, B. R. (1981). *N. Engl. J. Med.* **305**, 869–874.

Dautrevaux, M., Boulanger, Y., Han, K., and Biserte, G. (1969). *Eur. J. Biochem.* **11**, 267–277.

De Larco, J. E., and Todaro, G. J. (1978). *Proc. Natl. Acad. Sci. U.S.A.* **75**, 4001–4005.

De Larco, J. E., Reynolds, R., Carlberg, K., Engle, C., and Todaro, G. J. (1980). *J. Biol. Chem.* **255**, 3685–3690.

Fabricant, R. N., De Larco, J. E., and Todaro, G. J. (1977). *Proc. Natl. Acad. Sci. U.S.A.* **74**, 565–569.

Gill, G. N., and Lazar, C. S. (1981). *Nature (London)* **293**, 305–307.

Haigler, H., Ash, J. F., Singer, S. J., and Cohen, S. (1978). *Proc. Natl. Acad. Sci. U.S.A.* **75**, 3317–3321.

Holley, R. W., Bohlen, P., Fava, R., Baldwin, J. H., Kleeman, G., and Armour, R. (1980). *Proc. Natl. Acad. Sci. U.S.A.* **77**, 5989–5992.

Laemmli, U. K. (1970). *Nature (London)* **277**, 680–685.

Marquardt, H., and Todaro, G. J. (1982). *J. Biol. Chem.* (in press).

Nakanishi, S., Inoue, A., Kita, T., Nakamura, M., Chang, A. C. Y., Cohen, S. N., and Numa, S. (1979). *Nature (London)* **278**, 423–427.

Nexo, E., Hollenberg, M. D., Figueroa, A., and Pratt, R. M. (1980). *Proc. Natl. Acad. Sci. U.S.A.* **77**, 2782–2785.

Oakley, B. R., Kirsch, D. R., and Morris, N. R. (1980). *Anal. Biochem.* **105**, 361–363.

Ozanne, B., Fulton, J., and Kaplan, P. L. (1980). *J. Cell. Physiol.* **105**, 163–180.

Reynolds, F. H. Jr., Sacks, T. L., Deobagkar, D. N., and Stephenson, J. R. (1978). *Proc. Natl. Acad. Sci. U.S.A.* **75**, 3974–3978.

Reynolds, F. H. Jr., Todaro, G. J., Fryling, C., and Stephenson, J. R. (1981). *Nature (London)* **292**, 259–262.

Reynolds, R. K., Van de Ven, W. J. M., and Stephenson, J. R. (1978). *J. Virol.* **28**, 665–670.

Roberts, A. B., Lamb, L. C., Newton, D. L., Sporn, M. B., De Larco, J. E., and Todaro, G. J. (1980). *Proc. Natl. Acad. Sci. U.S.A.* **77**, 3494–3498.

Rosenberg, N., and Baltimore, D. (1976). *J. Exp. Med.* **143**, 1453–1463.

Scher, C. D., and Siegler, R. (1975). *Nature (London)*, **253**, 729–731.

Schreiber, A. B., Yarden, Y., and Schlessinger, J. (1981). *Biochem. Biophys. Res. Comm.* **101**, 517–523.

Scolnick, E. M., Howk, R. S., Anisowicz, A., Peebles, P., Scher, C., and Parks, W. P. (1975). *Proc. Natl. Acad. Sci. U.S.A.* **72**, 4650–4654.

Sherwin, S. A., Minna, J. D., Gazdar, A. F., and Todaro, G. J. (1981). *Cancer Res.* **41**, 3538–3542.

Todaro, G. J., and De Larco, J. E. (1978). *Cancer Res.* **38**, 4147–4154.

Todaro, G. J., Fryling, C., and De Larco, J. E. (1980). *Proc. Natl. Acad. Sci. U.S.A.* **77**, 5258–5262.

Tsukada, T., Nakai, Y., Jingami, H., Imura, H., Taii, S., Nakanishi, S., and Numa, S. (1981). *Biochem. Biophys. Res. Commun.* **98**, 535–540.

Twardzik, D. R., Sherwin, S. A., Ranchalis, J. E., and Todaro, G. J. (1982a). *Cancer Res.* (in press).

Twardzik, D. R., Todaro, G. J., Marquardt, H., Reynolds, F. H. Jr., and Stephenson, J. R. (1982b). *Science (Washington, D.C.)* (in press).

Witte, O. N., Rosenberg, N., Paskind, M., Shields, A., and Baltimore, D. (1978). *Proc. Natl. Acad. Sci. U.S.A.* **75**, 2488–2492.

14

Tumor Subpopulation Interactions

GLORIA H. HEPPNER

I. Introduction

Consideration of the concept "tumor heterogeneity" leads one to focus on the differences among tumors and among tumor subpopulations from the same tumor. The multitudinous ways in which tumor cells vary assume prominence in our thoughts. That individual cancers, whether or not of monoclonal origin, are mixed populations of neoplastic, as well as stromal, cells is an important fact to consider in the practice of cancer research. At the very least, it requires that an investigator address problems of tissue sampling and cell separation in the design of experimental

TUMOR CELL HETEROGENEITY

225

protocol. It also provides a ready source of the experimental variability that plagues all biologists, but especially those working with cancer. It is important, however, not to become so enamored by the concept of tumor heterogeneity as to lose sight of the tumor itself. Just as human societies are not characterized by the simple summing of their individual components, tumors are also more complex than a "roll call" of their subpopulations, however many there may be, would suggest. Like societies, tumors are interacting ecosystems in which the characteristics of the whole are influenced, but not limited, by the characteristics of the parts. In order to begin to understand this "tumor ecology" we have developed a model system consisting of a single tumor separated into cellular subpopulations that we then grow in various combinations to study interactions. We have found that the mechanisms of tumor subpopulation interaction are potentially great in number and often subtle.

II. Historical Perspective

Those of us who only recently have taken up the problem of tumor heterogeneity are becoming used to finding reference in the earlier literature to what we thought were new observations. The idea of tumor subpopulation interactions has a distinguished past. For example, Hauschka (1953) noted that two sublines isolated from the Krebs-2 tumor were more rapidly lethal than the parent stock and concluded that they "were apparently held in check by other elements in the parental population, and in spite of their greater virulence were unable to displace competitive variants." Masking of ascitic variants within a nonascitic tumor was shown by Klein and Klein (1956). Makino (1956) demonstrated growth interaction between two different rat sarcomas inoculated into the same host. Apparent growth interactions between sublines of the TA3 mammary tumor line were also reported by Nowotny and Grohsman (1973).

An especially important example of tumor subpopulation interaction, that between primaries and their metastases, has substantial experimental demonstration, as well as anecdotal observation. Inhibition of metastatic growth by primaries (Greene and Harvey, 1960, DeWys, 1972) and primary growth by metastases (Yuhas and Pazmiño, 1974), as well as stimulation of metastatic growth by primaries (Goldie et al., 1956), have been seen. Such effects have often been attributed to immunological mechanisms (Milas et al., 1974; Gorelik et al., 1978) but other explanations have not been explored vigorously.

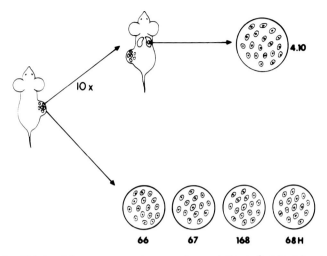

Fig. 1. Origin of five mammary tumor subpopulations. See text for details.

III. Our Model System

A. Derivation of the Subpopulations

The derivation of the model system which we use to study tumor subpopulation interactions is illustrated in Fig. 1. The system consists of five subpopulations obtained from a single mammary adenocarcinoma that arose spontaneously in a multiparous strain BALB/cfC$_3$H female mouse. Four of the subpopulations, designated as 66, 67, 168, and 68H, were developed from cells cultured from the autochthonous tumor. Line 67 was isolated by growing cells of the original monolayer culture on a gelatinized petri dish. Line 66 was isolated by isokinetic gradient centrifugation of tenth passage level monolayer cultures. Lines 168 and 68H were isolated by differential trypsinization of a second passage level monolayer culture. Our fifth subpopulation, designated 4.10, was isolated from a lung nodule metastatic from a subcutaneous implant of the tenth *in vivo* passage from the autochthonous tumor. Details of the isolation procedures have been published (Dexter *et al.*, 1978; Heppner *et al.*, 1978).

B. Characterization of the Subpopulations

Although their cellular morphology in monolayer culture is either polygonal (68H, 4.10) or spindle-shaped (66, 67, 168), all five lines are of epithelial origin by ultrastructural and antigenic criteria (Hager *et al.*, 1981b). They differ among themselves in karyotype and various *in vitro* growth characteristics, such as doubling time in monolayer and cloning efficiency in soft agar (Dexter *et al.*, 1978). They also differ in relative tumorigenicity; at subcutaneous inoculation of 10^5 cells the latency periods for the different subpopulations range from 2 weeks to approximately 3 months. The frequency of metastasis from subcutaneous implants to the lung is essentially zero for lines 67 and 68H, approximately 20% for 168, and 70% for 66. Line 4.10 originally metastasized at a very high frequency, but lost this capacity with prolonged passage. We have since derived a series of 4.10 variant lines that range in metastatic frequency from very low to essentially 100% (Miller, F., unpublished observations). This would seem to be another example of instability of the metastatic phenotype, as described by Doll *et al.* (1981).

In regard to the general question of stability, there is a marked difference among the five subpopulations. Although it is possible to clone out variants, such as drug-resistant clones, from lines 66, 67, 168, or 4.10 using classic selection and cloning procedures, only line 68H is unstable in general. Interestingly, this instability is only revealed after *in vivo* passage. Unlike what is seen with the other four subpopulations, tumors produced by 68H cells are extremely heterogeneous in culture. Indeed a whole series of new subpopulations has been isolated from a 68H tumor and shown to be unique by a combination of morphological, karyotypical, and growth characteristics (Hager *et al.*, 1981a). That these variants have origin in 68H rather than in the host in which the tumor was grown is evident from karyotyping; all of the line 68H variants have a female karyotype whereas the host was a male. Thus, line 68H is itself a model system for studying the origin of tumor heterogeneity.

The immunological characteristics of the five subpopulations are quite complex (Miller and Heppner, 1979). Although their parent tumor arose in a mouse carrying the murine mammary tumor virus (MuMTV), only line 68H strongly expresses MuMTV cross-reacting antigens, detectable by immunofluorescence, in its cell membranes. (All the lines exhibit some indication of the presence of MuMTV cytoplasmic antigens and genomic material.) Lines 68H, 66, 168, and 4.10 express other MuMTV-associated moieties, however, which render them either immunogenic or sensitive to an immune response directed against mammary tumor common antigens. Lines 66, 67, 168, and 4.10 express a "unique" antigen characteristic of individual mammary tumors. Line 68H does not express the unique antigen and 67 is negative for the common one.

Similar to what is discussed elsewhere in this volume, the five subpopulations are differentially sensitive to a variety of chemotherapeutic drugs

(Heppner *et al.*, 1978) and radiation (Leith *et al.*, 1979). These differences in sensitivity to therapeutic agents seem unrelated to differences in growth and behavioral characteristics.

The five subpopulations provide us with a variety of different characteristics which we can attempt to relate to the behavior of "whole" tumors. It is unlikely that they are identical representatives of cells originally within their parent tumors. The parent tumor was heterogeneous, however, as shown by morphology, karyotype, and expression of MuMTV antigens (Dexter *et al.*, 1978). It is also unlikely that the five subpopulations represent the only ones in the original tumor. We know from our studies with 68H that the number of subpopulations is potentially very great and, furthermore, may change with time. Indeed, a major problem in this area of research is quantitation of heterogeneity. Thus, though our approach barely begins to address the complexity of the real situation, we hope it provides insight into the types of relationships among tumor subpopulations on which the "tumor society" is maintained.

IV. Growth Interactions between Tumor Subpopulations

A. Growth Interactions Detected *in Vivo*

A major difficulty in designing experiments in which tumor subpopulations coexist is distinguishing the individual components in mixtures quantitatively. This is an especially difficult problem *in vivo* because of the additional complications provided by stromal components. In order to avoid this difficulty we have used an experimental protocol in which cells of individual subpopulations are injected subcutaneously into opposite sides of the same, syngeneic mouse (Fig. 2). Growth of the subpopulations in this "bilateral" configuration is compared to single implant growth and to growth when paired with self. Using this protocol we have found that (1) 68H tumor growth is stimulated by 168 tumors, (2) 168 tumor growth is slowed by 68H tumors, (3) 168 tumor growth is slowed by 4.10 tumors, and (4) 66 and 67 mutually interact to inhibit each other's growth (Miller *et al.*, 1980).

We have chosen one of the above interactions, namely, that between 4.10 and 168, to explore the responsible mechanisms. Our results suggest that the host immune response is playing a major role (Miller *et al.*, 1980). Thus, irradiation of the host with 400 R 2 days prior to tumor implantation prevents the interaction from occurring. The immunological relationships between 168 and 4.10 also suggest an immunological basis. Line 4.10 cells

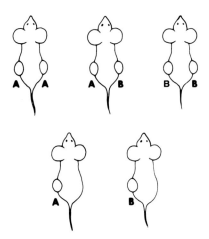

Fig. 2. *In vivo* protocol to detect tumor subpopulation interactions.

are highly immunogenic against challenge with either 168 or 4.10 tumors. This is true whether the immunization is done with 4.10 cells alone or with a mixture of 4.10 and 168 cells. Line 168 cells, however, are unable to immunize effectively against either 4.10 or themselves. Our explanation for the growth interaction between 4.10 and 168 tumors is the induction of immunity to 168 cells by the 4.10 tumors. In this view the host is a partner in the maintenance of a ''balance'' between the two subpopulations.

B. Growth Interactions Detected *in Vitro*

One easily identified marker that can be used to distinguish subpopulation 68H is expression of MuMTV cell membrane antigen. We have taken advantage of this marker in experiments in which we mixed together 68H and 168 cells, in varying proportions, and cultured the mixtures in monolayer. The doubling time of 68H cells growing alone in these experiments was up to twice as long as that of 168 cells alone. Growth rates of the mixed cultures were determined by standard techniques. The proportion of MuMTV expressing cells in the mixtures was determined at intervals and used to calculate the growth rate of that component of the culture. A potential weakness of these experiments is the possibility that expression of MuMTV antigen by 68H, or lack of expression by 168 cells, might be altered by exposure to the other subpopulation and so the number of antigen expressing cells would not be an accurate reflection of the number of 68H cells. However, we have no evidence of any subpopulation interactions influencing MuMTV antigen expression, even under conditions of antigen induction by IUdR (J. C. Hager, unpublished observations). Assuming then that expression of MuMTV antigen can be used as a marker for 68H cells in coculture with 168 cells, the major result of these experiments was that the proportion of 68H cells in the coculture remained constant, even after trypsinization and passage of the monolayer (Heppner *et al.*, 1980). Thus, even though 68H and 168 cells grew at markedly different rates alone, they grew at the same rate together. Depending on the conditions of the experiment, this rate was either that of 68H alone or 168 alone, meaning that either 68H cells grew faster or 168 cells slower in the mixture than when they were growing alone.

As can be imagined these coculture experiments were very cumbersome and, furthermore, did not lend themselves readily to investigation of mechanism. We devised another *in vitro* protocol to overcome these drawbacks. This protocol, which is indicated in Fig. 3, physically separates the two cell types and thus eliminates the possibility of cell contact mechanisms that may have played a role in the growth interactions seen in the coculture experiments. In the new protocol cells of two subpopulations were plated on individual cell culture cover slips and grown in combination in common petri dishes. Control experiments indicated that cells do not wander from one cover slip to another, at least in the time frame of these experiments, generally 3 days. The results of these experiments show that certain subpopulations can influence the growth of others, but unlike the coculture experiments the direction of the influence is always negative. Specifically 168 or 66 cells can inhibit growth of other subpopulations but 68H, 67, and 4.10 cells generally cannot (Heppner *et al.*, 1980). To some extent the growth inhibitory activity of cover slip grown cells can be mimicked with cell culture medium conditioned by 168 cells. The

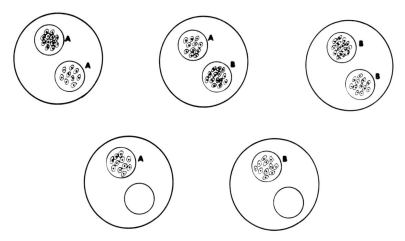

Fig. 3. *In vitro* protocol to detect tumor subpopulation interactions.

inhibitory activity can be removed from the medium by a 0.2 μ filter or by centriguation at 108,000 g for 30 minutes and is extremely labile. It is produced by cultures that are mycoplasma-free according to accepted criteria. Its spectrum of activity includes a variety of mammary tumor cells, even MCF-7 human breast cancer cells, but does not extend to cells of other origin (Miller and Heppner, 1980). Not all mammary tumor cells are affected. We have been frustrated in our attempts to further characterize the growth inhibitory activity because of its lability and because 168 cultures are not stable in regard to its production. However, it would appear that it is not responsible for the stimulatory growth interaction with 68H cells in coculture and so represents yet another way in which subpopulations can interact.

V. Drug Sensitivity Interactions between Tumor Subpopulations

A. Sensitivity Interactions Detected in Vivo

The demonstration that tumor subpopulations can influence each other's growth suggests that such interactions may influence other characteristics as well. Examples from the literature have been mentioned above in Section II. We have chosen to investigate possible interactions influencing sensitivity to chemotherapy because of their significance in the design of drug sensitivity assays, as well as influence on treatment response. For these experiments we have used the same types of protocols employed in the growth interaction studies.

One drug to which our subpopulations are differentially sensitive is cyclophosphamide (CY). Line 168 is relatively more sensitive to this agent than is line 4.10 (Heppner et al., 1978). Using the bilateral protocol illustrated in Fig. 2, we tested whether the sensitivity to CY of either 168 or 4.10 tumors is influenced by the presence of the other subpopulation. Syngeneic mice were injected subcutaneously with both subpopulations or the same subpopulation on opposite sides and treated with varying doses of CY, beginning 2 days after tumor implantation and continuing for 4 weeks on a weekly basis. The sensitivity of 168 tumors was unaffected by the presence of 4.10. At a dose of drug to which there was a clear difference in sensitivity between 168 and 4.10 tumors alone, namely, 50 mg/kg/week, the sensitivity of 4.10 tumors to CY was enhanced by the presence of 168 tumors (Miller et al., 1981). This enhanced sensitivity depended on the response of 168 tumors to drug because at lower doses, to which 168 tumors did not respond, the response of 4.10 tumors was not altered. Unlike the growth interaction between 4.10 and 168 tumors (see Section IV,A), irradiation of the hosts prior to tumor implantation did not negate the ability of 168 tumors to enhance the sensitivity of 4.10 tumors to CY.

CY must be metabolized to an active form(s), a process generally considered to be performed by the microsomal enzymes of the liver. We wondered whether the differential sensitivity, and the interaction in sensitivity, of 168 and 4.10 tumors to CY might somehow be related to drug metabolism. To test this, we carried out standard LD_{50} determinations in mice bearing either both 168 and 4.10 tumors or two implants of either 168 or 4.10 tumors. The experiments were done when the tumors were, on the average, 20 mm² in surface area. The results clearly showed that CY is more lethal in mice bearing 168 or 168 plus 4.10 tumors than in mice bearing 4.10 tumors alone. Toxicity in tumor-free mice is intermediate (Miller *et al.*, 1981). Thus, 168 tumors enhance activation of CY which, we hypothesize, allows the drug to be more effective against 4.10 tumors than it is when 168 tumors are not present. Because 4.10 tumors are sensitive to high doses of CY, we think that 168 tumors are, in effect, increasing the drug dose. Whether the 168 tumors do this through an effect on the host or whether they can activate directly CY themselves is uncertain. Line 168 cells are somewhat sensitive, and more so than 4.10 cells, to CY *in vitro* suggesting that they can metabolize CY. However, this *in vitro* sensitivity requires a high concentration of CY and a long time of exposure.

B. Sensitivity Interactions Detected *in Vitro*

Using methods similar to those we have described for interactions influencing growth (IV,B), we have used the cover slip protocol (Fig. 3) to search for interactions influencing drug sensitivity *in vitro*. Most of our work has been with methotrexate (MTX), which we had previously shown to be differentially effective against our subpopulations (Heppner *et al.*, 1978). We have plated subpopulations that differ in sensitivity to MTX on separate cover slips and grown them together in common petri dishes in varying concentrations of drug. As with the CY experiments, the direction of the results has been the enhancement of the sensitivity of the relatively MTX-insensitive subpopulation in the presence of the sensitive subpopulation as shown by a shift to the left of the concentration–response curve for the less sensitive subpopulation. This interaction does not occur with all combinations of sensitive and insensitive subpopulations, suggesting that some nonspecific toxicity or media-depletion factor is not responsible. The transfer of sensitivity is MTX-concentration dependent; no interaction is seen at very low or very high concentrations where the sensitive population is unaffected or the insensitive population alone affected, respectively. Inhibition of MTX activity by thymidine inhibits the enhanced sensitivity of the insensitive subpopulation. Since our various subpopulations have similar abilities to transport MTX, regardless of sensitivity to this drug, it would appear that the basis for the interaction lies beyond the level of drug uptake.

Whatever the mechanism of transfer of MTX sensitivity, it must involve a diffusable mediator. It is clear, however, that other types of cellular interactions could influence sensitivity to chemotherapy. For example, one well characterized interaction is the transfer of thioguanine (TG) sensitivity (Loewenstein, 1979). TG sensitivity can be transferred from sensitive to resistant cells by a mechanism involving cell contact. TG-resistant cells that are deficient in the enzyme hypoxanthine-guanine phosphoribosyl transferase and thus unable to produce TG nucleotide can receive this metabolite through contact with some TG-sensitive cells (Corsaro and Migeon, 1977). The ability to transfer is thought to involve formation of gap junctions (Pitts and Simms, 1977) so that not all TG-resistant cells can be recipients nor all TG sensitive cells donors. Bonnie Miller has shown that all our subpopulations (which are sensitive to TG) can transfer that sensitivity to a TG-resistant clone of line 66. The efficiency of transfer as measured by the optimum density of the interactive populations varies from line to line with 66 itself being the most efficient and line 168 the least. This transfer is only seen when the donors and recipients are in contact; it is not seen with the cover slip protocol.

VI. Conclusions

The most compelling conclusion from our work, indeed perhaps from the work presented in this entire symposium, is that tumors are mixed cell populations, the understanding of which requires concepts and techniques appropriate to population biology rather than clonal analysis. Even though the majority of tumors may be monoclonal in origin (Fialkow, 1976), a "clone is not forever" and both phenotypic and genetic mechanisms create extensive diversity within tumor cell populations. Some of this heterogeneity can be described in terms of tumor geography and cell cycle concepts (Weiss, 1980). Other aspects are due apparently to the evolution of distinct tumor cell subpopulations. Experimental focus on this latter type of heterogeneity has been on the isolation and description of tumor subpopulations with the implication that their isolated behavior is reflective of their behavior in the tumor "group." The second conclusion from our work is that this idea is too simple. The characteristics of isolated subpopulations are not necessarily those of the same subpopulations when grown as mixtures. In order to appreciate the significance of cellular heterogeneity in any given phenotype, one must ask whether that phenotype is maintained in tumors and, if not, what governs its regulation. Finally, what is the effect of the removal of a "governing" subpopulation on the phenotype of the remaining cells? For example, will surgical removal of a primary tumor influence the drug sensitivity of metastases?

A third conclusion from our work is that there are numerous ways by which tumor subpopulation interactions may occur. When we began our work we expected to find rather specific mechanisms of cellular communication of the sort that apparently operate in embryogenesis or the immune system. Instead we found a whole spectrum of mechanisms—some mediated by host and some by tumor, some involving cell contact, and some operating over a distance—which can serve to influence the tumor ecosystem. Although more specific mechanisms may also be important, it is clear that our original concept was naive. Tumor subpopulation interactions can occur for any of a complex array of immunological, biochemical, physiological, nutritional, and other reasons. How we make use of these interactions in experimental design and clinical application is an enormous challenge.

Acknowledgments

This work is a collaborative effort with my colleagues Drs. Fred and Bonnie Miller. Their role is gratefully acknowledged. I also wish to acknowledge the support from Concern Foundation and from the National Cancer Institute, Grant CA-27419.

References

Corsaro, C. M., and Migeon, B. E. (1977). *Proc. Natl. Acad. Sci. U.S.A.*, **74**, 4476–4480.
DeWys, D. (1972). *Cancer Res.* **32**, 374–379.
Dexter, D. L., Kowalski, H. M., Blazar, B. A., Fligiel, Z., Vogel, R., and Heppner, G. H. (1978). *Cancer Res.* **38**, 3174–3181.
Doll, J., Poste, G., Fidler, I. H. (1981). *Proc. Natl. Acad. Sci. U.S.A.* **78**, 6226–6230.
Fialkow, P. J. (1976). *Biochim. Biophys. Acta.* **458**, 283–321.
Goldie, H., Walker, M., Kelley, L., and Gaines, J. (1956). *Cancer Res.* **16**, 553–558.
Gorelik, E., Segal, S., and Feldman, M. (1978). *Int. J. Cancer,* **21**, 617–625.
Greene, H. S. N., and Harvey, E. K. (1960). *Cancer Res.* **20**, 1094–1100.
Hager, J. C., Fligiel, S., Stanley, W., Richardson, A. M., and Heppner, G. H. (1981a). *Cancer Res.* **41**, 1293–1300.
Hager, J. C., Russo, J., Ceriani, R. L., Peterson, J. A., Fligiel, S., Jolly, G., and Heppner, G. H. (1981b). *Cancer Res.* **41**, 1720–1730.
Hawschka, T. S. (1953). *J. Natl. Cancer Inst.* **14**, 723–736.

Heppner, G. H., Dexter, D. L., DeNucci, T., Miller, F. R., and Calabresi, P. (1978). *Cancer Res.* **38,** 3758–3763.

Heppner, G. H., Miller, B., Cooper, D. N., and Miller, F. R. (1980). *In* "Cell Biology of Breast Cancer" (C. M. McGrath, M. J. Brennan, and M. A. Rich, eds.), pp. 161–172. Academic Press, New York.

Klein, G., and Klein, E. (1956). *Ann. N. Y. Acad. Sci.* **63,** 640–661.

Leith, J. T., Zeman, E. M., Glicksman, A. S., and Heppner, G. H. (1979). *Proc. Am. Assoc. Cancer Res.* **20,** 28.

Loewenstein, W. R. (1979). *Biochim. Biophys. Acta.* **560,** 1–65.

Makino, S. (1956). *Ann. N. Y. Acad. Sci.* **63,** 818–830.

Milas, L., Hunter, N., Mason, K., and Withers, H. R. (1974). *Cancer Res.* **34,** 61–71.

Miller, B. E., and Heppner, G. H. (1980). *Proc. Am. Assoc. Cancer Res.* **21,** 38.

Miller, B. E., Miller, F. R., Leith, J., and Heppner, G. H. (1980). *Cancer Res.* **40,** 3977–3981.

Miller, B. E., Miller, F. R., and Heppner, G. H. (1981). *Cancer Res.* **41,** 4378–4381.

Miller, F. R., and Heppner, G. H. (1979). *J. Natl. Cancer Inst.* **63,** 1457–1463.

Nowotny, A., and Grohsman, J. (1973). *Int. Arch. Allergy* **44,** 434–440.

Pitts, J. D., and Simms, J. W. (1977). *Exp. Cell Res.* **104,** 153–163.

Weiss, L. (1980). *In* "Cell Biology of Breast Cancer" (C. M. McGrath, M. J. Brennan, and M. A. Rich, eds.), pp. 189–205. Academic Press, New York.

Yuhas, J. M., and Pazmiño, N. H. (1974). *Cancer Res.* **34,** 2005–2010.

15

Cell Differentiation in Neoplasia

CLEMENT L. MARKERT

I. Introduction

Neoplasms are generally initiated by the transformation of a single normal cell into a neoplastic cell. The neoplastic cell then multiplies, making the neoplasm evident. In metazoans like ourselves, many different kinds of neoplasms have been recognized, certainly several hundred. Neoplasms can arise from nearly every kind of normal cell. Particularly prone to neoplastic transformation are stem cells or those cells in which division is common. Nondividing cells like nerve cells or striated muscle cells virtually never undergo neoplastic transformation. Neoplasms, once developed, undergo further cell differentiation to produce a variety of cell types, clonally related, but phenotypically distinct.

Many of the characteristics of the normal cell of origin are retained during neoplastic development but new characteristics are acquired and many of the original differentiated characteristics of the normal cell do disappear or are greatly reduced in expression. The initiation and development of a neoplasm represent a change in the pattern of gene function within the cell as compared to the normal cell from which the neoplasm arose. The phenotype of the neoplastic cell must represent the functioning genotype. There is seldom evidence for truly novel genetic expression in

TUMOR CELL HETEROGENEITY

237

tumor cells. They can only make abnormal use of the normal cell genome. The only known exceptions are those cases in which a viral genome has been inserted into the host cell genome and is expressed in the production of virally encoded proteins. But even these viral proteins are generally variant homologues of normal host cell proteins (Weinberg, 1980).

A useful way of describing neoplastic development is to represent such development as a misprogramming of normal gene function (Markert, 1968). Thus, neoplasms are diseased expressions of normal processes of cell differentiation. In these neoplastic programs of gene function, the individual genes are normal but the particular pattern of gene function is abnormal. Although we recognize that malignant neoplasms cause serious disease in the host organism, it is important to realize that the cancer cell itself is not a diseased biological cell. Quite the contrary: it has a phenotype that makes it unusually successful in growing and proliferating in many cellular environments and in resisting external attacks on it. In many ways it represents the most successful type of cell differentiation that the organism can produce as measured by individual cell multiplication and survival (Markert, 1977).

II. Comments on Normal Processes of Cell Differentiation

If the normal processes of cell differentiation have gone awry in the production of a malignant, or neoplastic, cell, what then are the normal processes of cell differentiation that might be subject to abnormal deviations?

Developmental biologists have examined the processes of cell differentiation for many years and now realize that the differential regulation of gene function is the most central feature of metazoan development. Unfortunately, we still do not know how genes are regulated in groups to function or not to function, nor do we know how the level of function, that is, the frequency of transcription, is determined for each gene. Nevertheless, whatever the mechanisms may be, they will surely be the same in both normal and neoplastic cells. This assertion applies both to the initial event in neoplastic transformation and to the subsequent cellular differentiation that occurs within the developing tumor mass, and particularly after metastasis to new tissue environments.

Let us examine some of the basic information on normal cell differentiation that has been acquired by developmental biologists before taking up specific cases of neoplastic transformation. Cell differentiation may be based on genetic or epigenetic events or a combination of both. By "genetic," I mean changes in the DNA and by "epigenetic," I mean alterations in the functional activity of the DNA without change in structure. Embryologists have sought to identify the genetic, chromosomal, or nuclear basis for the cytoplasmic phenotype of cells during embryonic development by two major techniques: nuclear transplantation and tissue transplantation. When patches of cells from an early amphibian embryo are transferred to new locations in the embryo, they readily adapt and continue development in accord with their new location. However, as embryonic development progresses, the plasticity of transferred groups of cells diminishes until finally, at advanced stages of development, they are unresponsive to the new environments and continue to differentiate in accord with their original locations and not in accord with their new cellular environments (Spemann, 1938; Waddington, 1948).

From such experiments, we can conclude that normal cellular differentiation in the embryo requires a precisely structured environment that changes through time in an ordered fashion to provoke the required sequence in patterns of gene function that lead to fully "adult" cells. Embryonic cells can only take one step at a time and each step must be in the proper sequence to reach the terminal adult stage of differentiation. Since these transplantation experiments involve the transposition of groups of cells, rather than individual cells, it might be argued that as the transferred group matures, it creates its own stable cellular environment which in effect isolates the transplant from the surrounding cellular environment. Thus, the issue of whether the differentiative changes are truly genetic or are simply based on epigenetic environmental influences is not easily settled by such experiments.

We can, however, examine the genome itself by nuclear transplantation experiments, and such experiments have been carried out in many laboratories (Briggs, 1977; Diberardino, 1980; Du Pasquier and Wabl, 1977; Gurdon, 1974; McKinnell, 1978; Markert and Ursprung, 1963, Ursprung and Markert, 1963). The evidence demonstrates that the nuclei of early amphibian, and now in mammalian embryos (Illmensee and Hoppe, 1981), are totipotent. Transplantation of the nucleus from an early embryonic cell to a previously enucleated egg will frequently enable the egg to develop into a completely normal adult individual. However, nuclei taken from progressively older and more differentiated embryonic cells exhibit a declining ability to replace the egg nucleus and to generate normal development. Finally, at some late stage in development, the transplanted nuclei, although provoking cell division and sometimes abnormal embryonic development, fail to give rise to normal adults. There are a few exceptions to this generalization, but the overwhelming mass of evidence from nuclear transplantation suggests that the nuclei do become irreversibly differentiated, at least by the test of transplantation. Since the chromosomes can replicate many times after nuclei of such differentiated cells are transplanted into an egg, we are nearly compelled to believe that the DNA itself has been altered in some fashion (Markert and Ursprung, 1963). Nothing is left from the original transplanted nucleus except the molecules that replicate; that leaves the DNA, but the DNA is incapable of supporting normal development.

The leading example of programmed changes in DNA during cell differentiation is presented by lymphocytes (Early and Hood, 1981) and this example, so surprising in itself, may serve as a model for other types of cell differentiation. Possible chemical changes in the DNA are most clearly illustrated by the methylation of cytosine residues. This methylation can be correlated with cell differentiation (Jones and Taylor, 1980). However, if programmed cell-specific changes in the DNA do occur during normal cell differentiation, such changes must be subtle and difficult to identify. Against this general background of experience with normal cell differentiation, I should now like to discuss several specific cases that may be informative with respect to both normal and abnormal cell differentiation.

As embryonic development proceeds, the number of pathways of differentiation that are available to any cell is progressively reduced until finally, only a single pathway to one type of terminally differentiated adult cell remains open. There are exceptions to this dogmatic generalization. One exception is provided by Wolffian lens regeneration in certain species of amphibia (Yamada, 1967; Reyer, 1954; Uriel, 1976). Removal of the lens from an eye of these amphibians leads to the regeneration of a new lens, but the new lens is derived from the pigmented layer of the iris and is not derived from the epidermis as was true for the original lens. Moreover, in this formation of a new lens, a section of the pigmented layer of the iris undergoes dedifferentiation, loses its pigment and many of the specific enzymes characteristic of the pigmented cells, and then redifferentiates into lens cells with a conspicuously different repertory of functioning genes. Among the products of these genes are the crystallins, proteins found in the lens but not in the iris. Wolffian lens regeneration is a clear case of dedifferentiation and redifferentiation in an entirely new direction. It is also important to note that the embryonic histories of the pigmented iris and the original lens are quite different. The acquisition of the new cellular phenotype by the regenerated lens cells does not necessarily mean that genetic changes have not occurred in some part of the genome—but the new phenotypes do demonstrate that dramatically different patterns of gene function can be elicited even from terminally differentiated adult cells, patterns of gene function that lead to perfectly normal cells, albeit of a very different type. This change in cell differentiation is provoked in the adult eye simply by a change in the environment of the pigmented cells of the iris.

On the chromosomal level, perhaps the most dramatic instance of a reversal of normal patterns of gene function attributable to a given chromosome occurs during the formation of oocytes in the mammalian ovary. Mammalian female cells exhibit the phenomenon of X-inactivation, that is, one of the two X chromosomes is inactivated at random in each cell at a very early stage in embryonic development. Thereafter, all of the descendent cells of each cell maintain the same X in the inactive form. Thus, primordial germ cells also have only one active X and this has been demonstrated experimentally. During embryonic development of the ovary, at about 14 days of gestation in the mouse, both X's are again active in oocytes. After meiosis, each ovum contains only one X, but it is active. The reactivation of a previously inactive X chromosome during oogenesis demonstrates that a chromosome can be maintained in an inactive form through many generations of cell division and then restored to full activity (Gartler et al., 1975; Migeon and Jelalian, 1977). It is difficult to imagine any change in the DNA that could provide a basis for such alternate reversible states. The phenomenon appears to be epigenetic and could be extended, hypothetically, to account for all of the patterns of gene inactivation (or activation) during normal cell differentiation. Thus, both Wolffian regeneration and X-inactivation, in their various expressions, suggest an epigenetic basis for cellular differentiation, whereas the evidence from nuclear transplantation suggests a genetic basis. We all know of the recent work demonstrating that DNA rearrangements occur in the differentiation of the cells of the immune system and these lead to the production of different immunoglobulins. This evidence, too, suggests, if generalized, that cell differentiation may involve changes in the DNA, in the structure of chromosomes, and, therefore, be based on genetic rather than epigenetic events.

The subtle restrictions on the capacity of cells to differentiate and the roles of the cellular environment in provoking particular types of differentiation are well illustrated by the behavior of parthenogenetic embryos. In mammals, it is possible to provoke the egg to develop without being fertilized (Graham, 1974; Steinhardt et al., 1974). In fact, this phenomenon occurs without outside intervention with a very high frequency in certain strains of mice (Eppig et al., 1977). However, none of these parthenogenetically produced embryos ever succeed in developing all the way to term. They usually die at some early stage in development. However, it is possible to rescue such parthenogenetic embryos by combining them with a normal embryo to make a chimeric mouse. Such chimeras develop to term, mature normally, and the parthenogenetic cells are evident in the various tissues and organs of the chimeric individual. In fact, cells of parthenogenetic origin can even give rise to gametes and result in the production of a second generation of mice (Stevens, 1978). Evidently, there is no intrinsic cellular deficiency in the parthenogenetic embryos that precludes normal development on the part of any particular cell. What is absent in the embryonic parthenotes is the necessary intercellular environment within the parthenogenetic embryo that will allow the cells of the embryo to participate effectively in the formation of a new individual. The nature of this deficiency is completely unknown, but what these experiments demonstrate to us is that environments in the embryo are subtle, precise, and powerful in directing the course of normal cell differentiation.

In response to the sequence of cellular environments to which cells are exposed during embryonic life, the differentiated cells express only a small part of their total genome, perhaps about 10%, the vast majority of structural genes remaining silent. It seems possible to suppose that a deficient or mutant gene that is not expressed in any particular type of differentiated cell would be irrelevant to the normal function and perhaps differentiation of such a cell. In fact, we know that mutant genes are expressed in only a restricted number of differentiated cell types. For example, a deficiency in the structural gene for the enzyme tyrosinase will prevent the formation of functioning enzyme molecules and lead to the condition we know as albinism in which the individual forms no melanin pigment. In other respects, the cells of such individuals appear to be perfectly normal.

III. Cell Differentiation and Neoplasia

Pigment cells clearly require a certain pattern of gene expression in order to become pigment cells. If the genetic makeup of potential pigment cells is abnormal, they may proceed to make pigment but then transform into malignant cell types such as melanomas. This is well illustrated by certain hybrid fish, hybrids between swordtails and platyfish. Such hybrid fish almost always develop numerous melanomas derived from their macromelanophores (Gordon, 1951; Anders, 1967). The other cells of such fish, even other kinds of pigment cells, appear to be normal and are not prone to malignant transformation. Melanomas are not common in either of the two species of fish used to make the hybrid. Thus, perfectly normal genomes, normal in each of the two species, when put together in a hybrid, produce an abnormal pattern of gene function that confers on cells of the macromelanophore phenotype, and only on them, a melanoma phenotype. The transformation of the macromelanophore into a melanoma is clearly due to the abnormal chromosomal makeup of the cell, but this abnormal chromosomal makeup is expressed only after numerous normal steps in cell differentiation have occurred, all of which steps may be due to epigenetic events.

One of the most dramatic experiments on the nature of neoplastic cell differentiation occurred when Brinster (1974), Mintz and Illmensee (1975), and Stewart and Mintz (1981) injected teratocarcinoma cells into the blastocyst cavity of normal embryos. Mintz and co-workers obtained chimeric mice in which many normal cells, including gametes, were derived from the teratocarcinoma cells. The teratocarcinomas of mice may be produced in two ways. They arise spontaneously in a small fraction of embryos in certain strains of mice; they may also be produced by transferring early mouse embryos into the testis or under the kidney capsule where the embryo continues to develop but in a very disorganized fashion that frequently generates a teratocarcinoma. Such teratocarcinomas contain stem cells that continually divide; some of the cells differentiate into recognizable adult types of cells that cease to divide and are nonmalignant but the stem cells continue to multiply as undifferentiated highly malignant cells. Placing such cells into the blastocyst cavity enables them to occupy sites in the embryo that elicit from the teratocarcinoma cells normal cellular differentiation, including the formation of gametes. Thus, the initial cancer cell has been transformed into a normal cell by subjecting it to the powerful cellular environments of the embryo. Such teratocarcinomas appear to have been epigenetically produced. It is very difficult to imagine any genetic basis for an initial malignant transformation that can be so readily reversed by transplanting the teratocarcinoma cells into an embryo. The evidence discussed so far suggests that normal cell differentiation and abnormal cell differentiation, resulting in neoplasms, can be produced by two distinct mechanisms: by genetic changes in the DNA and also by epigenetic changes which do not affect the structure of the DNA.

Normal cell differentiation appears to be such a fastidious, demanding process that it is easy to imagine many mistakes that would lead to abnormal programs of gene function. Probably such cellular aberrations are common in the development of an individual but the vast majority of such abnormal changes would surely be of no benefit to the cell, would probably prove lethal to the cell, or certainly would not confer on the cell that particular constellation of properties that enables a docile, normal, disciplined cell to become neoplastic. Cell death is a very common phenomenon both in the embryo and in the adult (Saunders, 1966). Some cell death is programmed and essential for normal development but much of the cell death appears random. It appears likely to me that a large fraction of this cell death is due to aberrations in the programs of gene function, nearly all such aberrations being deleterious to the cell in which they occur. In fact, the transformation of a normal cell into a truly successful neoplastic cell must be an exceedingly rare event. We are composed of about ten trillion cells and yet only one out of four of us will ever produce a clinically evident malignant neoplasm. We all have numerous small, benign neoplasms and so abnormal cell differentiation is common, but successful malignant differentiation is exceedingly rare. In those adult cells that do not normally divide, such as nerve cells and muscle cells, a reprogramming of gene function that would lead to a neoplastic phenotype would pass completely unnoticed unless combined simultaneously with those cellular changes required to initiate and sustain cell division. A single nondividing cancer cell would have no clinical significance and would not be recognized. Cell division is indispensable for the amplification of the malignant phenotype so that it may be clinically recognized, but it is not basic to the neoplastic transformation itself.

Once a malignant neoplasm has developed and begins to metastasize, the metastasizing cells enter new cellular environments. Such environments pose new challenges to the survival of the cancer cell and, at the same time, may provoke or select for new forms of differentiation in the malignant cell (Cairns, 1975). Doubtless, a great many metastasizing cancer cells die because they are not able to respond to the challenge of the new cellular environments in which they find themselves. The ability to respond to a particular cellular environment depends upon the preceding state of cell differentiation which, in its turn, depends on the particular pattern of gene function in that cell. Thus, a sequence of differentiative transformations is to be expected in neoplastic cells as they metastasize and invade new cellular environments. It is the basic evolutionary story: variation and survival of the fittest. Only in this case, it is the neoplastic cell that is changing and being selected for those characteristics that confer an advantage in multiplying in the various cellular environments of the host.

IV. Conclusions

Our basic problem in examining both neoplastic development and normal cell differentiation lies in discovering the mechanism by which specific programs of gene function are brought into effect in a cell. The vast increase in our knowledge of the molecular genetics of cells is very pleasing, but it is not likely to tell us much about the regulation of gene function during the course of cell differentiation, normal or abnormal. What are the mechanisms by which a cell responds to its environment by the activation of hundreds or thousands of new genes at specified levels of activity while suppressing the activity of many other genes? It seems likely to me that these mechanisms represent higher orders of interaction of the genetic material, entire chromosomes or at least large segments containing many genes. Topographic relationships among chromosomes in the interphase nucleus are at present in a "black box," but such relationships may be exceedingly important for determining patterns of gene function. Each pattern of gene function clearly is dependent on, and stems from, the preceding pattern of gene function. All routes of change are not equally available to cells in different states of differentiation. The history of the cell as expressed in the successive states of differentiation through which the cell has passed places rigid restrictions on the capacity of the cell to embark upon any new course of development. Perhaps this is why gross changes in chromosome composition are associated with many types of malignant transformation. Hybrid genomes, trisomies, deletions, rearrangements, and insertion of viral or normal nucleotide sequences into abnormal locations in the DNA all affect the structure and possibly the topography of chromosomes with respect to each other, leading to specific new programs of gene function some of which may prove to be neoplastic.

The basic problems of cell differentiation can be approached either through the study of normal cells or abnormal cells. When we understand differentiative processes in one cell type, we will surely understand them in the other. Perhaps the study of cancer cells will prove to be the most efficient route for understanding cell differentiation. At least the economic and scientific resources invested by our society in research on neoplastic development is far greater than allocated to the study of normal development. I see no a priori basis for preferring one route over the other, but successful solution of the problems of cell differentiation, when that occurs, will be one of the great achievements of biological science and enable us to regulate and control cell behavior, both normal and abnormal.

References

Anders, F. (1967). Tumour formation in platyfish-swordtail hybrids as a problem of gene regulation. *Experentia* **23**, 1–9.

Briggs, R. (1977). Genetics of cell type determination. *In* "Cell Interactions in Differentiation" (L. Saxen and L. Weiss, eds.), pp. 23–43. Academic Press, New York.

Brinster, R. L. (1974). The effect of cells transferred into the mouse blastocyst on subsequent development. *J. Exp. Med.* **140**, 1049–1056.

Cairns, J. (1975). Mutation selection and the natural history of cancer. *Nature (London)* **255**, 197–200.

Diberardino, M. A. (1980). Genetic stability and modulation of metazoan nuclei transplanted into eggs and oocytes. *Differentiation* **17**, 17–30.

Du Pasquier, L., and Wabl, M. R. (1977). Transplantation of nuclei from lymphocytes of adult frogs into enucleated eggs. *Differentiation* **8**, 9–19.

Early, P., and Hood, L. (1981). Mouse immunoglobulin genes. *Gen. Eng.* **3**, 257–288.

Eppig, John J., Kozak, Leslie P., Eicher, Eva M., and Stevens, Leroy C. (1977). Ovarian teratomas in mice are derived from oocytes that have completed the first meiotic division. *Nature (London)* **269**, 517–518.

Gartler, S. M., Andina, R., and Gant, N. (1975). Ontogeny of X-chromosome inactivation in the female germ line. *Exp. Cell Res.* **91**, 454–457.

Gordon, M. (1951). Genetic and correlated studies of normal and atypical pigment cell growth. *Growth Symp.* **10**, 153–219.

Graham, C. F. (1974). The production of parthenogenetic mammalian embryos and their use in biological research. *Biol. Rev.* **49**, 399–422.

Gurdon, J. B. (1974). "The Control of Gene Expression in Animal Development." Oxford Univ. Press, London and New York.

Illmensee, K., and Hoppe, P. C. (1981). Nuclear transplantation in Mus musculus: Developmental potential of nuclei from preimplantation embryos. *Cell* **23**, 9–18.

Jones, P. A., and Taylor, S. M. (1980). Cellular differentiation, cytidine analogs and DNA methylation. *Cell* **20**, 85–93.

McKinnell, Robert Gilmore (1978). "Cloning Nuclear Transplantation in Amphibia." Univ. of Minnesota Press, Minneapolis, Minnesota.

Markert, C. L. (1968). Neoplasia: a disease of cell differentiation. *Cancer Res.* **28**, 1908–1914.

Markert, C. L. (1977). Cancer: the survival of the fittest (keynote address). *In* "Cell Differentiation and Neoplasia" (Grady F. Saunders, ed.), pp. 9–22. Raven, New York.

Markert, C. L., and Ursprung, H. (1963). Production of replicable persistent changes in zygote chromosomes of *Rana pipiens* by injected proteins from adult liver nuclei. *Develop. Biol.* **7**, 560–577.

Migeon, B. R., and Jelalian, K. (1977). Evidence for two active X chromosomes in germ cells of females before meiotic entry. *Nature (London)* **269**, 242–243.

Mintz, B., and Illmensee, K. (1975). Normal genetically mosaic mice produced from malignant teratocarcinoma cells. *Proc. Natl. Acad. Sci. U.S.A.* **72**, 3585–3589.

Reyer, R. W. (1954). Regeneration of the lens in the amphibian eye. *Q. Rev. Biol.* **29**, 1–46.

Saunders, J. W., Jr. (1966). Death in embryonic systems. *Science (Washington, D.C.)* **154**, 604–612.

Spemann, H. (1938). "Embryonic Development and Induction." Yale Univ. Press, New Haven, Connecticut.

Steinhardt, R. A., Epel, D., Carroll, E. J., Jr., and Yanagimachi, R. (1974). Is calcium ionophore a universal activator for unfertilised eggs? *Nature (London)* **252**, 41–43.

Stevens, Leroy C. (1978). Totipotent cells of parthenogenetic origin in a chimeric mouse. *Nature (London)* **276**, 266–267.

Stewart, T. A., and Mintz, B. (1981). Successive generations of mice produced from an established culture line of euploid teratocarcinoma cells. *Proc. Natl. Acad. Sci. U.S.A.* **78**, 6314–6318.

Uriel, J. (1976). Retrodifferentiation and the myth of Faust. *Cancer Res.* **36**, 2469–2475.

Ursprung, H., and Markert, C. L. (1963). Chromosome complements of *Rana pipiens* embryos developing from eggs injected with protein from adult liver cells. *Dev. Biol.* **8**, 309–321.

Waddington, C. H. (1948). The genetic control of development. *Symp. Soc. Exp. Biol.* **2**, 145–154.

Weinberg, R. A. (1980). Integrated genomes of animal viruses. *Ann. Rev. Biochem.* **49**, 197–226.

Yamada, T. (1967). Cellular and subcellular events in Wolffian lens regeneration. *Curr. Top. Dev. Biol.* **2**, 267–283.

16

Embryologic Microenvironment in the Regulation of Cancer Cells

G. BARRY PIERCE AND ROBERT S. WELLS

I. Introduction

For generations, pathologists have used the appearance of cells in tumors as a means of identifying the type of tumor and of establishing prognosis. Tumors composed of cells that closely resemble normal cells usually behave in a benign manner, whereas those that appear embryonic (blastomas) or undifferentiated (carcinomas and sarcomas) have the capacity for rapid growth, invasion, and metastasis, and are considered to be malignant. Pathologists are aware of tumors in which undifferentiated and differentiated cells are admixed, and prognosis is assessed on the basis of the least differentiated elements of those tumors. Among the useful contributions from this conference has been the observation that morphological variation is only one type of tumor cell heterogeneity, and that one population of cells in a tumor may influence another (Poste *et al.*, 1981; see Chapters 9 and 14).

Morphological heterogeneity is an important form of tumor cell heterogeneity, however, and was originally attributed to varying degrees of de-

TUMOR CELL HETEROGENEITY

differentiation of normal differentiated cells that had responded to a carcinogenic stimulus. This idea was proposed long before anything was known of tissue renewal and is probably incorrect (Pierce *et al.*, 1978).

II. Stem Cells, Differentiation, and Tumor Cell Heterogeneity

It is now established, for one tumor, that normal stem cells responsible for tissue renewal are the targets in carcinogenesis, and give rise to malignant stem cells (Stevens, 1967). The normal stem cells and malignant stem cells are equally undifferentiated (Pierce *et al.*, 1967). It has also been shown that normal cells in culture and their spontaneously transformed counterparts closely resemble each other ultrastructurally (Wilson and Franks, 1972). In breast and colon, normal and malignant stem cells are equivalent in terms of differentiation, making it unnecessary to postulate dedifferentiation to account for the undifferentiated appearance of tumor cells (Pierce *et al.*, 1977). The morphological heterogeneity of cells of tumors is the result of differentiation of a few of the progeny of malignant stem cells (Pierce *et al.*, 1978). This is usually enough to allow histotypic diagnosis but the prognosis depends on the presence and number of the undifferentiated, malignant cells. This whole scheme is illustrated in squamous cell carcinoma in which there are vast areas of undifferentiated malignant tissue in which a few islands of recognizable squamous epithelium are found. It has been shown that these squamous pearls originate by differentiation from the undifferentiated malignant cells, and that as they differentiate they lose their malignant attributes (Pierce and Wallace, 1971).

It can be concluded that a carcinoma is a caricature of the normal process of tissue renewal in the sense that many undifferentiated cells that carry the malignant phenotype are produced in relationship to the number that differentiate and are benign (Pierce *et al.*, 1978). Squamous cell carcinoma was not the first tumor in which differentiation of malignant stem cells was demonstrated. The first was in 1959, when it was shown by direct means that embryonal carcinoma cells differentiated into the mature tissues of teratocarcinomas (Pierce and Dixon, 1959). Then it was demonstrated that the mature cells derived from the cancer cells were not malignant; they were benign, functional, and incapable of forming a tumor (Pierce *et al.*, 1960). These observations were confirmed by cloning experiments in which teratocarcinomas with their heterogeneous tissue types were produced by transplanting single embryonal carcinoma cells *in vivo* (Kleinsmith and Pierce, 1964).

It is of some interest that the demonstration of differentiation of malignant cells should have been made in teratocarcinoma because the leukemologists were aware of the stem cell nature of leukemias in the mid-1950s (Makino, 1956). It was not until the spleen colony forming assay was developed by Till and McCulloch (1961) that the tools became available to study differentiation in them.

Whereas the earlier experiments on teratocarcinoma indicated that morphological heterogeneity of this tumor was the result of differentiation, the cloning experiments indicated that this type of heterogeneity was compounded by the number of stem lines in the tumor. There were at least four stem lines, and each cloned stem cell line had its own capacity for differentiation. This is illustrated in Table I. The tissue types present in the parent tumor are listed as are four of 42 cloned tumors derived from the parent tumor. These were chosen because they illustrate such wide

TABLE I

Incidence (Percentage) of Differentiated Tissues, Growth Rate, and Embryoid Body Production of Several Clones[a]

Tissues present	Stock teratocarcinoma (14)[b]	Clones			
		NRS-Cl 9 (10)[b]	NRS-Cl 18 (7)[b]	NRS-Cl 35 (8)[b]	NRS-Cl 38 (10)[b]
Embryonal carcinoma	100	100	100	100	100
Astrocytes	100	100	100	100	100
Ependyma	100	100	100	100	100
Simple glands	76	40	14	100	60
Trophoblast	39	20	29	100	40
Squamous epithelium	79	10	0	75	0
Mesenchyme	71	30	14	100	60
Cartilage	50	0	14	25	40
Bone	7	0	14	25	30
Smooth muscle	57	0	0	38	30
Striated muscle	43	0	0	25	30
Notochord	0	0	0	0	10
Ciliated epithelium	71	30	14	88	40
Visceral yolk sac	100	100	0	100	100
Parietal yolk sac	79	10	29	50	70
Growth rate (days)	28	35	33	54	37
Embryoid bodies	Two-layered	Two-layered	None	Three-layered	Three-layered

[a] Material reprinted with permission from *Cancer Research* **24**(9), 1547, October, 1964.

[b] Number of tumors from at least five generations.

differences in growth rates, ability to form embryoid bodies, and differentiated tissues that we assumed that they represented different stem lines. Each of these stem lines could be maintained and did not revert to either the parental or sibling phenotypes (Kleinsmith and Pierce, 1964).

III. Interaction between Tumor Cells and Their Environment

To gain further information on the heterogeneity of tumors, we turned to a malignant melanoma of the hamster that usually metastasized to the lungs as pigmented tumors, but occasionally as amelanotic tumors. These amelanotic metastases when transplanted always gave rise to amelanotic tumors. The pigmented tumor was cloned to determine if it contained melanotic and amelanotic cells. A slowly growing, deeply pigmented clone was isolated as was another, an amelanotic clone that grew about four times faster than the pigmented one (Gray and Pierce, 1964). With this tremendous disparity in growth rates, why did the amelanotic clone not quickly dominate, resulting in a pure amelanotic tumor? Or why did it not grow as a black and white tumor?

If the parental tumor were maintained subcutaneously, it remained melanotic. If transplanted intraperitoneally for three generations, amelanotic cell lines resulted. Two factors were apparently operative: The first was the selective pressures of the environment of the subcutaneous space versus that of the intraperitoneal space. The second was the interaction of pigmented and slow-growing cells of the tumor on the unpigmented fast-growing ones. This smacked of a chalone-like effect of the pigmented on the amelanotic cells. It turned out that Klein and Klein (1956) had observed a similar phenomenon in studies of ascites conversion of a lymphoma. When they injected a mixture of 5% ascites-positive cells with 95% ascites-negative cells, the heterogeneous cell suspension would not form an ascites when injected intraperitoneally. We interpreted those results in the light of developmental biology, i.e., a critical number of cells of like propensity must be present for a differentiation (or a phenotype) to be expressed. These ideas obviously relate to the problems of latency, dormancy, and progression, and indicate that small numbers of cells from malignant tumors are responsive to their environment, and only after achieving a threshold number can they express their malignant potential.

Heppner *et al.* (1978) and Heppner (1982) have studied heterogeneity in a variety of tumors and have demonstrated in elegant fashion how one population of drug-sensitive cells of a tumor can influence drug resistance of another population. Poste *et al.* (1981) have recently shown the influence of cells capable of metastasizing on those incapable of forming metastases, and vice versa. How is this achieved? Does it require cell–cell contact and metabolic cooperation? Does it require cell contact and a humoral factor or does it require a humoral factor alone?

Clearly, people studying heterogeneity from many different approaches are all beginning to focus on precisely the same question. How does the intimate environment of one population of cancer cells effect another?

Brinster (1974) demonstrated this phenomenon in an experiment that clearly demonstrated that the microenvironment provided by the blastocyst could control malignant expression of an embryonal carcinoma cell. In this experiment single embryonal carcinoma cells were injected into blastocysts of an autologous strain and the injected embryos were transferred into the uteri of foster mothers. Among the offspring borne was an animal that exhibited coat color markings of the cancer strain and embryo strain. The microenvironment of the blastocyst had been able to regulate the embryonal carcinoma cell to the point that it behaved as a normal embryonic cell and some of its offspring must have formed neural crest cells that migrated to the skin and ultimately formed pigment cells (Brinster, 1974). Mintz and Illmensee (1975) confirmed the observations and, using isoenzyme markers, determined the percentage of cancer derived cells in many of the tissues of the chimeric animal. Papaioannou *et al.* (1975) also confirmed Brinster's observation and showed that if clumps of 20 or more cancer cells were injected into the blastocyst animals with tumors were born. This indicated a limit to the number of cells that the blastocyst could control. Then Illmensee (1978) reported that some blastocysts containing only a single embryonal carcinoma cell occasionally gave rise to tumors in the chimeric mice suggesting that embryonal carcinoma cells were heterogeneous in their response to the blastocyst. Papaioannou *et al.* (1979) have had similar experiences.

IV. Control of Tumor Cell Growth by the Blastocyst

Since all the work on tumor cell heterogeneity discussed above indicated the importance of microenvironments on the control of malignant expression, we saw an opportunity in the Brinster experiments to study the phenomenon in controlled situations. We decided to determine how the blastocyst regulated embryonal carcinoma. To this end, an assay simpler in protocol than that of producing chimeric mice was required (Pierce *et al.*, 1979). We decided to base the assay on a comparison of the incidence of tumors produced when embryonal carcinoma cells were cloned alone, versus that obtained when embryonal carcinoma cells were injected into blastocysts and the blastocysts were transplanted into animals. For an additional positive control, embryonal carcinoma cells were injected into the perivitelline space of blastocysts and these blastocysts were then injected into animals and their capacity to form tumors was measured.

Two (402A$\overline{\text{x}}$ and 247) of three embryonal carcinomas tested in this assay were controlled to a significant degree by the environment of the blastocoel, but they were not controlled when injected in the perivitelline space (Pierce et al., 1982). The third tumor (F9) was not controlled when injected into the blastocoel. We have no explanation for this apparent aberrant observation other than 247 and F9 are each derived from OTT6050 and demonstrated again the phenomenon of tumor cell heterogeneity.

The idea that the blastocyst could control embryonal carcinoma cells fits with what is known about embryonic differentiation. Embryonic induction depends on specific stimuli (usually known) acting on competent responding cells (Grobstein, 1959). Embryonal carcinoma cells are believed to be competent to respond to whatever inductive signals effect inner cell mass cells. This would appear to be borne out by the data. When L1210 leukemia, sarcoma 180, and B16 melanoma were tested in the blastocyst, they were not controlled, observations construed as negative evidence compatible with the idea that there is specificity to the reaction of the blastocyst and embryonal carcinoma (Pierce et al., 1982).

C1300 neuroblastoma showed evidence of control when tested in the tumor assay, but since neurulation follows blastulation by 96 hours or less, we interpret the data to the effect that the tumor cells, which are derived from neural crest cells, may be regulated at the time of neural crest cell differentiation (Pierce et al., 1982). Parietal yolk sac carcinoma cells were not controlled by the blastocyst (Pierce et al., 1982). This was surprising because distal endoderm (the normal counterpart of parietal yolk sac carcinoma cells) first appears in the very late blastula. We have no explanation for this disparate observation.

We conclude on the basis of these observations that embryonal carcinoma is controlled by the blastocyst, and although not proved the data are compatible with the idea that there may be specificity for this reaction (Pierce et al., 1982).

It was decided to examine the manner in which the blastocyst controlled tumorigenicity of embryonal carcinoma. Since the blastocyst is composed of trophectoderm, inner cell mass, and blastocoel fluid, it is conceivable that any one or any combination of these components might be required to exert control. On the basis of preliminary data, it was decided to explore the effect of trophectoderm. To this end, a technique was devised to inject a cell into the blastocoel, cut off the inner cell mass, and test whether or not the resultant trophectodermal vesicle could control colony formation by the contained cell (Pierce and Wells, 1982, in preparation).

Control of colony formation is an assay based on the ability of the blastocoel to control colony formation of embryonal carcinoma cells *in vitro* as an alternative to tumor formation *in vivo* (Wells, 1982). Briefly, the incidence of colonies from embryonal carcinoma cells cultured individually in microculture wells was compared to that of embryonal carcinoma cells injected into blastocysts which were then cultured under the same conditions. Tumor line 247 was chosen as the test cell because it was controlled equally well in the colony forming and tumor forming assays.

Colony formation of single 247 cells was controlled by trophectodermal vesicles to the same degree as it was in the intact blastocyst. About 10% of cells in vesicles formed colonies in relationship to about 35% for the controls (unpublished). To ensure that cells were not lost or killed by the techniques of injection, it was decided to rescue them after 2 hours in the vesicle and compare colony-forming ability of rescued embryonal carcinoma cells to that of cells not exposed to trophectoderm. Two hours was chosen for this experiment because it was known from studies of the role of cell cycle in blastocyst control of embryonal cancer that cells rescued from intact blastocysts at 2 hours had not been controlled (Wells, 1982).

The 247 cells were rescued from the vesicles by immunosurgery (Solter and Knowles, 1975). This technique depends on the observation that trophectodermal cells are joined together by tight junctions which exclude macromolecules (including immunoglobulins) from the blastocoel or from trophectodermal vesicles. Thus, trophectoderm can be killed in a cytotoxic immune reaction whereas inner cell mass cells or an embryonal carcinoma cell injected into the blastocoel would be spared.

Colony-forming ability of controls explanted as usual was about 40% and that of 247 cells rescued from the blastocyst was about 30%. In view of the extensive technical procedures employed this difference was considered within experimental error. The conclusion was reached that trophectoderm controlled colony formation of embryonal carcinoma cells (Pierce and Wells 1981, in preparation).

Additional positive controls are needed to interpret the results of these experiments. For instance, it is possible that isolated microenvironments such as that of a trophectodermal vesicle (trophectodermis interconnected by tight junctions) might lack essential nutrients required for survival of a cell in the 24-hour interval prior to attachment and hatching of the trophectodermal vesicle. L1210 leukemia cells which are not controlled by the blastocyst will be used for the additional control.

At this point we can be sure that the tumor-forming ability of embryonal carcinoma is controlled by the blastocyst, and there are enough positive control lines that lived successfully in the blastocyst *in vivo* (L1210, S180, F9, and PYS) to ensure that we are not dealing with a starvation phenomenon as a result of the structure of the blastocyst, or some mechanism whereby the blastocyst destroys foreign cells. Preliminary experiments suggest that the injected embryonal carcinoma cell preferentially localizes on the inner cell mass. We are doing high resolution electron microscopy to see if the 247 cells form gap junctions and metabolically cooperate with inner cell mass cells. This adherence of inner cell mass and cancer cell is obviously of great importance if the cancer cell is to be incorporated into the embryo to form a chimeric animal. On the other hand, if trophectoderm controls embryonal carcinoma cells enclosed in vesicles, the control in the blastocyst may be mediated by metabolic cooperation via trophectoderm, and inner cell mass, or embryonal carcinoma may be controlled by some stimulus in blastocoel fluid that was synthesized by trophectoderm. Possibly, blastocoel fluid by itself can regulate embryonal carcinoma cells unattached to inner cell mass and the preferential attachment of the cells to the inner cell mass is only important if the cell is to be incorporated into the embryo. Since the blastocyst contains $1 \times 10^{-4} \mu l$ of fluid, it has been necessary to modify our usual tissue culture techniques to analyze the fluid directly because with them we can only keep embryonal carcinoma cells alive in about $2 \mu l$ of fluid. A means has been devised to clone cells in fractions of microliters of fluid using the micromanipulator. A cell is placed in these droplets under 5% CO_2 in air and 100% humidity. At this time we do not know the results of either the studies in metabolic cooperation or the effect of blastocoel fluid by itself, but we are expecting the worst and believe that probably a combination of fluid and cells may be required for ultimate control.

V. Summary

In conclusion, a technique has been devised to test the response of embryonal carcinoma to the microenvironment created by the isolated trophectoderm of the blastocyst. Evidence to date, which is not perfectly controlled, suggests that trophectoderm controls colony-forming activity of embryonal carcinoma cells. If true, it means that trophectoderm also controls inner cell mass, and if the reaction is specific as these preliminary data would suggest and if the activity is diffusible it may ultimately be possible to inject the diffusible material into individuals harboring metastasis with these tumors in hopes of a noncytotoxic therapy for cancer.

Acknowledgments

The authors wish to acknowledge the expert technical assistance of Alan Jones, James E. Caldwell, and Andrea Lewellyn.

This research was supported in part by a gift from R. J. Reynolds Industries, Inc., and by Grants #CD-81 from the American Cancer Society and #CA-15823 from the National Cancer Institute.

References

Brinster, R. L. (1974). *J. Exp. Med.* **140,** 1049–1056.

Fidler, I. J. (1982). "The Heterogeneity of Metastatic Properties in Malignant Tumor Cells and Regulation of the Metastatic Phenotype," *Tumor Cell Heterogeneity: Origins and Implications* (A. H. Owens, Jr., D. S. Coffey and S. B. Baylin, eds.). Academic Press, New York.

Gray, J. M., and Pierce, G. B. (1964). *J. Natl. Cancer Inst.* **32,** 1201–1210.

Grobstein, C. (1959). *In* "The Cell" (J. Brachet and A. E. Mirsky, eds.), Vol. I, pp. 437–496. Academic Press, New York.

Heppner, G. H. (1982). "Tumor Subpopulation Interactions," *Tumor Cell Heterogeneity: Origins and Implications* (A. H. Owens, Jr., D. S. Coffey, and S. B. Baylin, eds.). Academic Press, New York.

Heppner, G. H., Dexter, D. L., DeNucci, T., Miller, F. R. and Calabrisi, P. (1978). *Cancer Res.* **38,** 3758–3763.

Illmensee, K. (1978). *In* "Genetic, Mosaics and Chimeras in Mammals" (L. Russel, ed.), pp. 3–25. Plenum, New York.

Klein, G., and Klein, E. (1956). *Ann. N.Y. Acad. Sci.* **63,** 640–661.

Kleinsmith, L. J., and Pierce, G. B. (1964). *Cancer Res.* **24,** 1544–1551.

Makino, S. (1956). *Ann. N.Y. Acad. Sci.* **63,** 818–830.

Mintz, B., and Illmensee, K. (1975). *Proc. Natl. Acad. Sci. U.S.A.* **72,** 3585–3589.

Papaioannou, V. E., McBurney, M. W., Gardner, R. L., and Evans, R. L. (1975). *Nature (London)* **258,** 70–73.

Papaioannou, V. E., Evans, E. P., Gardner, R. L., and Graham, C. F. (1979). *J. Embryol. Exp. Morphol.* **54,** 277–295.

Pierce, G. B., and Dixon, F. J. (1959). *Cancer* **12,** 573.

Pierce, G. B., and Wallace, C. (1971). *Cancer Res.* **31,** 127–134.

Pierce, G. B., and Wells, R. S. (1982), in preparation.

Pierce, G. B., Dixon, F. J., and Verney, E. L. (1960). *Lab Invest.* **9,** 583–602.

Pierce, G. B., Stevens, L. C., and Nakane, P. K. (1967). *J. Natl. Cancer Inst.* **39,** 755–773.

Pierce, G. B., Nakane, P. K., Martinez-Hernandez, A., and Ward, J. M. (1977). *J. Natl. Cancer Inst.* **58,** 1329–1345.

Pierce, G. B., Shikes, R., and Fink, L. M. (1978). "Cancer: A Problem of Developmental Biology." Prentice-Hall, Englewood Cliffs, New Jersey.

Pierce, G. B., Lewis, S. H., Miller, G. J., Moritz, E., and Miller, P. (1979). *Proc. Natl. Acad. Sci. U.S.A.* **76,** 6649–6651.

Pierce, G. B., Pantazis, C. E., Caldwell, J. E., and Wells, R. S. (1982). *Cancer Res.,* in press.

Poste, G., Doll, J., and Fidler, I. J. (1981). *Proc. Natl. Acad. Sci. U.S.A.* **78,** 6226–6230.

Solter, D., and Knowles, B. B. (1975). *Proc. Natl. Acad. Sci. U.S.A.* **72,** 5565–5569.
Stevens, L. C. (1967). *J. Natl. Cancer Inst.* **38,** 549–552.
Till, J. E., and McCulloch, E. A. (1961). *Radiat. Res.* **14,** 213–222.
Wells, R. S. (1982). *Cancer Res.,* in press.
Wilson, P. D., and Franks, L. M. (1972). *Br. J. Cancer* **26,** 380–387.

PART V

Genetic Mechanisms

17

Mechanisms of Multistage Carcinogenesis and Their Relevance to Tumor Cell Heterogeneity

I. BERNARD WEINSTEIN, ANN D. HOROWITZ, PAUL FISHER, VESNA IVANOVIC, SEBASTIANO GATTONI-CELLI, AND PAUL KIRSCHMEIER

I. Introduction

The subject of tumor cell heterogeneity deals with a fundamental problem in cancer biology that has broad implications with respect to cancer

TUMOR CELL HETEROGENEITY

diagnosis, clinical manifestations of the disease, and the strategy of cancer therapy. The speakers during the first part of this symposium have dealt with this subject largely as it relates to fully evolved malignant tumor cells. We believe, however, that a complete understanding of the mechanisms responsible for tumor cell heterogeneity will require greater knowledge of the early events in the evolution of a normal cell into a tumor cell and of the complex process by which environmental (exogenous) factors interact with host (endogenous) factors in the multistep carcinogenic process. The stages of initiation, promotion, and progression in a multistep carcinogenic process are shown diagramatically in Fig. 1 (for detailed reviews of these aspects see Foulds, 1969; Berenblum, 1975; Peto, 1977; Scherer and Emmelot, 1979; Slaga *et al.*, 1978; Weinstein *et al.*, 1979; Weinstein, 1981).

The early stages in the origin of cancer cells provide at least two sources of heterogeneity. The first is that in the experimental animal, and in some situations in humans, tumors have a multifocal rather than a unifocal origin. This is quite apparent in experimental liver carcinogenesis where the multifocal hyperplastic nodules show considerable heterogeneity even at very early stages of the carcinogenic process (Scherer and Emmelot, 1979; Slaga *et al.*, 1978). This heterogeneity may reflect the heterogeneity of the initial target cells and/or stochastic events in the interaction between carcinogenic agents and individual target cells. A second source of heterogeneity relates to the multistep nature of the carcinogenic process. Thus, even a tumor arising from a single clone of initiated cells may display heterogeneity depending on the degree to which individual cells within the tumor cell population have moved through various stages of tumor promotion or progression. It is of interest that even in cell culture systems the *in vitro* transformation of a well-defined population of

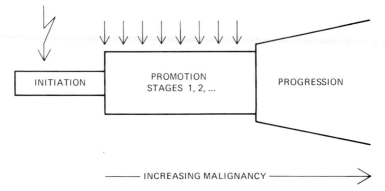

Fig. 1. Schematic diagram of multistage carcinogenesis.

cells by a pure strain of oncogenic virus or by a single pure chemical carcinogen often proceeds through multiple steps, and when individual transformed clones obtained from a single experiment are carefully compared to each other they may differ considerably in terms of their phenotypes. In addition, the prolonged serial passage of clones of transformed cells, and the exposure of these clones to tumor promoters, can enhance their progression (for review of these aspects see Fisher *et al.*, 1979; Barrett and Ts'o, 1978; Colburn *et al.*, 1979; Morris, 1981). Thus, the tendency of tumors to generate variant cell populations and to undergo progression in their phenotypes may have its origins in the early phases of the carcinogenic process. Since analogous phenomena are seen in cell culture systems, studies on the mechanism of action of carcinogens and tumor promoters and of progression of the transformed phenotype in cell culture systems may provide important clues to the basis of tumor cell heterogeneity.

There has been a tendency to think of multistage carcinogenesis and tumor progression as a series of successive mutations and selections, eventuating in the clonal outgrowth of a fully malignant tumor. This may, however, be a gross oversimplification. As discussed elsewhere (Weinstein *et al.*, 1980), we think that a more suitable model is the multistage process that occurs during normal embryologic development, in which new stem cell populations emerge and develop into specialized cells and tissues. There is considerable evidence that the successive stages in carcinogenesis may involve qualitatively different events, that they can be enhanced or inhibited by quite different types of environmental and host factors, and that at least the early stages are often reversible (Slaga *et al.*, 1978; Weinstein *et al.*, 1980).

One of the most instructive experimental models of multistage carcinogenesis has been the system of two-stage mouse skin carcinogenesis, which has been incisively analyzed by Berenblum (1975), Van Duuren (1969), Boutwell (1974), Hecker (1975), and others. These studies clearly defined two qualitatively different stages, initiation and promotion, and indicated that each stage can be brought about by quite different types of agents. Recent studies indicate that the process of tumor promotion can also be divided into at least two phases (Boutwell, 1974; Slaga *et al.*, 1980). Elsewhere, we have contrasted the various properties of initiators and promoters (Weinstein *et al.*, 1980). Tumor promoters can be defined as compounds that have very weak or no carcinogenic activity when tested alone, but markedly enhance tumor yield when applied repeatedly following a low or suboptimal dose of a carcinogen (initiator). At the biochemical level, it appears that the major difference between initiators and promoters is that initiators (or their metabolites) bind covalently to cellular DNA, but this is not the case for tumor promoters (Weinstein *et al.*, 1979, 1980). Later we will review evidence that the initial site of action of the phorbol ester tumor promoters is cell membranes.

The two-stage mouse skin carcinogenesis system has served as a valuable paradigm for studies on multistage aspects of carcinogenesis in several other tissues and species. Evidence that liver cancer, bladder cancer, colon cancer, and breast cancer proceed via stages analogous to initiation and promotion has been reviewed elsewhere (Slaga *et al.*, 1978; Weinstein, 1981). The concept of promotion appears to be particularly relevant to the role of reproductive factors and hormones in the causation of human breast cancer (Weinstein, 1981).

II. Tumor Promoters and Multifactor Interactions

A. Effects of Promoters in Cell Culture

Within the past few years cell culture systems have provided a wealth of information on the action of 12-O-tetradecanoyl phorbol-13-acetate (TPA) and related phorbol ester tumor promoters (for detailed reviews see Weinstein *et al.*, 1980; Blumberg, 1980, 1981; Diamond *et al.*, 1980). These compounds can exert highly pleiotropic effects on the growth, function, and differentiation of a variety of cell types. We have found it convenient to classify these effects into three categories: (1) mimicry and enhancement of transformation, (2) modulation of differentiation, and (3) membrane effects (Weinstein *et al.*, 1980).

A number of the cell culture effects of the phorbol ester tumor promoters led us to suggest that they act by binding to and usurping the function of membrane-associated receptors that are normally utilized by an endogenous growth factor (Weinstein *et al.*, 1977; Lee and Weinstein, 1978; Weinstein *et al.*, 1980). In this sense, tumor promotion induced by the phorbol esters may be closely related to the more general phenomenon of hormonal carcinogenesis. We have recently found, for example, that when rodent fibroblast cultures are infected with an oncogenic adenovirus, or exposed to X-ray, and then grown in the presence of epidermal growth factor (EGF), this growth factor enhances cell transformation to an extent comparable to that obtained with TPA (Fisher *et al.*, 1981). Like TPA, EGF also enhances the *in vitro* progression of adenovirus transformed rat embryo fibroblasts (Fisher *et al.*, 1979). Subsequent studies have indicated that EGF also markedly enhances the *in vitro* transformation of murine granulosa cells by the Kirsten strain of murine sarcoma virus (Harrison and Auersperg, 1981). One could readily imagine, therefore, that in the intact animal the endogenous level of EGF (or related growth factors), and/or the responsiveness of a given tissue to endogenous growth factors, would be important host factors in determining whether exposure of that tissue to a chemical, physical, or viral agent will eventuate in neoplasia. Exogenous or endogenous growth factors might also influence tumor progression and the development of variant cell populations in fully established tumors.

B. Studies on Phorboid Receptors.

Utilizing [^{3}H]phorbol dibutyrate, Blumberg and colleagues have obtained direct evidence for specific high affinity saturable "phorboid receptors" in membrane preparations from chick embryo fibroblasts and mouse epidermis (Driedger and Blumberg, 1980; Delclos et al., 1980). Our laboratory (Weinstein et al., 1980; Horowitz et al., 1981) and others (Shoyab and Todaro, 1980) have confirmed and extended the evidence for the existence of membrane-associated phorboid receptors in a variety of cell types. In general, the abilities of a series of phorbol esters to compete with [^{3}H]PDBu for binding to cell surface receptors correlates with their known potencies in cell culture and with their activities as tumor promoters on mouse skin (Driedger and Blumberg, 1980; Delclos et al., 1980; Shoyab and Todaro, 1980; Horowitz et al., 1981). These results provide evidence that the phorboid receptors mediate the biological action of the phorbol esters. As discussed below, it appears that the phorboid receptors also mediate the TPA-like effects of a new class of tumor promoters, teleocidin and structurally related indole alkaloids. Although the putative endogenous ligand for the phorboid receptors has not yet been identified, we have partially purified a factor present in normal serum that inhibits [^{3}H]PDBu receptor binding (Horowitz et al., 1981, 1982). Studies are in progress to determine the possible physiological significance of this factor.

What might be the normal function of phorboid receptors and their putative endogenous ligand? We have postulated that this receptor system could play a role during embryogenesis by enhancing the outgrowth of new stem cell populations (Weinstein et al., 1980; Weinstein, 1981). In the adult this same system might enhance stem cell replication during hyperplasia, wound healing, and regeneration. In all these situations it might be necessary to transiently inhibit terminal differentiation so as to expand the proliferative population. Subsequently this system might be inactivated to allow terminal differentiation to proceed and to return the tissue to a stable state of tissue renewal. During tumor promotion aberrant stem cells (generated during initiation) might undergo preferential clonal expansion as a result of excessive stimulation of the phorboid receptor system. This model has obvious implications in terms of the normal control of proliferation of stem cell populations and the possible role of endogenous host factors in tumor promotion, progression, and the generation of tumor cell heterogeneity. If our hypothesis is correct, then it might be possible to develop analogues of the phorbol esters that could be used as pharmacologic agents to enhance normal tissue repair or to enhance the repletion of tissues with stem cells following trauma, radiation, or drug toxicity. Alternatively, it might be possible to design agents that would block the phorboid receptors and thus protect the host from certain endogenous or exogenous agents that affect promotion or progression.

C. Teleocidin and Other Indole Alkaloids

Until recently, the phorbol esters were the only class of skin tumor promoters that showed marked structure–function specificity and that were active at nanomolar concentrations. The recent discovery by T. Sugimura and colleagues that teleocidin and certain other indole alkaloids are as potent as TPA in inducing ornithine decarboxylase in mouse skin, and in acting as tumor promoters on mouse skin, is, therefore, extremely interesting (Fujiki *et al.*, 1979, 1981). In collaborative studies we have found that, like TPA, nanomolar concentrations of teleocidin and dihydroteleocidin induce a rapid increase in 2-deoxyglucose uptake, induce arachidonic acid release and prostaglandin synthesis, and inhibit EGF-receptor binding in cell culture (Umezawa *et al.*, 1981). Other cell culture effects shared by teleocidin and TPA include induction of adhesion and terminal differentiation of HL-60 cells (Nakayasu *et al.*, 1981); inhibition of differentiation of Friend erythroleukemia cells (Fujiki *et al.*, 1979), of B-16 melanoma cells (Fisher *et al.*, 1982) and human myoblasts (Fisher *et al.*, 1982); and induction of choline release from cellular phospholipids of HeLa cells (Sakamoto *et al.*, 1981; Fisher *et al.*, 1982).

Although the chemical structures of these indole alkaloids are quite different from those of the phorbol esters (Fig. 2), the fact that they induce similar effects on mouse skin and in cell culture, and act in the same concentration range, suggested that these indole alkaloids might act by binding to the phorboid receptors. Indeed, we have found that teleocidin is a potent inhibitor of the binding of [^{3}H]PDBu to membrane receptors (Umezawa *et al.*, 1981). These results prompted us to build molecular models of TPA and teleocidin and to search for structural similarities that might explain the apparent affinities of these two types of compounds for the same set of receptors (Weinstein, I. B., Horowitz, A. D., and Jeffrey, A., unpublished studies). Both compounds are amphipathic since they both have hydrophobic and hydrophilic domains (Fig. 2). In the case of the

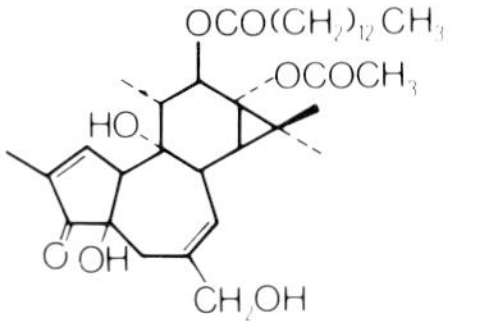

TPA

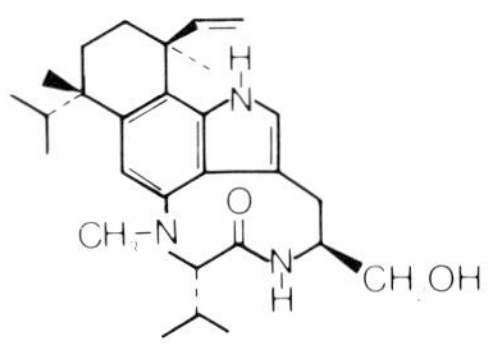

Teleocidin

Fig. 2. Structures of TPA and teleocidin.

phorbol esters there is evidence that all of the biologically active compounds have a highly hydrophobic residue on the 12 position, although the precise chemical structure of this residue is not critical. Presumably this region of the molecule is required for a relatively nonspecific hydrophobic interaction with a region on the phorboid receptor, or the adjacent lipid microenvironment. The saturated six-membered ring of teleocidin might play an analogous role. Extensive structure–activity studies of the phorbol esters on mouse skin and in cell culture (for review see Weinstein *et al.*, 1977; Yamasaki *et al.*, 1981) indicate that the region of the molecule containing the 3-keto, 4-OH, and 6-CH$_2$OH residues displays marked structural and steric specificity. Our model building studies indicate that the nine-membered lactam region of teleocidin, which also contains both a keto residue and a -CH$_2$O residue (Fig. 2), can assume a conformation remarkably similar to the corresponding region present in the biologically active phorbol esters. We postulate, therefore, that these regions of the phorbol esters and indole alkaloids form highly specific chemical bonding and/or steric interactions with the phorboid receptors. Additional compounds are being examined to obtain further data relevant to this hypothesis. Information of this type could make it possible to rationally design compounds that would either act as agonists or blockers of the phorboid receptor system.

D. Membrane Effects of Certain Complete Carcinogens

Since with repeated applications benzo[*a*]pyrene (BP) and certain other polycyclic aromatic hydrocarbon (PAH) carcinogens can act as complete carcinogens on mouse skin (Berenblum, 1975; Burns and Albert, 1980), we have recently studied the possibility that PAHs might induce effects on membranes and membrane receptors similar to those induced by the phorbol ester tumor promotors (Ivanovic and Weinstein, 1981, 1982). We have found that the exposure of C3H 10T1/2 cells to a nontoxic dose of BP (10^{-6} M) causes a delayed but marked inhibition of EGF–receptor binding (Ivanovic and Weinstein, 1981). The ability of PAH carcinogens to induce the cytochrome P_1-450 system and several other drug metabolizing enzymes is apparently mediated by the binding of these compounds to a specific cytosol receptor protein, the Ah receptor (also called the TCDD receptor) (Okey *et al.*, 1979; Poland *et al.*, 1979). We found a good correlation between the abilities of a series of PAHs to inhibit EGF binding to 10T1/2 cells and published data on the affinities of these compounds for the Ah receptors. Therefore, we have hypothesized that the binding of certain PAHs to the Ah receptor induces a pleiotropic program that includes not only increases in certain drug metabolizing enzymes, but also changes in membrane structure and function that are similar to those induced by the phorbol ester tumor promoters (Ivanovic and Weinstein, 1981). Consistent with this hypothesis are data that, like the phorbol esters, PAH carcinogens also induce ornithine decarboxylase (O'Brien, 1976) and induce the release of arachidonic acid from membrane phospholipids (Levine and Ohuchi, 1978). The effects of both tumor promoters and certain carcinogens on cell membranes may have a bearing on designing new strategies of cancer chemoprevention. The glucocorticoid hormones are extremely effective inhibitors of tumor promotion on mouse skin (Belman and Troll, 1972; Viage *et al.*, 1977). They are also potent antagonists of some of the membrane-related effects of both TPA and BP (Ivanovic and Weinstein, 1981) suggesting that their antitumor promoting action is exerted at the level of cell membranes. We think that it is likely that the inhibitor effects of certain retinoids on carcinogenesis is also exerted at this level. These and similar agents might also be used to limit the development by tumors of heterogeneous subpopulations.

E. Chemical–Viral Interactions

There are several examples in which initiating carcinogens, tumor promoters, or other chemical and physical agents interact synergistically with viruses in the carcinogenic process, both *in vivo* and in cell culture (for review see Fisher and Weinstein, 1979; Fisher *et al.*, 1979). Indeed, it seems likely that certain human cancers may be due to interactions between chemical agents and types of viruses which alone would have little or no oncogenic potential. This appears to be the case for liver cancer in Africa, nasopharyngeal cancer in Asia, and Burkitt's lymphoma in Africa (for review see Weinstein, 1981).

It appears that the primary effects of the phorbol ester tumor promoters result from alterations in cell surface membrane structure and function (Weinstein *et al.*, 1980). It is of interest, therefore, that current evidence suggests that the transforming proteins coded for by several tumor viruses act at or near the cell surface membrane. These findings suggest that alterations in membrane function play a central role not only during the process of carcinogenesis, but also during maintenance of the tumor cell phenotype in cells transformed by chemicals or oncogenic viruses. Certain aspects of tumor cell heterogeneity may also have their origin in membrane-related changes.

It is unfortunate that in the past researchers concerned with cancer etiology have been polarized into two camps, those in search of viruses as causes of human cancer and those concerned with chemical carcinogens. We suspect that much greater progress will be made if one takes the view that certain human cancers result from complex interactions between viruses and chemicals, and that the final pathways by which both classes of agents produce cell transformation are quite similar.

III. Host Genes Involved in Carcinogenesis

In contrast to oncogenic viruses, carcinogens and tumor promoters cannot introduce new genetic information into cells. During the transformation process they must, therefore, call on genes already present in the target cells to bring about and maintain the transformed state. A major challenge in carcinogenesis research is to identify the cellular gene(s) involved in radiation and chemical carcinogenesis and to compare their sequences, state of integration, and/or expression in normal and carcinogen-transformed cells. Elsewhere, we have discussed the hypothesis that chemical carcinogenesis may involve rearrangements or amplification of specific cellular genes rather than random point mutations (Weinstein *et al.*, 1980; Weinstein, 1981).

Studies of the RNA acute leukemia and sarcoma viruses have led to the concept that these viruses arose by the recombination of RNA leukemia viruses with specific *onc* genes (also called *sarc* genes or proto-oncogenes) endogenous to normal vertebrate species (for review see Bishop, 1980). Infection of cells by sarcoma viruses leads to the integration of the virul *onc* genes into aberrant sites in the host genome, where they are expressed at high levels and thus lead to the transformed state. The proviral DNAs of murine retroviruses are flanked by long terminal repeat sequences (LTR) of about 600 base pairs (bp). There is evidence that these sequences contain strong promoter signals for controlling transcription and that they might also play a role in gene transposition (Hayward *et al.*, 1981; Dhar *et al.*, 1980; Blair *et al.*, 1981).

It is possible that the cellular homologues of *onc* or LTR sequences are involved in the transformation of cells by nonviral agents. We have postulated that in higher organisms DNA damage induced by chemicals or radiation might trigger alterations in the state of integration and/or switch-on of the constitutive expression of these genes, in the absence of a virus vector. In collaboration with Dino Dina and colleagues at the Albert Einstein College of Medicine we have recently carried out a series of experiments to test this hypothesis (Gattoni *et al.*, 1982; Kirschmeier *et al.*, 1982). The results of these studies are described below.

A. Studies of Cellular *onc* Genes in Normal and Transformed Murine Cells

We utilized a cloned DNA fragment *pmos-1* representing a portion of the *onc* gene (*v-mos*) of Moloney murine sarcoma virus (Mo-MSV) as a probe to determine whether or not transformation of rodent cells by chemical carcinogens or radiation is associated with alterations in the state of integration or transcription of the normal cellular sequence (*c-mos*) that is homologous to the *v-mos* gene (Oskarsson *et al.*, 1980; Jones *et al.*, 1980). Figure 3 shows the results obtained when the DNAs of various normal and transformed murine cell lines were cleaved with the restriction enzyme *Sac*I, separated by gel electrophoresis, transferred onto nitrocellulose filters and hybridized to the ^{32}P-labeled *pmos-1* probe, according to the procedure of Southern (1975). All the cell lines examined contained a major DNA fragment of approximately 7 kb which hybridized to *pmos-1* DNA. A second minor fragment was often also observed. The size of the major *SAC*I fragment is in good agreement with the physical map of the *c-mos* locus in BALB/c mice obtained by Oskarsson *et al.*, (1980). We have performed this type of analysis on a total of 24 different normal and transformed murine or rat cell lines and tissues (Gattoni *et al.* 1982). The results obtained with all the murine cells were identical to those shown in Fig. 3. DNA from a cell line derived from a rat hepatoma or DNAs from polyoma virus transformed rat cell lines gave results identical to those obtained with normal rat cell lines (Gattoni *et al.*, 1982). Thus, it appears that normal development and differentiation, prolonged serial passage, or transformation induced by radiation, chemical carcinogens, polyoma virus, or spontaneously are not associated with gross rearrangements of the *c-mos* sequences in cellular DNA.

There is increasing evidence that the transcriptional activity of a number of genes is associated with their 5-methylcytosine (5-MeC) content,

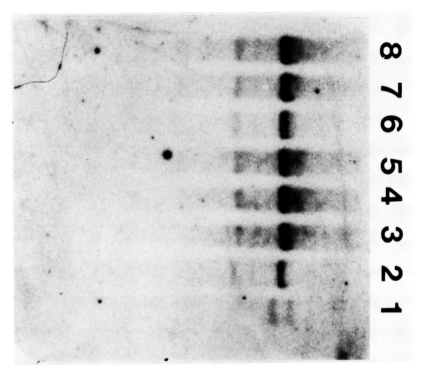

Fig. 3. Restriction endonuclease analysis of mouse *c-mos* sequences. DNA from various mouse cell lines was isolated, samples (20 µg) were digested with *Sac*I and electrophoresed in a 1.0% "submarine" agarose gel. After blotting onto a nitrocellulose filter (18) hybridization to ^{32}P-labeled *pmos-1* DNA was performed. (For additional details, see Gattoni *et al.,* 1982.)

although other factors also play a role in the control of transcription (van der Ploeg and Flavell, 1980; Cohen, 1980; Jones and Taylor, 1980). Analysis of methylation patterns in DNA takes advantage of the fact that certain restriction enzymes that have a CpG dinucleotide as part of their recognition site will not cleave this sequence if it contains 5-MeC. The restriction endonuclease *Hpa*II (recognition site 5'CCGG3') is particularly useful since, although its action is blocked by methylation of the second C residue in the recognition sequence, the activity of the isoschizomer *Msp*I is not affected by this methylation (van der Ploeg and Flavell, 1980). Therefore, we used this pair of enzymes in parallel studies to obtain information on the extent of methylation of *c-mos* sequences in normal and transformed murine cells. All DNAs were cleaved with *Sac*I to generate a major *c-mos* containing fragment of approximately 7 kb. One set of DNAs was then cleaved with *Hpa*II while the other was cleaved with *Msp*I. The patterns obtained by hybridization to ^{32}P-labeled *pmos-1* DNA indicate that the *c-mos* sequences are hypermethylated in all cell lines, since *Msp*I always gave a lower molecular weight set of fragments than did *Hpa*II (Gattoni *et al.*, 1982). To confirm and extend these results we repeated the same type of experiment using *EcoR*I rather than *Sac*I as the methylation insensitive restriction endonuclease (Gattoni *et al.*, 1982). The DNA of normal C3H 10T1/2 cells and those of two carcinogen transformed cell lines were digested in parallel with *EcoR*I + *Hpa*II or *EcoR*I + *Msp*I (Fig. 4). When digested with only *EcoR*I, all three DNA samples generated a unique *c-mos* fragment of about 15 kb. Additional cleavage with *Hpa*II or *Msp*I provided evidence that in all three DNA samples this fragment was hypermethylated. During the course of these studies we obtained indirect

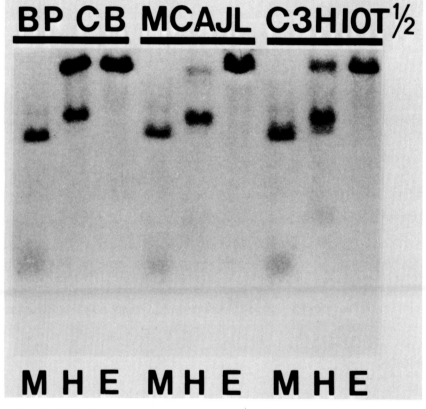

Fig. 4. DNAs from three mouse cell lines C3H 10T1/2, C3H 10T1/2 J.L. #3 (MCA-transformed), and C3H 10T1/2 C.B. #2 (BP-transformed) were digested with *Eco*R, *Eco*RI + *Hpa*II, and *Eco*RI + *Msp*I, electrophoresed, and blot hybridized to the ^{32}P-labeled *pmos-1* DNA. (For additional details, see Gattoni *et al.*, 1982.)

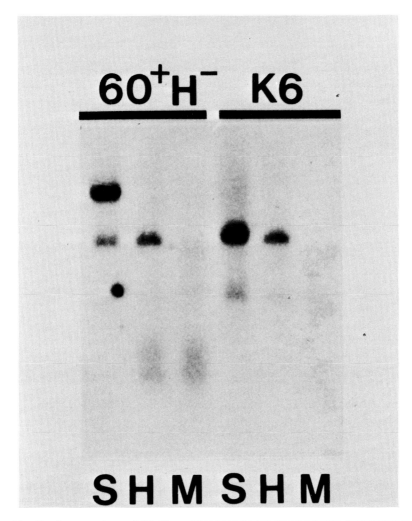

Fig. 5. A comparison of ^{m}CpG modifications in exogenous *v-mos* sequences and endogenous *c-mos* sequences of rat cells. DNAs from two transformed rat cell lines, 60$^+$H$^-$ (transformed by Mo-MSV) and K$_6$ (transformed by polyoma virus), were digested with *Sac*I, *Sac*I + *Hpa*II, and *Sac*I + *Msp*I, electrophoresed, and blot hybridized to ^{32}P-labeled *pmos-1* DNA as described in the legend to Fig. 3. S, *Sac*I; H, *Sac*I + *Hpa*II; M, *Sac*I + *Msp*I. (For additional details, see Gattoni *et al.,* 1982.)

evidence that the *c-mos* sequence in both normal and transformed murine cells contains not only C^mCGG sequences but also ^mCCGG sequences (Gattoni *et al.*, 1982).

To determine the state of methylation of an exogenously acquired *v-mos* sequences we used the Mo-MSV transformed rat cell line 60^+H^- (Graiser *et al.*, 1980). As a control we used a polyoma virus transformed rat cell line. As shown in Fig. 5, when the DNA from the 60^+H^- line was cleaved with *Sac*I it yielded fragments of 5.4 and 4.0 kb that hybridized with the *pmos-1* probe, whereas the normal rat cell DNA contained only a 4.0 kb fragment. The 5.4 kb fragment in 60^+H^- represents the exogenous *v-mos* sequence. Additional cleavage of the DNA with *Hpa*II and *Msp*I showed that the 5.4 fragment containing the *v-mos* sequence was completely digested by both enzymes. On the other hand, the 4.0 kb fragment containing the *c-mos* sequence was insensitive to *Hpa*II and completely digested by *Msp*I (Fig. 5). These results indicate that the integrated *v-mos* sequence is undermethylated when compared to the *c-mos* sequence, even when these two sets of sequences are present in the same cell.

The above evidence indicating that the *c-mos* sequences are extensively methylated in both normal and transformed C3H 10T1/2 cells suggested that they are not transcriptionally active. To obtain direct evidence on this question we analyzed the RNA of these cells for the presence of transcripts homologous to our probe. The polyadenylated fraction [poly(A^+)] of total cellular RNA was subjected to agarose gel electrophoresis, blotted, and hybridized to ^{32}P-labeled *pmos-1* sequences, by the method described by Thomas (1980). We found that the poly(A^+) RNA obtained from normal mouse tissues (brain, liver, spleen, kidney) or from cell lines transformed by various agents other than Mo-MSV contained no detectable RNA homologous to the *pmos-1* probe (Gattoni *et al.*, 1982). As expected, the poly(A^+) RNA obtained from the cell line 60^+H^- which was transformed by Mo-MSV was strongly positive. We estimate that our method was sensitive enough to detect as little as 0.1 copy of the related mRNA per cell.

B. Studies on the Expression of Poly(A^+) RNA Containing LTR-Like Sequences

In a second set of studies we have pursued an alternative approach to identifying retrovirus-related genes that might be involved in radiation and chemical carcinogenesis. Several types of evidence indicate that the LTR regions of retrovirus genomes play a crucial role in controlling transcription,and the specific sequences involved are present in the *U3* portion of the LTR sequence (Dhar *et al.*, 1980). The R region of the LTR defines the site of initiation (at the 5′ end) of viral RNA synthesis, and the U5 region represents the portion of the LTR sequence that is present at the 5′ terminus of the mature viral RNA (Dhar *et al.*, 1980). The LTR sequence also has structural features similar to transposable elements of bacteria, suggesting that LTR sequences might also be involved in gene transposition (Hayward *et al.*, 1981; Dhar *et al.*, 1980). They could act, therefore, as mobile promoters capable of initiating the transcription of sequences adjacent to sites into which they might become integrated (Hayward *et al.*, 1981). Consistent with this possibility are recent studies indicating that the insertion of the LTR sequence of an avian leukosis virus into the host cell DNA activates transcription of a flanking host *onc* sequence designated *c-myc* and that this is responsible for the induction of lymphomas (Hayward *et al.*, 1981). Normal murine cells contain DNA sequences homologous to the LTR sequence of murine retrovirus proviral DNA (Dhar *et al.*, 1980). These findings suggest that if damage to cellular DNA caused the rearrangement and/or activation of endogenous LTR sequences this could lead to the constitutive expression of host sequences (*onc* or other genes) whose products might be capable of inducing cell transformation. In theory, these events could occur in the absence of a replicating leukemia virus.

To test this hypothesis we have examined whether there are differences between normal C3H 10T1/2 cells and C3H 10T1/2 cells transformed by radiation or chemical carcinogens in terms of the expression of RNA species containing sequences homologous to a probe prepared to the LTR sequence of Mo-MSV (Kirschmeier *et al.*, 1982). The poly(A$^+$) RNA fraction was purified from these cells, separated by gel electrophoresis, and then hybridized by the "Northern" blotting technique to a ^{32}P-labeled DNA probe for LTR sequences.

Figure 6 indicates that with the poly(A$^+$) RNA from normal C3H 10T1/2 cells there was negligible hybridization to the LTR probe (lane f). On the other hand, the poly(A$^+$) RNA from five different transformed C3H 10T1/2 cell lines (Fig. 6, lanes a–e) showed appreciable hybridization to this probe. At least five distinct poly(A$^+$) RNA species ranging from about 38 to 18 S were detected in the transformed lines. We have analyzed a total of eight transformed cell lines that were originally derived from normal C3H 10T1/2 following exposure to chemical carcinogens, or radiation and all of these displayed RNAs homologous to the LTR probe, yielding profiles similar to those shown in Fig. 6. With both an early and late passage clone of normal C3H 10T1/2 cells there was always undetectable or only slight hybridization to this probe. On the other hand, we have found that the exposure of normal C3H 10T1/2 cells to either bromodeoxyuridine or 5-azacytidine for 48 hours induced the expression of a series of

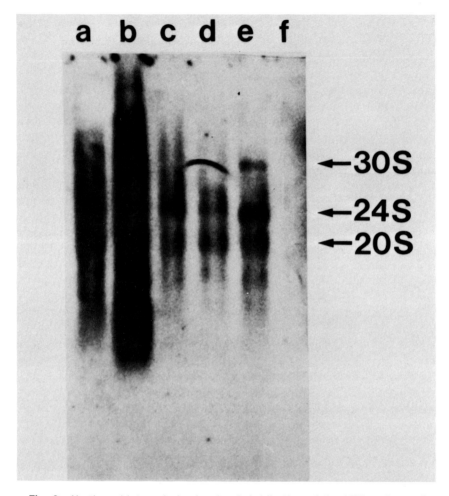

Fig. 6. Northern blot analysis showing hybridization of the LTR probe to the poly(A+) RNA from normal, transformed, and drug-induced murine cells. The gels contained poly(A+) RNAs from the following cell lines: lane a, C3H 10T1/2 JL#2 (UV-transformed); lane b, C3H 10T1/2 CB#2 (benzo[a]pyrene transformed); lane c, C3H 10T1/2 JL#1 (X-ray transformed); lane d, C3H 10T1/2 CB#1 (X-ray transformed); lane e, C3H 10T1/2 JL#3 (methylcholanthrene transformed); and lane f, normal C3H 10T1/2. Poly(A+) RNA was isolated from these cells, denatured with 50% formamide-6% formaldehyde at 65°C and separated on a 0.8% agarose gel containing 6% formaldehyde and 20 mM morpholinopropane sulfonic acid at pH 7.0. The RNA was then transferred to nitrocellulose sheets (BA 85, Schleichler and Schuell) and hybridized to a ^{32}P-labeled LTR probe. (For additional details, see Kirschmeier, *et al.,* 1982.)

poly(A$^+$) RNAs that were homologous to the LTR probe and were similar in size to those found in the transformed C3H 10T1/2 cell lines (Kirschmeier *et al.*, 1982). Thus, it seems that what is unusual in the transformed cells is the constitutive expression of these transcripts rather than the presence of LTR-containing DNA sequences that are unique to the transformed cells.

The poly(A$^+$) RNA transcripts detected with the LTR probe in the transformed C3H 10T1/2 cell lines could originate from endogenous murine retrovirus genomes and/or from the expression of host genes unrelated to the retroviruses but flanked by LTR sequences. Therefore, we performed a set of experiments to determine whether these transcripts contained, in addition to LTR-like sequences, sequences homologous to the known retrovirus genes *gag, pol, env*, and, the *U3* region of the LTR sequence, utilizing the appropriate ^{32}P-labeled DNA probes. We found that when a probe for the *gag-pol* region of murine retroviruses was hybridized to the poly(A$^+$) RNA of carcinogen transformed C3H 10T1/2 cell lines there was hybridization to the 30–38 S RNAs, but there was no detectable hybridization to the lower molecular weight RNAs (24–18 S) detected with the LTR probe (Kirschmeier *et al.*, 1982). The probe to the *env* region also hybridized to RNAs of about 30–38 S, and in addition to an RNA of about 24 S, but it did not hybridize to the 20–18 S RNAs detected with the LTR probe in transformed C3H 10T1/2. We also utilized a probe specific to the *U3* region of the LTR sequence. This region is usually contained in virally related messages since it is just proximal to the viral polyadenylation site (Dhar *et al.*, 1980). We found that the *U3* probe was homologous to the 30 and 24 S RNAs present in carcinogen-transformed derivatives of C3H 10T1/2. However, the 20 and 18 S transcripts recognized by the total LTR probe did not hybridize to the probe specific for the *U3* region of the LTR. No significant hybridization was detected with either the *gag, pol, env*, or *U3* probes and the poly(A$^+$) RNA from normal C3H 10T1/2 cells (Kirschmeier *et al.*, 1982).

Table I summarizes some of the results of the above studies. Although normal C3H 10T1/2 cells do not contain appreciable levels of poly(A$^+$) RNAs homologous to the LTR probe, all the transformed C3H 10T1/2 cell lines contain a series of poly(A$^+$) RNAs ranging in size from about 38 to 18 S. The results obtained with the additional probes suggest that the 30–38 S poly(A$^+$) RNAs present in the transformed cells are transcripts of endogenous retroviral genome(s). The 24 S RNA may represent a specific mRNA for the viral envelope glycoprotein. Although the 20 and 18 S transcripts that we have detected in transformed C3H 10T1/2 cells contain sequences homologous to LTR they do not appear to be due to transcription of known endogenous MuLV genomes. We suspect that these tran-

TABLE I

Summary of Northern Blots

Source of RNA	Probe used											
	LTR			gag-pol			ENV			U3		
	a[a]	b	c	a	b	c	a	b	c	a	b	c
C3H 10T1/2 Normal	−	−	−	−	−	−	−	−	−	−	−	−
C3H 10T1/2 JL#2	+	+	+	+	−	−	+	+	−	+	+	−
C3H 10T1/2 CB#1	+	+	+	+	−	−	+	+	−	+	+	−
C3H 10T1/2 UR#1	+	+	+	+	−	−	+	+	−	+	+	−
C3H 10T1/2 UR#2	+	+	+	+	−	−	+	+	−	+	+	−

[a] The molecular weight classes a, b, and c indicate size of RNA that hybridizes with the respective probe. a, RNAs that are about 30–38 S; b, RNAs that are about 24 S; c, RNAs that are about 18–20 S. For typical profiles see Fig. 6. Cell line JL#2 was transformed by uv light, CB#1 by benzo[a]pyrene, UR#1 by methylcholanthrene, and UR#2 by methylcholanthrene. For additional details see Kirschmeier *et al.* (1982).

scripts reflect the expression of nonvirally related host sequences that utilize virally related LTR sequences as promoters. Southern blot analyses indicate that the genome of normal C3H 10T1/2 cells contains over 30 copies of LTR sequences (Kirschmeier *et al.*, 1982). It is possible that some of these flank host sequences that are unrelated to the MuLVs. We are currently analyzing whether the transformation of C3H 10T1/2 cells is associated with changes in the state of integration and/or methylation in one or more of these endogenous sequences.

IV. Summary

It seems likely that the tendency of established tumors to display progression to a more malignant phenotype and to develop highly variable subpopulations may have its origins in the early events in the carcinogenic process. There is considerable evidence that carcinogenesis is a multistep process resulting from a complex interaction between multiple factors, both environmental and endogenous. A number of environmental chemicals initiate the carcinogenic process by generating metabolites that bind covalently to cellular DNA. On the other hand, recent studies on the mechanism of action of certain tumor promoting agents indicate that they probably act by binding to specific cell surface receptors, thus altering membrane structure and functions. Presumably, these alterations in membrane properties lead indirectly to changes in the expression of genes controlling growth and differentiation. In collaborative studies we have found that the indole alkaloid tumor promoter teleocidin may act via the same receptor system. Evidence has been obtained that certain polycyclic aromatic hydrocarbon carcinogens can induce, via more indirect mechanisms, alterations in cell membranes that are somewhat similar to those produced by the phorbol ester tumor promoters. We suspect that changes in membrane structure and function may also be responsible for a number of aspects of tumor cell heterogeneity.

In contrast to oncogenic viruses, chemical carcinogens and tumor promoters cannot introduce new genetic information. They must, therefore, act through genes already present in the target cell. We have carried out a series of experiments to test the hypothesis that these host genes share homology with specific nucleic acid sequences present in some of the known retroviruses. In one set of experiments we used a cloned DNA containing a portion of the transforming sequence (the *onc* gene *v-mos*) of Moloney murine sarcoma virus (Mo-MSV). This provided a probe which is homologous to an *onc* gene (*c-mos*) normally present in many vertebrate species. However, after examining a number of normal rodent cell types and rodent cells transformed by either chemical carcinogens or radiation we found no evidence that transformation by these agents was associated with rearrangement of the *c-mos* sequence within the cell genome. In addition, in all of the normal and transformed cells the *c-mos* sequence was hypermethylated and transcriptionally silent. These results are in sharp contrast to the situation in cells transformed by Mo-MSV in which the exogenous *v-mos* sequence is integrated at new sites within the host genome, is undermethylated, and is extensively transcribed. In related studies, we have found that another onc gene, *c-ras*, also fails to show any evidence for rearrangement in carcinogen or radiation transformed C3H 10T1/2 cells (unpublished studies). Since there is evidence that eukaryotic cells can contain at least 15 *onc* genes (Bishop, 1980) our results do not rule out the possibility that onc genes other than *c-mos* and *c-ras* may play a role in the transformation of murine cells by chemicals or radiation. Additional studies utilizing probes to other onc genes are required to evaluate this possibility.

In contrast to the negative results obtained with the *c-mos* probe, we have discovered an interesting difference between normal and transformed C3H 10T1/2 cells by utilizing a probe homologous to the long terminal repeat (LTR) sequence of Mo-MSV. Whereas normal C3H 10T1/2 cells do not express significant amounts of poly(A^+) RNAs homologous to this probe, C3H 10T1/2 cell lines transformed by chemical carcinogens or radiation expressed significant amounts of RNA containing LTR-like sequences. Results obtained with additional probes suggest that this is not simply due to the switch-on of endogenous RNA leukemia viruses in these transformed cells. Studies are in progress to determine whether the constitutive expression of these RNAs in transformed cells is associated with gene rearrangements, demethylation of endogenous DNA sequences, or other mechanisms. The fact that we have observed the expression of these RNAs in all of the transformed C3H 10T1/2 cell lines that we have examined thus far (Kirschmeier *et al.*, 1982), and that LTR sequences play a key role in the mechanism of cell transformation by an avian leukosis virus (Hayward *et al.*, 1981), suggests that our findings may be relevant to the process of cell transformation induced by chemicals and radiation. Further studies are required to determine at which stage in the multistep carcinogenic process the switch-on of these RNA transcripts occurs and whether or not they code for functions necessary for maintenance of the transformed state. It will also be of interest to determine to what extent tumor progression and tumor cell heterogeneity are associated with alterations in the expression of endogenous *onc* genes and/or the function of LTR sequences.

Acknowledgments

This research was supported by DHS, NCI Grants CA 021111 and CA 02656. The authors wish to acknowledge the valuable collaboration with T. Sugimura and H. Fujiki of the National Cancer Center Research Institute, Tokyo, and K. Umezawa of the Cancer Institute, Tokyo, in the studies on teleocidin and related indole alkaloids. We also appreciate the valuable role of Dino Dina and colleagues at the Albert Einstein College of Medicine, Bronx, New York, in the studies on *c-mos* and LTR sequences. We thank Patricia Kelly for assistance in preparing this manuscript. Paul Kirschmeier was a recipient of a postdoctoral fellowship from the Daymon-Runyon Walter Winchell Cancer Fund and A. Horowitz has a fellowship from the Dupont Company.

References

Barett, J. C., and Ts'o, P.O.P. (1978). Evidence for the progressive nature of neoplastic transformation *in vitro*. *Proc. Natl. Acad. Sci. U.S.A.* **75**, 3761–3765.

Belman, S., and Troll, W. (1972). The inhibition of Croton Oil-promoted mouse skin tumorigenesis by steroid hormones. *Cancer Res.* **32**, 450–454.

Berenblum, I. (1975). Origin of the concept of sequential stages of skin carcinogenesis. *In* "Cancer: A Comprehensive Treatise" (F. F. Becker, ed.), pp. 323–344. Plenum, New York.

Bishop, J. M. (1980). The molecular biology of RNA tumor viruses: A physician's guide. *N. Engl. J. Med.* **303**, 675–682.

Blair, D. G., Oskarsson, M., Wood, T. G., McClements, W. L., Fischinger, P. J., and Vande Woude, G. F. (1981). Activation of the transforming potential of a normal cell sequence: A molecular model for oncogenesis. *Science (Washington, D.C.)* **212**, 941–943.

Blumberg, P. M. (1980). *In vitro* studies on the mode of action of the phorbol esters, potent tumor promoters. Part 1. *CRC Crit. Rev. Toxicol.* **8**, 153–197.

Blumberg, P. M. (1981). *In vitro* studies on the mode of action of the phorbol esters, potent tumor promoters. Part 2. *CRC Crit. Rev. Toxicol.* **8,** 199–238.

Boutwell, R. K. (1974). The function and mechanism of promoters of carcinogenesis. *CRC Crit. Rev. Toxicol.* **2,** 419–443.

Burns, F. J., and Albert, R. E. (1982). Mouse skin papillomas as early stages of carcinogenesis. *J. Am. Coll. Tox.* **1,** 29–45.

Cohen, J. C. (1980). Methylation of milk-borne and genetically transmitted mouse mammary tumor virus proviral DNA. *Cell,* **19,** 653–662.

Colburn, N. H., Former, B. F., Nelson, K. A., and Yuspa, S. J. (1979). Tumor promoter induces anchorage independence irreversibly. *Nature (London)* **281,** 589–591.

Delclos, K. B., Nagle, D. S., and Blumberg, P. M. (1980). Specific binding of phorbol ester tumor promoters to mouse skin. *Cell* **19,** 1025–1032.

Dhar, R., McClements, W. C., Enquist, L. W., and Vande Woude, G. G. (1980). Nucleotide sequences of integrated Moloney sarcoma provirus long terminal repeats and their host and viral junctions. *Proc. Natl. Acad. Sci. U.S.A.* **77,** 3937–3941.

Diamond, L., O'Brien, T. G., and Baird, W. M. (1980). Tumor promoters and the mechanism of tumor promotion. *Adv. Cancer Res.* **32,** 1–74.

Driedger, P. E., and Blumberg, P. M. (1980). Specific binding of phorbol ester tumor promoters. *Proc. Natl. Acad. Sci. U.S.A.* **77,** 567–571.

Fisher, P. B., and Weinstein, I. B. (1979). Chemical-viral interactions and multistep aspects of cell transformation. *In* "Molecular and Cellular Aspects of Carcinogen Screening Tests" (R. Montesano, H. Bartsch, and L. Tomatis, eds.), *IARC Sci. Publ.* **27,** 113–131.

Fisher, P. B., Bozzone, J. H., and Weinstein, I. B. (1979). Tumor promoters and epidermal growth factor stimulate anchorage-independent growth of adenovirus transformed rat embryo cells. *Cell* **18,** 695–705.

Fisher, P. B., Mufson, R. A., Weinstein, I. B., and Little, I. B. (1981). Epidermal growth factor, like tumor promoters, enhances viral and radiation-induced cell growth. *Carcinogenesis* **2,** 183–188.

Fisher, P. B., Mufson, R. A., Miranda, A. F., Fujiki, H., Sugimura, T., and Weinstein, I. B. (1982). Phorbol ester tumor promoters and teleocidin have similar effects on cell transformation, differentiation and phospholipid metabolism. *Cancer Res.* (in press).

Foulds, L. (1969, 1975). "Neoplastic Development," Vols. 1 and 2. Academic Press, New York.

Fujiki, H., Mori, M., Nakayasu, M., Terada, M., and Sugimura, T. (1979). A possible naturally occurring tumor promoter, teleocidin B from *Streptomyces. Biochem. Biophys. Res. Commun.* **90,** 976–983.

Fujiki, H., Mori, M., Nakayasu, M., Terada, M., Sugimura, T., and Moore, R. E. (1981). Indole alkaloids: Dihydroteleocidin B, teleocidin, and lyngbyatoxin A as members of a new class of tumor promoters. *Proc. Natl. Acad. Sci. U.S.A.* **78,** 3872–3876.

Gattoni, S., Kirschmeier, P., Weinstein, I. B., Escobedo, J., and Dina, D. (1982). Cellular moloney murine sarcoma ("c-mos") sequences are hypermethylated and transcriptionally silent in normal and transformed rodent cells, *Mol. Cell. Biol.* **2,** 42–51.

Graiser, M. Soeller, W., and Dina, D. (1980). Isolation and characterization of phenotypic revertants from Moloney sarcoma virus-transformed cells. *In* "Animal Virus Genetics" (B. Fields, and R. Jaenish, eds.). pp. 569–579. *ICN-UCLA Symp. Mol. Cell Biol.* Vol. XVIII. Academic Press, New York.

Harrison, J., and Auersperg, N. (1981). Epidermal growth factor enhances viral transformation of granulosa cells. *Science (Washington, D.C.)* **213,** 218–219.

Hayward, W. S., Neel, B. G., and Astrin, S. M. (1981). Activation of a cellular *onc* gene by promoter insertion in ALV-induced lymphoid leukosis. *Nature (London)* **290,** 475–480.

Hecker, E. (1975). Cocarcinogens and cocarcinogenesis. *In* "Handbuch der Allgemeinen Pathologie"(E. Grundmann, ed.), Vol. IV/6, pp. 651–676. Springer-Verlag, Gerswulste, Tumors II, Berlin and New York.

Horowitz, A. D., Greenebaum, E., and Weinstein, I. B. (1981). Identification of receptors for phorbol ester tumor promoters in intact mammalian cells and of an inhibitor of receptor binding in biologic fluids. *Proc. Natl. Acad. Sci., U.S.A.,* **78,** 2315–2319.

Horowitz, A. D., Greenebaum, E., and Weinstein, I. B. (1982). Inhibition of phorbol ester-receptor binding by a factor from human serum. *Mol. Cell. Biol.* **2,** 545–553.

Ivanovic, V., and Weinstein, I. B. (1982). Benzo[*a*]pyrene and other inducers of cytochrome P_1-450 inhibit binding of epidermal growth factor to cell surface receptors. *Carcinogenesis* (in press).

Ivanovic, V., and Weinstein, I. B. (1981). Glucocorticoids and Benzo[*a*]pyrene have opposing effects on EGF receptor binding. *Nature (London)* **293,** 404–406.

Jones, M., Bosselman, R. A., vande Horn, F. A., Bern, A., Fan, H., and Verma, I. M. (1980). Identification and molecular cloning of Moloney mouse sarcoma virus-specific sequences from uninfected mouse cells. *Proc. Natl. Acad. Sci. U.S.A.* **77,** 2651–2655.

Jones, P. A., and Taylor, S. M. (1980). Cellular differentiation, cytidine analogs and DNA methylation. *Cell* **20,** 85–93.

Kirschmeier, P., Gattoni, S., Dina, D., and Weinstein, I. B. (1982). Carcinogen and radiation transformed C3H 10T1/2 cells contain RNAs homologous to the LTR sequence of a murine leukemia virus. *Proc. Natl. Acad. Sci. U.S.A.* **79,** 273–277.

Lee, L. S., and Weinstein, I. B. (1978). Tumor promoting phorbol esters inhibit binding of epidermal growth factor to cellular receptors. *Science (Washington, D.C.)* **202,** 313–315.

Levine, L., and Ohuchi, I. (1978). Stimulation by carcinogens and promoters of prostaglandin production by dog kidney (MDCK) cells in culture. *Cancer Res.* **38,** 4142–4146.

Morris, A. G. (1981). Neoplastic transformation of mouse fibroblasts by murine sarcoma virus: A multi-step process. *J. Gen. Virol.* **53,** 39–45.

Nakayasu, M., Fujiki, H., Mori, M., Sugimura, T., and Moore, R. E. (1981). Teleocidin, lyngbyatoxin A and their hydrogenated derivatives, possible tumor promoters, induce terminal differentiation in HL-60 cells. *Cancer Lett.* **12,** 271–277.

O'Brien, T. G. (1976). The induction of ornithine decarboxylase as an early, possibly obligatory, event in mouse skin carcinogenesis. *Cancer Res.* **36,** 2644–2653.

Okey, A. B., Bondy, G. P., Mason, M. E., Kahl, G. F., Eisen, H. J., Guenther, T. M., and Nebert, D. W. (1979). Regulatory gene product of the Ah locus. Characterization of the cytosolic inducer-receptor complex and evidence for its nuclear translocation. *J. Biol. Chem.* **254,** 11636–11648.

Oskarsson, M., McClements, W. L., Blair, D. G., Maizel, J. V., and Vande Woude, G. F. (1980). Properties of a normal mouse cell DNA sequence (sarc) homologous to the src sequence of Moloney sarcoma virus. *Science (Washington, D.C.)* **207,** 1222–1224.

Peto, R. (1977). Epidemiology, multistage models and short-term mutagenicity tests. *In* "Origins of Human Cancer" (H. H. Hiatt, J. D. Watson, and J. A. Winston, eds.), Vol. IV, pp. 1403–1428. Cold Spring Harbor, New York.

Poland, A., Greenlee, W. F., and Kende, A. S. (1979). Studies on the mechanism of action of the chlorinated dibenzo-*p*-dioxins and related compounds. *Ann. N. Y. Acad. Sci.,* **320,** 214–230.

Sakamoto, H., Terada, M., Fujiki, H., Mori, M., Nakayasu, M., Sugimura, T., and Weinstein, I. B. (1981). Stimulation of prostaglandin production and choline turnover in HeLa cells by lynbyatoxin A and dihydroteleocidin B. *Biochem. Biophys. Res. Commun.* **102**, 100–107.

Scherer, E., and Emmelot, P. (1979). The multihit concept of tumor cell formation and its bearing on low dose risk assessment. *In* "Environmental Carcinogenesis" (P. Emmelot, and E. Kriek, eds.), pp. 303–318. Elsevier/North Holland Biomedical Press, Amsterdam.

Shoyab, M., and Todaro, G. J. (1980). Specific high affinity cell membrane receptors for biologically active phorbol and ingenol esters. *Nature (London)* **288**, 451–455.

Slaga, T. J., Sivak, A., and Boutwell, R. K., eds. (1978). "Carcinogenesis, Vol. 2: Mechanisms of Tumor Promotion and Cocarcinogenesis." Raven, New York.

Slaga, T. J., Fisher, S. M., Nelson, K., and Gleason, G. L. (1980). Studies on the mechanism of skin tumor promotion: Evidence for several stages in promotion. *Proc. Natl. Acad. Sci. U.S.A.* **77**, 3659–3663.

Southern, E. (1975). Detection of specific sequences among DNA fragments separated by gel electrophoresis. *J. Mol. Biol.* **98**, 503–517.

Thomas, P. S. (1980). Hybridization of denatured RNA and small DNA fragments transferred to nitrocellulose paper. *Proc. Natl. Acad. Sci. U.S.A.* **77**, 5201–5205.

Umezawa, K., Weinstein, I. B., Horowitz, A., Fujiki, H., Matsushima, T., and Sugimura, T. (1981). Similarity of teleocidin B and phorbol ester tumor promoters in effects on membrane receptors. *Nature (London)* **290**, 411–413.

van der Ploeg, L. H. T., and Flavell, R. A. (1980). DNA methylation in the human β-globin locus in erythroid and nonerythroid tissues. *Cell* **19**, 947–958.

Van Duuren, B. L. (1969). Tumor promoting agents in two-stage carcinogenesis. *Prog. Exp. Tumor Res.* **11**, 31–68.

Viage, A., Slaga, T. J., Wigler, M., and Weinstein, I. B. (1977). Effects of anti-inflammatory agents on mouse skin tumor promotion, epidermal DNA synthesis, phorbol ester-induced cellular proliferation, and production of plasminogen activator. *Cancer Res.* **37**, 1530–1536.

Weinstein, I. B. (1981). Studies on the mechanism of action of tumor promoters and their relevance to mammary carcinogenesis. *In* "Cell Biology of Breast Cancer" (C. M. McGrath, M. J. Brennan, and M. A. Rich, eds.), pp. 425–450. Academic Press, New York.

Weinstein, I. B., Wigler, M., and Pietropaolo, C. (1977). The action of tumor promoting agents in cell culture. *In* "Origins of Human Cancer" (H. H. Hiatt, J. D. Watson, and J. D. Winston, eds.), pp. 751–772. *Cold Spring Harbor Conf. Cell Proliferation, IV.* Cold Spring Harbor Labs., Cold Spring Harbor, New York.

Weinstein, I. B., Yamasaki, H., Wigler M., Lee, L. S., Fisher, P. B., Jeffrey, A. M., and Grunberger, D. (1979). Molecular and cellular events associated with the action of initiating carcinogens and tumor promoters. "Carcinogens: Identification and Mechanisms of Action" (A. C. Griffin and C. R. Shaw, eds.), pp. 399–418. Raven, New York.

Weinstein, I. B., Mufson, R. A., Lee. L. S., Fisher, P. B., Laskin, J., Horowitz, A., and Ivanovic, V. (1980). Membrane and other biochemical effects of the phorbol esters and their relevance to tumor promotion. *In* "Carcinogenesis: Fundamental Mechanisms and Environmental Effects" (B. Pullman, P. O. P. Ts'o, and H. Gelboin, eds.), pp. 543–563. R. Reidel Publ., Amsterdam, Holland.

Yamasaki, H., Weinstein, I. B., and Van Duuren, B. L. (1981). Induction of adhesion of erythroleukemia cells: A rapid screening method for plant diterpene tumor promoters. *Carcinogenesis,* **2**, 537–543.

18

Relationships among Neoplastic Transformation, Somatic Mutation, and Differentiation

PAUL O. P. TS'O

I. Introduction

Since the pioneering work of Berwald and Sachs (1963, 1965) much effort has been made to develop adequate and useful mammalian cell systems for the study of the basic mechanism of neoplastic transformation in chemical carcinogenesis. The study of neoplastic transformation *in vitro* allows the analysis of the basic mechanisms of carcinogenesis at the level of cell biology and then downward to the level of molecular biology. Thus, the study of carcinogenesis can be investigated concerning the damage to genes at the DNA level and concerning the alteration of gene expression at the mRNA level.

TUMOR CELL HETEROGENEITY

In addition to the above "reductionalistic" approach, there is a new development for the study of different cell types from various tissues (i.e., fibroblast versus epithelial cells versus hematopoietic cells), as well as the study of cell types obtained from various differentiation stages and age of animals. This is a promising "constructionalistic" approach which links carcinogenesis to the differentiation process, such as embryonic development and aging.

II. *In Vitro* Neoplastic Transformation as a Model for the Study of Carcinogenesis

The first and most fundamental issue is whether the *in vitro* study of neoplastic transformation can provide the basic understanding of carcinogenesis in animals or men. Clearly, certain aspects of carcinogenesis, such as immunological defense and hormonal control, would not be easily investigated through a study of cells in culture. Nevertheless, the transformation of cells observed in tissue culture can have the same characteristics or can be governed by the same principles as the transformation of cells in the intact host. However, we need to choose the experimental system very carefully. In our laboratories (Barrett *et al.*, 1977; Barret *et al.*, 1978 a,b; Barrett and Ts'o, 1978) we have chosen the early culture of Syrian hamster embryo fibroblasts as pioneered by Berwald and Sachs (1963, 1965), DiPaolo (DiPaolo and Donovan, 1967; DiPaolo *et al.*, 1969; DiPaolo *et al.*, 1971), and others. These cells are normal diploid cells and can maintain their karyotype in culture. In passaging, these fibroblasts will senesce with a very low rate of spontaneous transformation. Since the laboratory Syrian hamster is highly inbred, tumorigenicity can be studied quantitatively without immunological interference.

Two major observations from our laboratory and other laboratories indicate that *in vitro* neoplastic transformation, using Syrian hamster embryo fibroblasts, can serve as a reliable model for carcinogenesis:

A. First, several abnormal growth properties of transformed cells are closely associated with tumorigenicity. In this experiment, a variety of clonally devised cell lines with varying degrees of tumorigenicity were established (Barrett *et al.*, 1979). The heritable and abnormal growth properties were then quantitatively measured. A statistically significant correlation between certain abnormal growth properties, notably anchorage-independent growth (cloning efficiency in soft agar), and tumorigenicity of these cells was established (Table I). A much more extensive investigation using this approach is now near completion with cells transformed spontaneously, as well as by physical and chemical means.

TABLE I

Correlation among *in Vitro* Growth Properties and Tumorigenicity of Syrian Hamster Cell Lines

Growth parameters	Coefficient of rank correlation, τ^a
Cloning efficiency, semisolid agar	0.986^b
Fibrinolytic activity	0.754^c
Generation time, 1% serum	0.754^c
Cloning efficiency, liquid medium	0.638^c
Organization of intracellular actin	0.570^c
Saturation density, 10% serum	0.246
Generation time, 10% serum	0.062

[a] Computation of the Kendall coefficient of rank correlation, τ, between the TD_{50} of the cell lines and their respective growth properties was performed.
[b] Significantly correlated at the 99% confidence level ($p \leq 0.01$).
[c] Significantly correlated at the 95% confidence level ($p \leq 0.05$).

The data clearly indicate that certain heritable, abnormal cellular properties of these neoplastically transformed cells in culture can be correlated to their tumorigenicity in animals.

B. Second, progression in neoplastic transformation *in vitro* mimics the progression in carcinogenesis *in vivo*. One major characteristic of carcinogenesis observed by pathologists (Foulds, 1954, 1969, 1975) is the phenomenon of progression. Subpopulations of carcinogenic cells undergo a series of qualitative and quantitative changes, leading finally to neoplasia and malignancy. This process takes considerable time and many cell generations. Our work (Barrett *et al.*, 1977; Barrett and Ts'o, 1978) and other studies clearly demonstrate that such a process also occurs in *in vitro* neoplastic transformation. Therefore, the phenomenon of progression in carcinogenesis can be studied in *in vitro* neoplastic transformation.

III. The Relationship between Somatic Mutation and Neoplastic Transformation

Currently, one important hypothesis for carcinogenesis is the theory of somatic mutation which needs to be investigated first. The initial step was to establish an experimental system in which somatic mutation and neoplastic transformation of the same cell culture could be investigated simultaneously after perturbation (Barrett *et al.*, 1978a; Barrett and Ts'o, 1978). In the simultaneous studies of somatic mutation (point mutation) and neoplastic transformation, it is evident that while neoplastic transformation may be initiated by somatic mutation, somatic mutation is an inadequate biological model for the study of neoplastic transformation. One example of this problem is shown in Table II. Somatic mutation and neoplastic transformation of diploid SHE cells were examined concomitantly. Mutations, induced by B[a]P and MNNG, were quantitated at the HGPRT and the Na^+/K^+ ATPase loci and compared to phenotypic transformations measured by changes in clonal morphology and colony formation in agar. Both cellular transformations had characteristics distinct from the somatic mutations observed at the two loci. Morphological transformation was observed after an expression or detection time comparable to somatic mutation but at a frequency 25- to 540-fold higher. Transformants capable of colony formation in agar were detected at 10^{-5}–10^{-6} frequency, but not until 32–75 population doublings after carcinogen treatment. While this frequency of transformation is comparable to that of somatic mutations, the detection time required is much longer than the optimal expression time of conventionally studied somatic mutations. The main reason is that the type of somatic mutation chosen as a model system is the one in which the mutation of a single gene can be studied in a truncated manner, namely, involving a one-step change from wild type to mutant, without inducing a cascading effect in a cell which leads to further consequences. In this context, it is difficult to study a gene mutation that will lead subsequently to other mutations, which in turn will affect the original mutation. To the contrary, one characteristic of neoplastic transformation is a phenomenon of a cascading effect of many interrelated, highly coupled processes in the cell. Therefore, in using a highly simplified somatic mutation model (point mutation) to approximate the complex neoplastic transformation process, the information obtained is often in-

TABLE II

Comparison of Phenotypic Changes of SHE Cells

	Somatic mutation	Morphological transformation	Anchorage-independent growth[a]
Observed frequency (spontaneous)	$<10^{-6}$	$\sim 10^{-4b}$	$<1.4 \times 10^{-8}$
Observed frequency (carcinogen-treated)	10^{-5}–10^{-4}	10^{-3}–10^{-2}	10^{-5}–10^{-6}
Expression/detection time[c]	6–8	≤ 8	32–75

[a] As measured by colony formation in soft agar.
[b] Six spontaneous, morphologically transformed colonies were observed per ~62,000 control colonies examined.
[c] Population doublings.

adequate and inappropriate (Barrett and Ts'o, 1978). However, the major issue remains, can neoplastic transformation be initiated by a single gene mutation? If it can, what would be the nature of such a mutation? This issue is complicated by the phenomenon of neoplastic progression. This question, therefore, can only be answered separately for each of the various steps between substages during progression. Nevertheless, somatic genetic analysis of neoplastic transformation, particularly of the progression process, is a worthwhile enterprise.

IV. Somatic Genetic Studies of Neoplastic Transformation

The somatic genetics study of neoplastic transformation, especially on the phenomenon of progression, is a very complicated issue. However, at present, several definitive conclusions can be made and are described below.

A. The rate of spontaneous neoplastic transformation was analyzed by fluctuation analysis (Barrett *et al.*, 1981b). Several spontaneous transformation lines of Syrian hamster fibroblasts were developed in our laboratory from fibrinolytically active clones (Barrett *et al.*, 1977; Barrett and Ts'o, 1978). Upon prolonged culture, these clonal lines spontaneously generated soft agar positive (Aga^+) colonies, which were subsequently shown to be tumorigenic. It was further shown that acquisition of tumorigenicity of a culture can be strictly correlated to the appearance of the Aga^+ subpopulation. Through fluctuation analysis (Luria–Delbruck analysis), the rate of spontaneous neoplastic transformation leading to Aga^+ colonies was found to be about the same as that of spontaneous somatic point mutations. It was first thought that perhaps at least two steps were required in neoplastic transformation. The first step could be an initiation of an autosomal recessive mutation, while the second step would be another mutation to convert the original recessive mutation from a hemizygous state to a homozygous state. This hypothesis, while attractive at the time, was subsequently not supported by the following major observations (Barrett *et al.*, 1981b; Crawford, 1981).

1. It was found that these spontaneously transformed cells are aneuploid or nearly tetraploid; thus, it is very difficult to induce recessive mutations [including sex-linked, recessive mutations (HPRT locus)] in these cells. However, these cells can be induced to yield dominant mutations (Na^+/K^+ ATPase locus). Therefore, expression of recessive mutations in these cells is highly unfavorable.

2. As expected from the first observation, the frequency of Aga^+ colonies in these cultures cannot be increased through treatment by a variety

of mutagens and carcinogens. Therefore, while the apparent rate of the appearance of Aga$^+$ in this spontaneously transformed line mimics that of a spontaneous point gene mutation rate, the data do not support the hypothesis that this is the underlying mechanism in progression. Neither observation supports the hypothesis that neoplastic transformation is a manifestation of a dominant mutation.

B. At the same time, the chromosomal variability of this spontaneous line in culture was investigated. It was found that the spontaneous variation of karyotypes is very high, even after recloning. These results indicated that karyotypic heterogeneity with a high rate of nondisjunction is an intrinsic property of these cells. Quantitative calculations indicate that a high rate of nondisjunction, or a high tendency in karyotypic variability, could be an underlying mechanism of the spontaneous changes leading to the emergence of Aga$^+$ subpopulations.

C. The investigation for the nature of the mutation was expanded by two different approaches, with the underlying assumption that somatic mutation can be a major cause for neoplastic transformation.

1. The first approach was through intraspecies cell hybrids (Crawford, 1981), in which highly tumorigenic cells (BP6T) and the normal Syrian hamster fibroblasts were hybridized in culture. The results indicated that the Aga$^+$ property was immediately suppressed in the hybrid within several cell doublings after hybridization. But, the Aga$^+$ properties in the hybrid did reexpress upon further growth in culture after 10–25 cell doublings. The progenies from the hybrids exhibited a high degree of variability in the expression of Aga$^+$. The data revealed that the hybrid formation initially suppressed the Aga$^+$ property and that the Aga$^+$ property was then reexpressed upon segregation. This investigation again points to the importance of variability of chromosomes as an important aspect of neoplastic transformation.

2. The second approach was the investigation based on the effect of gene dose, or ploidy (Morry, 1980). In these experiments, clones of diploid ($2N$) cells and clones of tetraploid ($4N$) cells were selected, and were then separately treated by mutagens and carcinogens. The results clearly indicate that while diploid clones can be induced to neoplastic transformation, the tetraploid cells under an identical situation cannot be induced to exhibit any neoplastic properties. The experiments clearly indicate that if the response to perturbation is related to somatic mutation, then the response has to be due to a recessive mutation.

The conclusion in this investigation is that if chemically induced neoplastic transformation is initiated by somatic mutation under certain circumstances, the mutation has to be recessive in nature. At present the underlying mechanisms for the long period of progression are not yet clear, but this progression is most likely due to the occurrence of chromosomal variability, which may lead to two alternative consequences.

One possible consequence is the expression of the recessive autosomal mutation through a process of converting the hemizygous state into the homozygous state through karyotypic changes. However, there is another possible consequence. After the initial insult, which may or may not cause a mutation, chromosome variability is needed to express phenotypically the neoplastic characteristics by alteration of gene balances or the structure of the genetic apparatus. The only way to resolve this problem is to perturb experimentally the chromosome patterns of the cells in order to generate clones and populations having various chromosomal patterns in culture for further investigation. Experiments of this nature are currently in progress.

V. DNA as a Critical Target for Neoplastic Transformation

Although it may not be possible to directly investigate the exact involvement of somatic mutation in neoplastic transformation, experiments can be done to delineate whether DNA is a critical target in the cells, the perturbation of which alone will lead to neoplastic transformation. In this experiment, the most critical issue is to find means to perturb DNA only, and not any other macromolecules in the cell. This is usually not the case in a chemical transformation experiment, since the metabolically activated carcinogens may attack many types of molecules within the cell. Therefore, special experiments have to be designed. Over the past five years in our laboratory, three sets of DNA-specific perturbation experiments have been done.

A. Incorporation of 5-bromodeoxyuridine into DNA, followed by near-uv irradiation (Barrett *et al.*, 1979; Tsutsui *et al.*, 1979). This experiment leads to specific strand breaks in DNA where 5-bromodeoxyuridine has been incorporated. This experiment was done with both unsynchronized and synchronized cell culture, demonstrating the cell cycle dependence of such a perturbation. In fact, somatic mutation and neoplastic transformation can only be induced by such a treatment at S phase and is particularly more effective in the mid-S phase.

B. Perturbation by incorporation of tritiated thymidine, using tritiated uridine as a control (Lin *et al.*, 1982). This experiment clearly showed that with similar dosages of radiation, tritiated uridine did not induce somatic mutation and morphological transformation, while tritiated thymidine did induce both somatic mutation and neoplastic transformation of cells in culture.

C. Perturbation by DNase I encapsulated in liposomes (Zajac and Ts'o, 1980). The cells were treated by pancreatic DNase I encapsulated in phosphotidylserine liposomes. The treated cells exhibited DNA breaks, chromosome abnormalities, cell death, a certain type of somatic mutation, as well as neoplastic transformation after a prolonged period of progression. These data, based on a specific perturbation with DNase I, clearly indicate that damage to DNA as evidenced by single strand breaks can initiate neoplastic transformation.

The results of the above three sets of experiments reinforce each other in pointing to the conclusion that specific perturbation to DNA alone, possibly through strand breaks, is sufficient to initiate neoplastic transformation. However, through such a perturbation to DNA, cell killing can be observed within a few cell divisions, and somatic mutation can also be observed within 5–10 population doublings, the required time for expression. But neoplastic transformation as indicated by anchorage independent growth or tumorigenicity cannot be observed in this culture until 50–150 population doublings after the initial insult. What kind of cellular process requires an expression time of so many cell divisions? Apparently, this is one of the most challenging puzzles, and it becomes one of the crucial differences between neoplastic transformation and somatic mutation, even though both processes can be initiated by specific perturbation to DNA alone.

In view of the successful experiment described above concerning the specific and direct damage to DNA as the primary cause of the initiation of neoplastic transformation, initial investigations have now been made in our laboratory in order to find out whether perturbation which would *not* have led to DNA damage could lead to neoplastic transformation. In this case, we expect to dissociate somatic mutation from neoplastic transformation. In other words, we hope that agents can be identified which would lead to neoplastic transformation without inducing somatic mutation. Most recently, such a report has been given by Barrett *et al.* (1981a) concerning morphological transformation induced by estradiol.

VI. Relationship between Differentiation and Neoplastic Transformation

In our study of early embryonic fibroblasts, it was found that there exist cellular subpopulations having two of the growth properties of neoplastically transformed cells: lack of post confluence inhibition of cell division (CI⁻) and anchorage independence of growth (the Aga⁺ property) (Nakano and Ts'o, 1981). These properties are characteristic of neoplastic

TABLE III

Comparison of Cloning Ability of Various Normal and Transformed SHE Cells on Plastic Surfaces and Cell Mats and in Semisolid Agar

Cells	Cloning efficiency (%)			
	On plastic surfaces	On cell mats[a]	In soft agar	Diameter of colony on cell mat (mm)
BP12[b]	67.0	6.7	3.9	≈2
BP12B[b]	57.0	18.0	19.6	≈4
BP6[b]	82.5	33.5	42.0	≈4
BP6T[b]	84.5	49.6	85.0	≈6
SHE 21F CL2/1[c]	45.5	<0.0002	<0.0002	—
SHE 3P[d]	1.25	0.38	<0.001	≈1
SHE 4P[d]	1.38	0.13	<0.001	≈0.5
SHE 6P[d]	0.51	0.05	<0.001	≈0.5
SHE 7P[d]	0.26	<0.01	<0.001	—
SHE 8P[d]	0.30	<0.001	<0.001	—

[a] Incubation times on cell mats were 14 days for normal SHE cells and 7 days for transformed BP cells.

[b] All transformed SHE cells induced by benzo[a]pyrene treatment are described in Barrett et al., Cancer Res. **39**, 1504–1510 (1979).

[c] Spontaneously derived established clonal cell line of SHE cells that shows contact inhibition of cell growth.

[d] Approximately passage 3–8 (PDL undetermined) SHE 17F cells derived from 13-day gestation fetuses.

cells, as shown in Table III. These subpopulations decrease with increasing gestation period of the embryo as well as with continuing passage *in vitro*. Embryos at an earlier stage of gestation have a larger percentage of these types of cells. These properties can be seen in Tables IV and V. Furthermore, when these cells were grown on cell mat, it was found that they continued to lose the CI⁻ properties upon cell division and growth, even though these cells were originally selected for their ability to grow on cell mat. This finding indicates that the CI⁻ property is a transient property, and one that will be lost upon cell division and growth. The subpopulation having this CI⁻ property is not a permanent cell type but is a subpopulation of cells in a transitional stage. Careful investigation on the isolated clones suggests that these subpopulations did not lose proliferative capacity, but acquired the contact-inhibited phenotype or anchorage-dependent phenotype by cellular differentiation. The susceptibility of these subpopulations to become neoplastically transformed by MNNG was investigated by employing the clonally isolated embryonic fibroblasts lacking postconfluence inhibition of cell division (CI⁻). The isolated CI⁻

TABLE IV

Concomitant Quantitation of Cl⁻ Cells (Cell Mat Assay) and AD⁻ Cells (Agar Assay) during Serial Passage of SHE 30F Cells Derived from 13-Day-Old Embryos

		Cloning efficiency (%)		
Passage	PDL (no.)[a]	On plastic surfaces[b]	On cell mats[b]	In semi-solid agar[c]
2	1.1	2.50	0.16	0.008
3	4.7	0.64	0.04	0.002
5	8.5	1.04	<0.001	<0.0002
6	11.0	0.94	<0.001	<0.0002

[a] Population doublings were calculated from the number of initial cells per culture and number of cells obtained at time of subculture.
[b] Means of duplicate dishes.
[c] Each agar plate was inoculated with 5×10^5 cells. Data are means of triplicate dishes.

clones were divided into two portions: portion I was cultured on lethally irradiated cell mat to produce cultures enriched with Cl⁻ cells (0.6–4%) and portion II was cultured on plastic dishes to produce cultures depleted of Cl⁻ cells (0.02–0.2%) through rapid proliferation (Nakano et al., 1982). Upon MNNG treatment, the Cl⁻-enriched cultures exhibited twice as high a survival rate as the Cl⁻-depleted cultures (25% vs. 12%, respec-

TABLE V

Concomitant Quantitation of Cl⁻ Cells (Cell Mat Assay) and AD⁻ Cells (Agar Assay) during Serial Passage of SHE 50 Cells Derived from 10-Day-Old Embryos

		Cloning efficiency (%)			
Passage	PDL[a]	On plastic surfaces[b]	On cell mats[b]	In soft agar[c]	Diameter of colony on cell mat (mm)
Primary	0	0.23	3.66	—	1.0–2.0
1	0.3	0.25	3.00	—	1.0–2.0
2	1.0	1.25	0.88	0.014	0.5–1.0
3	1.6	1.17	0.16	0.006	0.5–1.0
4	3.3	0.91	0.02	0.003	<0.5
5	6.1	0.20	<0.0002	<0.0002	—

[a] Population doubling was calculated from number of initial cells per culture and number of cells obtained at time of subculture.
[b] Means of duplicate dishes.
[c] Each soft agar plate was inoculated with 5×10^5 cells. Data are means of triplicate dishes.

tively, at $10\mu M$). Based on clonal morphology assay and focus formation assay at the same MNNG dose or at equivalent biological survival dose, Cl^--enriched cultures were 10- to 20-fold higher in transformation frequency than the Cl^--depleted cultures; for cultures containing 4% Cl^- cells, these frequencies reached 20% and 0.2%, respectively. In continuous passage assay, 100% (9/9) of the Cl^--enriched cultures exhibited anchorage independent phenotypes in ~25 days whereas only 56% (5/9) of the Cl^--depleted cultures exhibited this transformation-associated phenotype in ~50 days. In contrast to the large difference in susceptibility to neoplastic transformation, both Cl^--enriched and Cl^--depleted cultures exhibited the same somatic mutation frequency (Na^+/K^+ ATPase locus) upon MNNG treatment. These results indicate that the NT susceptibility can be greatly influenced by differentiation and can be dissociated from somatic mutation; the less differentiated Cl^- cells can be transformed much more than the more differentiated Cl^+ cells. The relationship between differentiation and neoplastic transformation can be investigated in part by studying the propensity toward neoplastic transformation of cells prepared from tissues at various stages of differentiation (Bruce and Ts'o, 1980). The skin fibroblasts of 5- to 8-month-old Syrian hamsters (young adults) and 20-month-old Syrian hamsters (aging) were established in culture. These cells, together with the 12-day-old embryonic fibroblasts, exhibited an inverse relationship between average maximum population doubling (PDL) and age of the donor: embryo cells, 20.3 PDL; 6-month-old adults, 17 PDL; and 20-month-old adults, 10.8 PDL. These cells were treated with MNNG or B[a]P, passaged *in vitro,* and analyzed for neoplasia-related phenotypic changes. All treated adult cell cultures after 20–30 PDL contained morphologically distinct cells, which continued to proliferate while the control cultures senesced. However, the treated adult cell cultures only infrequently exhibited Aga^+ properties, and appeared to enter a second crisis period, in contrast to the treated embryonic cells which became neoplastically transformed and exhibited the Aga^+ property. Thus, carcinogenic treatment of adult hamster skin fibroblasts clearly can disrupt the senescence pattern, but only in rare cases does this lead to neoplastic transformation. These preliminary investigations further suggest that an inverse relationship exists between *in vivo* cellular age (age of donor animal) and frequency of neoplastic transformation *in vitro.*

We may ask the question, would the neoplastic transformation of cells from a young embryo be both qualitatively and quantitatively different from that of cells of aged animals? To provide a cellular model to study the basic mechanism relating carcinogenesis to development, and finally, to aging, we have considered this developmental process of the cells in three stages:

A. Cells that have full potential to replicate and have little constraint on replication, such as cells from embryos that replicate rapidly and seem to be non-contact-inhibited (Nakano and Ts'o, 1981).

B. Cells that have replicating potential but are constrained by other biological factors such as cell–cell contact, as is expected of a differentiating tissue.

C. Cells that now have lost their reproductive capability and cease to divide, as in a terminally differentiated tissue.

It is now apparent that we can develop from the fibroblast system these three cell types in different stages of development in culture. We can ask whether the neoplastic transformation of these three different cell types will involve similar or different processes or mechanisms. Apparently, we have to block the differentiation pathway for the embryonic cells to maintain them in a state of continuing replication without constraint, to achieve a state of neoplasia. Obviously, we have to reactivate the dormant reproductive capabilities in senescent cells to allow a continuation of cell division and an escape of senescence. Experiments are now in progress to answer the above questions.

In conclusion, investigation of the basic mechanisms of *in vitro* neoplastic transformation will go on through both a "reductionalistic" approach and a "constructionalistic" approach. In the former approach, investigations will be made at the molecular level using that information to describe the properties of the hertiable changes of cells observed in culture. In the latter approach, different cell types (in our laboratory both fibroblasts and hemopoietic tissues are being studied) at different stages of development in animals will be investigated *in vitro* by cell biology and molecular biology techniques. In this manner we hope to understand the basic mechanisms of carcinogenesis in the animal by a series of *in vitro* studies on different cell types obtained at different developmental stages as the first approximation. The current approach can be demonstrated in Figs. 1 and 2. Figure 1 depicts the progression of neoplastic transformation indicating the strong influence of developmental stages. At certain experimental stages (Stage I in the diagram) the rate of progression is fast and the frequency of transformation is high. Under an identical perturbation at an initiation, the progression can be relatively longer and the frequency of transformation can be comparatively much lower in cells obtained at another developmental stage (Stage II in the diagram). Figure 2 depicts the developmental process of the entire animal (or man). Cell cultures for *in vitro* studies can be obtained from the animals at different experimental stages for continuing passaging and perturbation. The cellular responses of these cells in culture after different types of perturbation

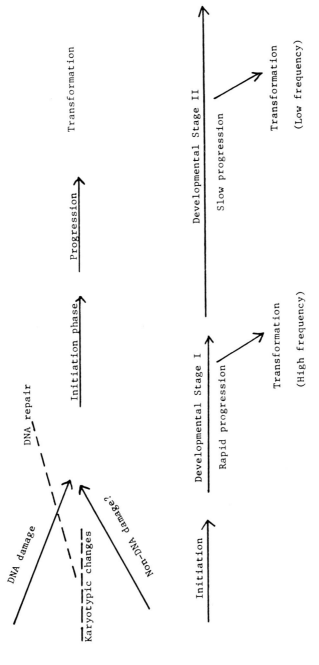

Fig. 1. The scheme of neoplastic transformation showing the influence of developmental stages.

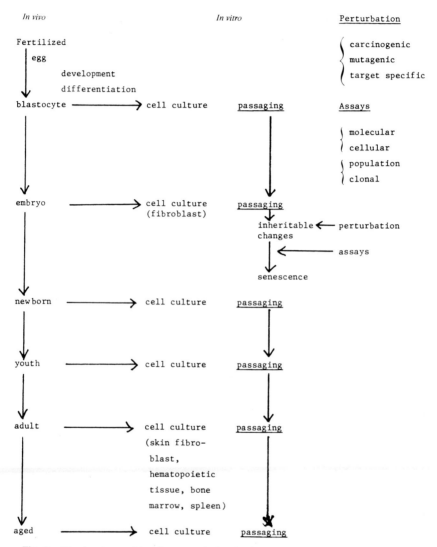

Fig. 2. The *in vivo* and *in vitro* correlation in the study of the developmental process of the entire animal.

can be assayed at the cell biology level or the molecular biology level. This experiment can be repeated for many cell types. Figure 2 provides the major strategy of the "constructionalistic" approach of trying to learn about the carcinogenesis mechanism at the cellular level and then the investigation extending to the whole animal.

Acknowledgments

This chapter is based on the results obtained from a collaborative effort of many scientists in the Division of Biophysics, School of Hygiene and Public Health, The Johns Hopkins University. Specifically, the contributions of the following colleagues are gratefully acknowledged: J. Carl Barrett, Sarah A. Bruce, Wai Nang Choy, Brian D. Crawford, Deborah L. Grady, Stanley Lin, David Morry, Robert K. Moyzis, Shuji Nakano, Masahide Takii, Takeki Tsutsui, and Maria Zajac. A critical reading of the manuscript by Khin Khin Gyi is also gratefully acknowledged.

References

Barrett, J. C., and Ts'o, P. O. P. (1978). *Proc. Natl. Acad. Sci. U.S.A.* **75**, 3297–3301.
Barrett, J. C., Crawford, B. D., Grady, Hester, D. L., Jones, P. A., Benedict, W. F., and Ts'o, P. O. P. (1977). *Cancer Res.* **37**, 3815–3823.
Barrett, J. C., Bias, N. E., and Ts'o, P. O. P. (1978a). *Mutation Res.* **50**, 121–136.
Barrett, J. C., Tsutsui, T., and Ts'o, P. O. P. (1978b). *Nature (London)* **274**, 229–232.
Barrett, J. C., Crawford, B. D., Mixter, L. O., Schechtman, L. M., Ts'o, P. O. P., and Pollack, R. (1979). *Cancer Res.* **39**, 1504–1510.
Barrett, J. C., Wong, A., and McLachlan, J. A. (1981a). *Science (Washington D.C.)* **212**, 1402–1404.
Barrett, J. C., Crawford, B. D., and Ts'o, P. O. P. (1981b). *In* "Advances in Modern Environmental Toxicology, Mammalian Cell Transformation by Chemical Carcinogenesis" (N. Mishra, V. Dunkel, and M. Mehlman, eds.), Vol. 1, pp. 467–501. Senate Press, Princeton, N.J.
Berwald, Y., and Sachs, L. (1963). *Nature (London)* **200**, 1182–1184.
Berwald, Y., and Sachs, L. (1965). *J. Natl. Canc. Inst.* **35**, 641–661.
Bruce, S. A., and Ts'o, P. O. P. (1980). *Eur. J. Cell Biol.* **22**, 552.
Crawford, B. D. (1981). Ph.D. Thesis, Johns Hopkins University.
DiPaolo, J. A., Donovan, P. J., and Nelson, R. (1969). *J. Natl. Cancer Inst.* **42**, 867–874.
DiPaolo, J. A., Nelson, P. J., and Nelson, R. (1969). *J. Natl. Cancer Inst.* **42**, 867–874.
DiPaolo, J. A., Nelson, R. L., and Donovan, P. J. (1971). *Cancer Res.* **31**, 3573–3583.
Foulds, L. (1954). *Cancer Res.* **14**, 327–339.
Foulds, L. (1969 and 1975). "Neoplastic Development," Vols. 1 and 2. Academic Press, London.
Lin, S. L., Takii, M., and Ts'o, P. O. P. (1982) *Radiat. Res.,* in press.
Morry, D. W. (1980). Ph.D. Thesis, Johns Hopkins University.

Nakano, S., and Ts'o, P. O. P. (1981). *Proc. Natl. Acad. Sci. U.S.A.* **78,** 4995–4999.

Nakano, S., Ueo, H., and Ts'o, P. O. P. (1982). Abstract, submitted to Am. Assoc. Cancer Res.

Tsutsui, T., Barrett, J. C., and Ts'o, P. O. P. (1979). *Cancer Res.* **39,** 2356–2365.

Zajac, M., and Ts'o, P. O. P. (1980) *Eur. J. Cell Biol.* **22,** 533.

19

Cell Population Studies during Epithelial Carcinogenesis

P. NETTESHEIM, G. R. BRASLAWSKY, V. E. STEELE, AND S. J. KENNEL

I. Introduction

Invasive cancer is the end product of a multiphasic cellular evolution which in humans and animals alike spans over months and years. Its induction phase, whether caused by single or multiple exposures to a carcinogen, may or may not be accompanied by measurable structural and biochemical changes, depending on the nature and severity of the insult. The cellular events triggered by and evolving from this insult during the ensuing months and years remain for the most part unnoticed. The purpose of our investigations is to map the development of neoplastic transformation during its "occult" phase. The model tissue in which we attempt to study neoplastic development is the mucosa of the conducting airways. The question to which we are attempting to obtain answers is: What phenotypic changes can be identified after the interaction of a carcinogen with the target cells has occurred that are characteristic for the cellular evolution of neoplastic disease?

Common to all full-fledged cancers is the breakdown of mechanisms that regulate normal growth and differentiation. The starting point of our investigations was the notion that early stages of this profound disruption of cell replication and differentiation may exist in the precursor cells destined to produce cancerous offspring, if we had means to detect them. Our approach was to examine *in vitro* alterations of growth behavior of tracheal epithelial cells exposed *in vivo* to carcinogen, with the expectation to detect qualitative as well as quantitative changes in growth capacity of cell populations undergoing neoplastic transformation (a process that we consider to develop over multiple cell generations).

What we intend to discuss in this chapter are results from three different phases of our work: (1) Alterations of growth capacity and escape from senescence or terminal differentiation are early events and markers of epithelial cells undergoing neoplastic transformation. These markers can be used to detect and quantitate different types of "carcinogen altered" cell populations and to analyze the dynamics of their evolution during the transformation process; (2) Shifts in modal distribution of DNA content commonly occur during the transition of cell populations from the preneoplastic to the neoplastic state; and (3) A cell surface antigen was found which reacts with several malignant epithelial cell lines of tracheal origin. The antigen also occurs on preneoplastic cells and may serve as a useful marker to study neoplastic development.

The emphasis in this discussion will be placed on those studies that are aimed at the analysis of neoplastic development as it occurs *in vivo;* tissue culture is used as a method of analyzing and quantitating the cellular events.

II. Alterations of *in Vitro* Growth Capacity—An Early Marker of Carcinogen-Altered Epithelial Cells Exposed *in Vivo* to Carcinogen

From the outset, it was essential to determine whether the neoplastic process, initiated *in vivo* in the tracheal epithelium, continues to develop when the carcinogen exposed epithelial cells are removed from the host and maintained in culture. If this occurred, then the *in vitro* analysis of developing preneoplastic and neoplastic cell populations during *in vivo* carcinogenesis would be feasible.

In a first series of studies (Marchok *et al.*, 1977, 1978), the epithelium of rat tracheas was exposed *in vivo* to known quantities of a carcinogenic polycyclic aromatic hydrocarbon utilizing the heterotopic tracheal transplant model (Kendrick *et al.*, 1974, Nettesheim *et al.*, 1977, Griesemer *et al.*, 1977). At the end of the exposure, the tracheas were removed from the hosts, cut into small pieces, and placed in culture under conditions that promote the outgrowth of the epithelium. These experiments showed that many epithelial cell cultures, derived from carcinogen exposed tracheas, differed in one fundamental aspect from epithelium of sham exposed tracheas: they were "immortal," i.e., many cultures escaped from senescence which most normal epithelial cells succumb to after 15–20 population doublings. Cell lines were established from these "carcinogen-altered" epithelial cells. When first tested for anchorage independent growth and oncogenicity in compatible hosts (Fig. 1), they were negative. However, after various lengths of time in culture, most of the cell lines became neoplastically transformed and gave rise to carcinomas upon inoculation into syngeneic recipients. These studies taught us two things: (1) Long before neoplastic (or transformed) cells develop in carcinogen-exposed epithelium, "carcinogen-altered" cells can be detected by their

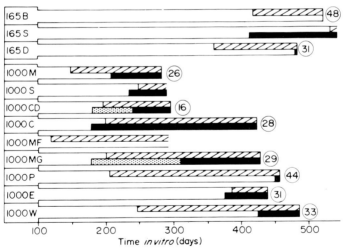

Fig. 1. Diagrammatic representation of time of appearance of growth in 0.33% agar (crosshatched areas) and tumorigenicity in the cell lines derived from DMBA-preexposed tracheas. Gray areas indicate when, upon inoculation into isogeneic hosts, the cell lines formed tumors that regressed or formed noninvasive keratinic cysts. Black areas indicate when cell lines formed invasive squamous cell carcinomas. Circled numbers are passage numbers at end of study. Numbers and letter on left are cell line designations. (From Marchok *et al.*, 1978.)

unlimited growth capacity. This is a fundamental biological change; the cells have escaped senescence. (2) The neoplastic process initiated *in vivo* continues to develop when such initiated tissues are placed *in vitro*. Since the immortalized cells are not neoplastic at early passages but become so at subsequent passages, we consider them to be preneoplastic, i.e., cells at an increased risk to become neoplastic. To put it another way, the carcinogen altered cells are the precursors of later developing neoplastic cells. Other investigators have also noticed marked changes in *in vitro* growth capacity during the transformation process in a variety of tissues. (Borland and Hard, 1974; Buoen *et al.,* 1975; Laerum and Rajewsky, 1975; Knowles and Franks, 1977).

In subsequent studies (Terzaghi and Nettesheim, 1979; Nettesheim *et al.,* 1982; Terzaghi *et al.,* 1982) attempts were made to analyze the observed phenomenon further and to quantitate the cell populations affected. The following questions were asked: (1) Are the carcinogen altered cells that can be recovered from carcinogen exposed tissues homogenous or heterogeneous populations, i.e., are different subclasses of carcinogen altered cells discernible? (2) Can they be quantitated? and (3) Do the population sizes change as a function of time after carcinogen exposure and as a function of carcinogen dose? A clonal assay was designed (Terzaghi and Nettesheim, 1979) for detection and enumeration of carcinogen-altered epithelial cells in order to study changes in the affected cell populations during tumor latency (or tumor induction time). This so-called epithelial focus assay (EF assay) is based on the earlier observation (Marchok *et al.,* 1977) that normal tracheal epithelium has only a very limited capacity to replicate *in vitro*. It takes advantage of the fact that after carcinogen exposure altered clonogenic cells develop in the epithelium which escape senescence.

At various times after exposure to the carcinogen, the epithelial lining of rat tracheas was removed and dispersed by enzymatic procedures and plated into culture dishes (Fig. 2). One month after plating, the number of proliferative epithelial foci was counted to obtain an estimate of the number of altered clonogenic units, called EFFU (epithelial focus forming units), in the recovered cell population. Under the conditions of the test, the existence of a proliferating epithelial focus (EF) at 1 month is already the first sign of the presence of an abnormally reproductive cell population. The EF are further examined for the degree of altered growth capacity by subculturing them. If an EF can be repeatedly subcultured, then it is designated an EF_s and the clonogenic unit from which it arose an $EFFU_s$. If the culture survives repeated subculturing and reaches cell line stage, it is tested for anchorage independent growth. If positive, the original EF from which the cell line is derived is designated $EF_{s,ag}+$ and the clono-

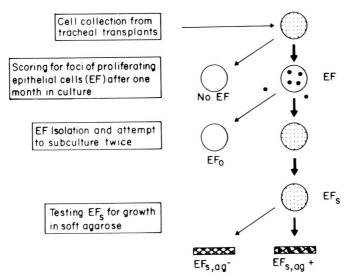

Fig. 2. Diagrammatic representation of sequential steps in the EF assay. Tracheas were exposed *in vivo* to 165 μg DMBA for 4 weeks, and cells were collected for *in vitro* culture immediately, 2, 4, or 8 months after exposure. Cells were then followed *in vitro* as diagrammed in order to score the number of epithelial cells per trachea with altered *in vitro* growth capacity (EF), to assess subculturability of isolated EF (EF$_s$), and to evaluate the capacity of EF$_s$ to grow in soft agarose (EF$_{s, ag+}$). (From Terzaghi and Nettesheim, 1979.)

genic unit from which the EF arose, EFFU$_{s,ag}$+. What the EF assay does is to enumerate the clonogenic units with altered growth capacity present in the exposed epithelium and to characterize these clonogenic units further by sequentially examining their progeny. Thus, based on the type of progeny they can generate, three abnormal types of clonogenic units can be distinguished in exposed tracheal epithelium: EFFU$_o$, EFFU$_{s,ag}$−, and EFFU$_{s,ag}$+ (The EFFU$_o$, as opposed to proliferative cells in unexposed adult rat tracheas, give rise to epithelial colonies which proliferate and expand for many weeks but they are not subculturable while epithelial colonies established from normal tracheas usually cease to proliferate after 2–3 weeks under the conditions of the EF assay). Data from one study using the EF assay are presented in Figs. 3 and 4. Epithelial cells were harvested from tracheas at various times after a brief exposure to carcinogen and the development of different types of carcinogen altered clonogenic units was monitored for 8 months. As is illustrated in Fig. 3, the number of tracheas containing altered clonogenic cells (EFFU) is roughly constant (80–90%) for at least 8 months after exposure. However, only about 40% of the tracheas contained EFFU$_s$ and only 15% contained

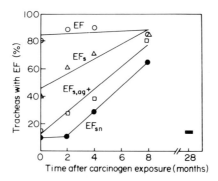

Fig. 3. Incidence of tracheas containing various types of "carcinogen-altered" cells as a function of time after carcinogen exposure. Carcinogen exposure was 165 μg of DMBA, delivered over 4 weeks. Abbreviations used are the same as those in the diagram of the EF assay (Fig. 2). EF_{sn}, cell populations obtained from subculturable EF, tumorigenic when injected into compatible hosts. Twenty tracheas per time point, ■, incidence of invasive and noninvasive carcinomas in 28 month tumor indication study. (From Nettesheim *et al.*, 1982.)

$EFFU_{s,ag}+$ immediately after exposure. During the subsequent exposure-free months, the proportion of tracheas containing these two types of abnormal clonogenic units steadily increased, reaching 70–80% at 8 months. The same trend was seen for tracheas harboring cells with oncogenic potential as measured by inoculation into compatible host animals. What is remarkable is that at the carcinogen dose used, only 10–15% of tracheas developed carcinomas when left intact in the host animals (Fig. 3). This is strong evidence indicating that only a fraction of the altered cells with neoplastic potential will ordinarily express that potential (unless permissive or promoting influences prevail; for further discussion of this observation, see Nettesheim *et al.*, 1982). Figure 4 summarizes data from the same experiment by displaying the shifts occurring within the various populations of altered clonogenic cells with time after exposure. The trends are essentially the same. At the end of exposure, all types of altered focus forming cells were present and with passage of time the proportion of subculturable and anchorage independent clonogenic units increased. The rate of the increase, particularly of the clonogenic units capable of producing anchorage independent progeny, was found to be carcinogen dose dependent (Terzaghi *et al.*, 1982). Detailed analyses of the potential and fate of these different focus forming units remain to be performed in the future. Two important aspects of these findings, which cannot be discussed here in all their implications, should be pointed out (for more complete presentation and discussion of these studies, see Nettesheim *et al.*, 1982): (1) After induction of the neoplastic process *in vivo*,

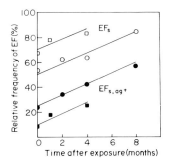

Fig. 4. Expansion of different carcinogen-altered cell populations as a function of time after cessation of carcinogen exposure. The data are from two separate experiments conducted more than 1 year apart. Carcinogen exposures are the same as those used in experiments summarized in Fig. 3. Data represent percentage of EF which are EF_s and percentage of EF_s which are $EF_{s, ag+}$. (From Nettesheim et al., 1982.)

the more severely altered clonogenic cells continue to increase in number for many months even though no further carcinogenic insults occur. (2) The continuous expansion of the severely altered cell compartments during the tumor latency period occurs not only in those tracheas that are developing tumors (after 18–28 months) but also in those that are not. This becomes apparent when comparing the number of tracheas developing tumors (10–15%) with the number of tracheas harboring clonogenic units with neoplastic potential ($EF_{s,ag}+$ and $EF_{s,n}$) in Fig. 3. This means that in the carcinogen exposed epithelium the number of clonogenic cells with neoplastic potential continues to increase even though this may not ever be overtly expressed in the form of a visible neoplasm during the lifetime of the animal. The key observation is that even at low carcinogen doses occult populations of cells endowed with neoplastic potential persist and expand.

III. Changes in DNA Content in Tracheal Epithelial Cell Populations during Neoplastic Development

We have searched for other quantifiable abnormalities in carcinogen altered cells. A number of epithelial cell populations derived from various *in vivo* and *in vitro* transformation studies were examined for changes in DNA content (Braslawsky et al., 1982a) as determined by incorporation of propidium iodide and quantitation of the dye–DNA complex using established methodologies of flow cytometry (Krishan, 1975). In four cases, measurements were made during the preneoplastic state as well as after conversion to the neoplastic state (see Table I). All of the cell lines had

TABLE I

Relative DNA Content of Transformed Tracheal Epthelial Cell Lines

Cell line	Passage level	Tumor-igenicity	Relative DNA content[a]
In vitro exposed MNNG			
2-10-1	48	+	6.0
	99	+	6.2
8-10-2	48	+	5.7
	77	+	5.9
8-1-2	7	−	6.3
	22	+	4.8
3F3	9	−	6.4
	32	+	3.9 . . . (6.1)
In vivo exposed DMBA			
1000W	8	−	5.0
	42	+	5.4
165D	9	−	3.3
	47	+	(3.3) . . . 5.9
165 (2-4) carcinoma	−	+	3.7
165 (3-5) carcinoma	−	+	6.5

[a] Peak channel number of the major G_1 peak of PI-stained cells using a Bio/Physics model 4801 (Ortho Instruments, Westwood, Mass.) flow cytometer. F-344 rat lymphocytes were used to standardize the instruments to channel #45 $\pm$ 3 channels for the G_1 peak. DNA content (triplicate experiments + SD) normalized against diploid rat lymphocyte DNA content. The numbers in parentheses indicate secondary or minor G_1 peaks (Braslawsky, 1982a).

hyperploid DNA values, as compared to freshly harvested rat tracheal epithelium or peripheral blood lymphocytes, regardless of which phase of neoplastic transformation they were in. Three of four cell lines showed a shift in the major DNA peak as they progressed from the preneoplastic to the neoplastic phase, suggesting the emergence of a new cell population. In the case of the cell line, 3F3, the new cell population had a modal G_1 DNA value of 3.9 as compared to that of the preneoplastic population of 6.4. A smaller subpopulation with a peak DNA value similar to that found during the preneoplastic phase persisted in the neoplastic population (Fig. 5). Cloning experiments confirmed the coexistence of two subpopulations in neoplastic phase 3F3 cell populations with different peak DNA values. In the case of cell line 165D (Fig. 6) conversion to the neoplastic state was associated with a shift of the G_1 peak to a higher value (from 3.3 to 5.9). However, a small subpopulation with the DNA value of the preneoplastic population again persisted into the neoplastic phase.

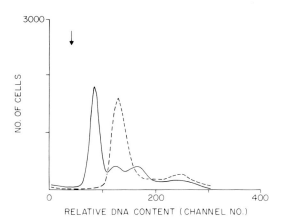

Fig. 5. DNA histogram of propidium iodide stained cells from cell line 3F3 at passage 7 (— — —) and passage 32 (———). Normal F-344 rat lymphocytes or freshly harvested tracheal epithelium established the diploid (G_1) peak (arrow). Nontumorigenic passage 7 shows 2 peaks, namely one at 6.4 c (G_1 peak) and one at 12.6 c (G_2 peak). Tumorigenic passage 32 shows 3 peaks namely at 3.9 c (G_1 peak), 6.0 c (G_1 peak) and 7.9 c (G_2 peak). (From Braslawsky et al., 1982a.)

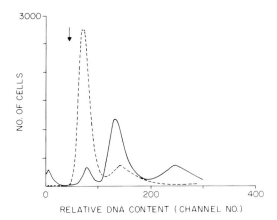

Fig. 6. DNA histogram of cell line 165D at passage 9 (— — —) and passage 47 (———). Non tumorigenic passage 9 shows a G_1 peak at 3.3 and a G_2 peak at 6.4. Tumorigenic passage 47 shows three peaks at 3.3 c, 5.9 c, and 11.9 c. (From Braslawsky et al., 1982a.)

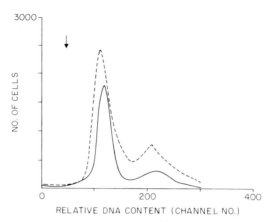

Fig. 7.   DNA histogram of cell line 1000W. Nontumorigenic passage 8 cells (— — —) show a G₁ peak at 5.0 c. Tumorigenic cells from passage 42 (———) show a G₁ peak at 5.4 c. (From Braslawsky et al., 1982a.)

Chromosomal analyses carried out on one of the cell lines before and after conversion to the transformed state supported the flow cytometry data, showing similar shifts in chromosome numbers. However, line 1000W indicates that changes in DNA content do not necessarily occur when a cell population progresses from the preneoplastic to the neoplastic phase (Fig. 7). We are currently conducting similar analyses of DNA profiles on carcinogen exposed primary cell cultures. In these studies, we have the opportunity to make DNA and chromosome measurements on primary epithelial cell cultures within a few weeks after they have been exposed to carcinogen. We know that as early as 2–3 weeks after carcinogen exposure, the growth rate of the exposed population is markedly increased over that of controls (Pai et al., 1982). This is the earliest sign of a carcinogen-induced effect, coinciding with the appearance of atypical epithelial foci which we have so far encountered.

IV. Tumor Associated Antigens in Preneoplastic and Neoplastic Tracheal Epithelial Cells

In the hope to develop a useful probe for the detection of transformed cells during the process of neoplastic development, a series of studies was conducted over the last several years aimed at identifying tumor associated antigens (Jamasbi and Nettesheim, 1977; Jamasbi et al., 1978; Braslawsky et al.,1981; Braslawsky et al., 1982b). The first indication that such antigens might occur rather commonly in chemically induced neoplasias of respiratory tract epithelium stemmed from tumor transplantation studies (Jamasbi and Nettesheim, 1977) in which induction of transplantation resistance was demonstrated by repeated transplantation of viable tumor cells (Table II). Subsequent studies have shown similar antigens appearing on respiratory tract epithelial cells transformed *in vitro* (Braslawsky *et al.*, 1981). In the course of these experiments, it was also demonstrated that appropriately immunized rats produce antibodies binding preferentially to the tumor cells used for immunization (Braslawsky *et al.*, 1981, 1982b) (Fig. 8). However, antisera not only reacted with the neoplastic epithelial cells used for immunization but also with antigens on other tracheal carcinoma cell lines (but not with normal liver, lung, kidney, brain, or spleen homogenates, or with primary cultures of freshly harvested tracheal epithelium). These results suggested

TABLE II

Demonstration of Cross-Reactivity among Rat Squamous Cell Carcinoma Tumor Lines as Determined by Induction of Transplantation Resistance

Recipients challenged with	Tumor takes in animals immunized against (%) [a]									
	BP_1	BP_2	BP_3	$DMBA_6$	MCA_7	Sarcoma	Fetal cells	Normal lung	Esophagus	Untreated
BP_1	0	60	100	90	60	90	90	90	ND[b]	100
BP_2	90	0	40	60	40	90	100	90	100	100
BP_3	100	40	0	60	40	ND	100	100	ND	100
$DMBA_6$	ND	20	40 ?[c]	0	0	0	10	60	ND	60
MCA_7	100	20	60	60	0	100	100	100	100	100
Sarcoma	100	100	90	60	90	0	100	90	ND	100

Note: Rats in each group were immunized against one tumor line and were challenged with $5 \times TD_{50}$ of the other tumor lines as well as the same line. Horizontally shaded squares indicate the existence of cross protection among the carcinoma lines and diagonally shaded squares indicate additional cross protection between $DMBA_6$ and sarcoma and between $DMBA_6$ and fetal antigens.

[a] 10 rats per group.

[b] Not done.

[c] Cross reactivity uncertain (Jamasbi and Nettesheim, 1977).

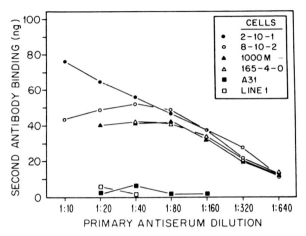

Fig. 8. Antibody binding activity of 2-10-1 immune rat serum for neoplastic rat tracheal epithelial cells (2-10-1, 8-10-2, 1000M, and 165-4-0), murine line 1 alveolar carcinoma cells, and murine A31 cell fibroblasts. Nonspecific binding was determined for each cell line by substituting normal F-344 rat serum for immune serum and was subtracted from the experimental results. (From Braslawsky *et al.*, 1982b.)

that the malignant tracheal cells have cell surface antigens that might serve as markers to trace the emergence of new cell populations during various stages of neoplastic development. However, the syngeneic immune response is complex and a major limitation of antisera is that one does not know against which one of potentially many antigenic determinants they are directed. Encouraged by the initial studies, we decided to develop monoclonal antibodies against the tumor associated antigens of one of the neoplastic tracheal cell lines. This was also an essential step in order to gain some understanding of what might be the basis of the cross-reactivity existing between different neoplastic cell lines. The results of five fusion experiments using syngeneic 2-10-1 immune spleen cells and murine myeloma cells are summarized in Table III. Spleen cells (10^8) were fused with myeloma cells (10^7) using polyethylene glycol 1640. After overnight incubation in complete growth medium, DME-20, the cells were distributed in microtiter plates containing selection medium (HAT medium) which allows only survival of hybridoma cells. During the second week of incubation the cultures were shifted to DME-20 and the culture supernatants were screened for antibody to 2-10-1. Positive hybrid cultures were selected, propagated, rescreened for antibody, and cloned. To date, four hybrid clones with antibodies against the malignant tracheal cell line 2-10-1 have been established. Serological recognition of cell surface antigens was achieved with the use of two different approaches: by

TABLE III

Hybridoma Production from Fusion with F-344 Tumor Immune Rat Spleen Cells to Murine P3 × 63Ag8 Parent (BALB/c) Myeloma Cells

	Transplantation resistant[a]	Immunized[b]	Tumor bearing[c]
Number of fusions	2	1	2
Hybridomas produced	1218	846	2076
Hybridoma-antibody positive			
First screen	14	9	0
Second screen	3	2	—

[a] Animals were resistant to challenge with 1×10^6 viable 2-10-1 cells. Transplantation-resistant rats were boosted with 1×10^7 X-irradiated (10,000 R) 2-10-1 cells (propagaged in 2% syngeneic rat serum) 4 days before fusion.

[b] Rats were immunized by 6 weekly injections of X-irradiated 2-10-1 cells, i.p. Cells were fused 4 days after last injection.

[c] Animals were inoculated with 1×10^6 viable 2-10-1 cells, i.m. One animal was sacrificed before the appearance of palpable tumor, the other animal sacrificed bearing a large tumor mass (Braslawsky et al., in preparation).

assessing the average level of antigen expression by a cell population and by measuring expression and density of antigen on individual cells within a population. The radiolabeled antibody binding test (ABT) is used to quantitate the amount of tumor associated antigen on various neoplastic and preneoplastic cell populations and to determine when during the process of neoplastic transformation these antigenic determinants appear. A fluorescent antibody binding test combined with flow cytometry is used to quantitate the amount of antigen on individual cells within the population as well as to enumerate the percentage of positive cells. The possibility exists in the future to sort cells on the basis of antigen content (or DNA content) in order to determine their role in neoplastic development. Table IV summarizes the binding activity of four monoclonal antibodies using the ABT. All four clones make antibodies against 2-10-1 but these antibodies also recognize an antigenic determinant on at least one other malignant tracheal cell line namely 1000M. They are not reactive, however, with line 1 cells (a mouse lung carcinoma). Figure 9 shows the flow cytometry data with antibodies from the same four hybridomas against the 2-10-1 and another malignant tracheal cell line, namely 8-10-2. The antibodies clearly recognize determinants on many of the 2-10-1 cells, but also on some of the 8-10-2 cells. Thus, together both studies suggest that at least three of the malignant tracheal cell lines share the same antigenic determinant.

We have since improved our techniques and find that almost 90% of the

TABLE IV

Summary of Binding Specificities of Hybridoma Antibodies

Target cells	Antibody source[a]	cpm	Binding ratio[b]
2-10-1	140-3C5	4391	5.85
	139-5E4	6376	8.49
	138-5H3(A)	7020	9.35
	140-5H3(B)	2695	3.59
100M	140-3C5	2352	3.13
	139-5E4	3376	4.50
	138-5H3(A)	3614	4.81
	140-5H3(B)	3066	4.08
Line 1	140-3C5	705	0.94
	140-5H3(A)	877	1.17

[a] Supernatants from cloned hybridoma cultures were precipitated and concentrated to approximately 1/25 the original volume with 50% saturated ammonium sulfate.

[b] Binding ratio: cell bound hybridoma antibody (cpm) divided by background binding (cpm). Background binding was determined using antifibrinogen monoclonal antibodies (Braslawsky et al., in preparation).

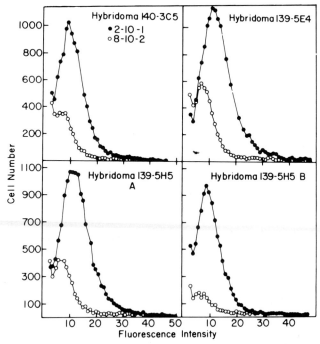

Fig. 9. Binding of monoclonal antibodies to cells from two malignant tracheal cell lines. Cells were stained by the fluorescent ABT using monoclonal antibody to 2-10-1 cells. Four monoclonal antibodies obtained from 50% ammonium sulfate precipitates of twice cloned rat–mouse hybrid cells were bound to either 2-10-1 (●) or 8-10-2 (○) cells. (From Braslawsky et al., in preparation.)

2-10-1 cells react with the antibodies directed against them and that cells from normal primary tracheal cultures may show a very low level of reactivity. Most recently, we have used the antisera as well as the hybridoma antibodies to determine whether the cell lines exhibit the antigenic determinant also during the preneoplastic phase, and have found that all those lines that are positive during the malignant phase are also positive during the premalignant phase. Thus, it seems that this antigen appears early during the transformation process. It will be necessary to go back to the early carcinogen-altered cells constituting the atypical epithelial foci in the primary cultures to determine when the antigen is first exhibited on these cells.

V. Summary

An assay was designed (EF assay) to analyze cell population changes in respiratory tract epithelium occurring *in vivo* during neoplastic development. The principal of this approach is based on the fact that carcinogen-exposed epithelial cells acquire different types of growth alterations which are expressed when the cells are placed in culture. As a function of time after exposure, cells appear which increasingly lose their normal growth restrictions. We are thus able to identify the progenitors of ultimate neoplastic cells in carcinogen-exposed epithelium at different stages of neoplastic transformation. For many months after the carcinogenic insult some of the "preneoplastic" cell populations increase in size. The data suggest that *in vivo* only a fraction of carcinogen altered cells may express their neoplastic potential fully. It appears that for long periods of time after carcinogen exposure, a spectrum of "carcinogen-altered" cells may persist undetected in the tissue, with different types and degrees of altered growth capacity and at increased risk to become neoplastic. Under what circumstances these cells will express their hidden neoplastic potential is uncertain. Proliferative or promotional stimuli may trigger expression.

Studies on the DNA content of preneoplastic cell populations and their malignant offspring suggest that the transition from the preneoplastic to the neoplastic state is often associated with changes in DNA content. Sometimes subpopulations of cells with different modal DNA distributions coexist in neoplastic cell cultures with one having the same DNA content as that of the preneoplastic population.

An antigenic marker has been found on neoplastic tracheal epithelial cells. Monoclonal antibody studies suggest that the same antigenic determinant may occur on cell surfaces of many tracheal carcinoma cells regardless of the transforming agent or the mode of transformation (*in vivo* or *in vitro*). The antigen was also found on preneoplastic cells and at barely detectable levels on normal tracheal epithelial cells. It is hoped that this antigen will be useful as a probe to study the cellular events during the process of neoplastic development.

References

Borland, R., and Hard, G. C. (1974). Early appearance of transformed cells from the kidneys of rats treated with a single carcinogenic dose of dimethylnitrosamine (DMN) detected by culture *in vitro*. *Eur. J. Cancer* **10**, 177–184.

Braslawsky, G. R., Steele, V. E., Kennel, S. J., and Nettesheim, P. (1981). Syngeneic immune response to rat tracheal epithelial cells transformed *in vitro* by *N*-methyl-*N*-nitro-*N*-nitrosoguanidine. *Br. J. Cancer,* **44**, 247–257.

Braslawsky, G. R., Flynn, K., Steele, V. E., and Nettesheim, P. (1982a). Changes in DNA content of rat tracheal epithelial cells during neoplastic progression *in vitro*. *Carcinogenesis* (submitted).

Braslawsky, G. R. Kennel, S. J., Steele, V. E. and Nettesheim, P. (1982b). Detection of tumor antigens by syngeneic antiserum on *in vitro* transformed tracheal epithelial cell line 2-10-1. *Int. J. Cancer* (submitted).

Braslawsky, G. R., Steele, V. E., Kennel, S. J., and Nettesheim, P. Binding of monoclonal antibody to tumorigenic and nontumorigenic phases of tracheal epithelial cell lines transformed *in vitro*. (in preparation).

Buoen, L. C., Brand, J., and Brand, K. G. (1975). Foreign-body tumorigenesis: *In vitro* isolation and expansion of preneoplastic clonal cell populations. *J. Natl. Cancer Inst.* **55**, 721–727.

Griesemer, R. A., Nettesheim, P., Martin, D. H., and Caton, J. E., Jr. (1977). Quantitative exposure of grafted rat tracheas to 7,12-dimethylbenz[*a*]anthracene. *Cancer Res.* **37**, 1266–1271.

Jamasbi, R. J., and Nettesheim, P. (1977). Demonstration of cross-reacting tumor rejection antigens in chemically induced respiratory tract carcinomas in rats. *Cancer Res.* **37**, 4059–4063.

Jamasbi, R. J., Nettesheim, P., and Kennel, S. J. (1978). Demonstration of cellular and humoral immunity to transplantable carcinomas derived from the respiratory tract of rats. *Cancer Res.* **38**, 261–267.

Kendrick, J., Nettesheim, P., and Hammons, A. S. (1974). Tumor induction in tracheal grafts: a new experimental model for respiratory carcinogenesis studies. *J. Natl. Cancer Inst.* **52**, 1317–1325.

Knowles, M. A., and Franks, L. M. (1977). Stages in neoplastic transformation of adult epithelial cells by 7,12-dimethylbenz[*a*]anthracene *in vitro*. *Cancer Res.* **37**, 3917–3924.

Krishan, A. (1975). Rapid flow cytofluorometric analysis of mammalian cell cycle by propidium iodide staining. *J. Cell Biol.* **66**, 181–193.

Laerum, O. D., and Rajewsky, M. F. (1975). Neoplastic transformation of fetal rat brain cells in culture after exposure to ethylnitrosourea *in vivo*. *J. Natl. Cancer Inst.* **55**, 1177–1187.

Marchok, A. C., Rhoton, J. C., Griesemer, R. A., and Nettesheim, P. (1977). Increased *in vitro* growth capacity of tracheal epithelium exposed *in vivo* to 7,12-dimethylbenz[*a*]anthracene. *Cancer Res.* **37**, 1811–1821.

Marchok, A. C., Rhoton, J. C., and Nettesheim, P. (1978). *In vitro* development of onco-genicity in cell lines established from tracheal epithelium preexposed *in vivo* to 7,12-dimethylbenz[*a*]anthracene. *Cancer Res.* **38,** 2030–2037.

Nettesheim, P., Griesemer, R. A., Martin, D. H., and Caton, J. E., Jr. (1977). Induction of preneoplastic and neoplastic lesions in grafted rat tracheas continuously exposed to benzo[*a*]pyrene. *Cancer Res.* **37,** 1272–1278.

Nettesheim, P., Terzaghi, M., and Klein-Szanto, A. J. P. (1982). Development and progres-sion of neoplastic disease. Morphologic and cell culture studies with airway epitheli-um. *In* "Mechanisms of Chemical Carcinogenesis" (C. C. Harris, ed.), Liss, New York. Keystone Conference, March 1981.

Pai, S. B., Steele, V. E., and Nettesheim, P. (1982). Quantitation of early cellular events during neoplastic transformation of tracheal epithelial cell cultures. *Carcinogenesis* (submitted).

Terzaghi, M., and Nettesheim, P. (1979). Dynamics of neoplastic development in carcinogen exposed tracheal mucosa. *Cancer Res.* **39,** 4003–4010.

Terzaghi, M., Nettesheim, P., and Riester, L. (1982). Effect of carcinogen dose on the dynamics of neoplastic development in rat tracheal epithelium. *Cancer Res.* (submit-ted).

20

Expression of Endogenous Oncogenes in Tumor Cells

U. G. ROVIGATTI, C. E. ROGLER, B. G. NEEL,
W. S. HAYWARD, AND S. M. ASTRIN

I. Introduction

This chapter will deal with two closely related topics. First, we will discuss the promoter insertion mechanism of viral oncogenesis, in which avian leukosis virus (ALV) has been shown to cause tumors in chickens by activating a cellular gene, the c-*myc* gene. Our second topic will be the expression of the human c-*myc* gene in cells of human lymphomas and leukemias.

When the avian leukosis viruses RAV-1 or RAV-2 are injected into day-old chicks, they cause bursal lymphomas 4–12 months after injection (Purchase and Burmester, 1978). These tumors metastasize to the liver, spleen, and/or kidney, killing the bird. There are a number of reasons why oncogenesis by the ALVs is probably different from the mechanism(s) employed by the acute oncogenic retroviruses such as Rous sarcoma virus (RSV) and avian myeloblastosis virus (AMV). The acute viruses cause tumor formation 2–3 weeks after injection of susceptible animals, transform appropriate target cells in culture, often have a single target tissue for tumor formation, and produce nonclonal tumors (Fishinger, 1979). These properties are explained by the fact that each of the acute viruses possesses a unique oncogene, a gene that causes neoplastic transformation, as demonstrated by the use of transformation defective mutants and temperature sensitive mutants (Weiss *et al.*, 1982). Thus, each infected cell can become transformed and contribute to the tumor mass. The ALVs, on the other hand, have a latent period of several months, have not been observed to transform cells in culture, are multipotent, producing occasional sarcomas and nephroblastomas as well as bursal lymphomas, produce clonal tumors, and do not appear to encode an oncogene in their genome. How then do these viruses cause malignant transformation of bursal cells?

We have recently documented three properties of ALV-induced lymphomas in the chicken: (1) the ALV provirus is integrated in nonrandom sites in the tumors and at least four common sites can be demonstrated using restriction endonuclease cleaved tumor DNA and appropriate probes; (2) new cellular transcripts, covalently linked to viral sequences, are present in the tumors; (3) in a majority of the lymphomas a cellular oncogene is expressed at a very high level (30- to 100-fold elevation as compared to nontumor cells). This endogenous oncogene is homologous to the transforming gene present in myelocytomatosis virus 29 (MC29) and it has been called c-*myc*. We have therefore proposed that the infecting ALV activates the transcription of c-*myc* by integrating next to it and providing a strong upstream promoter (the viral LTR). We have termed this mechanism oncogenesis by promoter insertion (Neel *et al.*, 1981; Hayward *et al.*, 1981). Since retroviruses integrate into the host genome without apparent specificity, ALV integration adjacent to the c-*myc* gene is probably a rare event. Thus, the tumors are clonal and there is a long latent period for tumor induction. Furthermore, we have recently analyzed the structures of the ALV proviruses integrated next to c-*myc* by cloning two junction fragments, corresponding to two out of four common regions of integration (Neel *et al.*, in preparation). These clones have been used for restriction enzyme analysis of 36 B cell lymphomas. The detailed analysis of these tumors is presented elsewhere (Astrin *et al.*, in preparation).

II. Results

A. Chicken B Cell Lymphomas

Here, we will illustrate the strategy that we have utilized in the restriction enzyme analysis and we will summarize the results obtained thus far.

Figure 1 shows a diagram of an ALV provirus with flanking cellular sequences and with the *Eco*RI restriction sites indicated. *Eco*RI cuts the ALV provirus four times and most importantly, it cuts inside the U3 sequences present in the LTRs at both ends of the provirus. These properties of the ALV allowed us to utilize the *Eco*RI digestion of tumor DNAs as a diagnostic test for ALV integration next to the c-*myc* gene. Such an event would create a new *Eco*RI restriction site next to c-*myc*. The resulting new *Eco*RI fragments obtained should contain both cellular sequences (c-*myc*, detected by myc probes) and viral U5 sequences (see Fig. 1).

As previously reported and shown in the leftmost lane of Fig. 2, normal cell DNA digested with *Eco*RI and analyzed by Southern blot yields a band of about 14 kb which hybridizes to a c-*myc* probe. In addition to this normal band, the four tumor sample DNAs also yield an extra band of MW less than 14 kb. Furthermore, in each case this new band is also detected by hybridization with a probe specific for viral U5 sequences (data not shown). We have extended this analysis to several ALV induced B cell lymphomas and we have found that in 30 out of 36 lymphomas an extra band is detected by *myc* probes. In each case, the extra *Eco*RI band is also detected by a viral U5 probe. Thus in 83% of the tumors, viral sequences are integrated adjacent to the c-*myc* gene. The presence of both the 14 kb band and a new smaller band in the tumors is explained by the fact that only one of the two copies of the c-*myc* gene present in the diploid genome is likely to be activated by promoter insertion, the other copy remaining unaltered. Of course, the phenotype induced by turning on c-*myc* expression is dominant.

We have found a few exceptions to the above pattern: (1) In tumor sample 22L (liver metastasis), two new bands are detected by *myc* probes

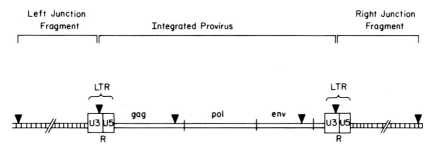

Fig. 1. Structure of the ALV provirus and the flanking cellular sequences. The arrows ▼ indicate *Eco*RI restriction sites. Notice the *Eco*RI cuts inside the LTRs thus leaving a small viral sequence attached to the right and left junction fragments. LTR, large terminal repeat; U3, unique 3′ sequence; U5, unique 5′ sequence; R, a sequence of approximately 20 nucleotides, which is present in viral RNA twice, once at the 3′ end and once at the 5′ end. (This sequence is contained within the probe we have designated as U5.)

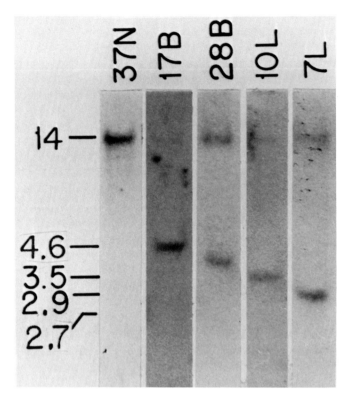

Fig. 2. Analysis of c-*myc* sequences present in normal and tumor cell DNA. Cellular DNA has been digested with *Eco*RI, and Southern blot analysis has been performed as previously described (Neel *et al.,* 1981; Hayward *et al.,* 1981; Astrin *et al.,* in preparation). Hybridization is to a radiolabeled c-*myc* probe. 37N is DNA from a normal bursa, 17B and 28B are two bursal lymphomas, and 10L and 7L are two liver metastases of different lymphomas. Notice that a common band corresponding to the normal DNA band is present at MW 14 kb. New bands corresponding to different integration sites (see Fig. 3) are present in each tumor sample.

after *Eco*RI digestion. This datum is probably best explained by the presence of two different clones of transformed cells in the liver. (2) In the lymphoma cell line RP9, the extra band detected by *myc* probes is not detected with the U5 probe. This situation is best explained by the integration next to c-*myc* of a defective provirus, missing the 3′ portion of the genome but still retaining *Eco*RI restriction sites. Or, alternatively, the ALV provirus may be integrated at the opposite end (3′) of c-*myc*. Preliminary data on the transcripts present in RP9 favor the first hypothesis. (3) In six of the 36 B cell lymphomas that have been analyzed, no new bands are detected by *myc* probes. In two of these cases, an RNA species has been detected that appears to contain viral U5 sequences as well as cellu-

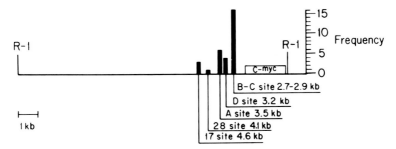

Fig. 3. Integration events adjacent to c-*myc* which result in production of a B cell lymphoma. The frequency of integration events is indicated in the abscissa, and the distance of the ALV integration site from the *Eco*RI site to the right of c-*myc* is indicated in the ordinate. This distance has been calculated from Southern blots similar to those shown in Fig. 2.

lar sequences. In all of these six cases, it is possible that new transcripts coding for different or unknown oncogene proteins are present.

As Fig. 3 shows, ALV proviral integration events cluster in five different regions to the left side of c-*myc*. These regions correspond to DNA stretches of 50 to 200 nucleotides into which proviruses integrate at different frequencies. All the integration regions lie in an area of 2 kb in front of the c-*myc* gene. The different features of these regions are presently being studied by sequence analysis (G. Gasic, personal communication).

We have also analyzed the sizes of the proviral inserts in 10 of the tumors. The sizes range from 0.4 to 7.4 kb. Since the size of an intact ALV provirus is 7.9 kb, it is evident that the proviruses integrated next to *myc* are defective. Preliminary data are consistent with the idea that those proviruses are defective in the 5' region of their genome, since they are missing a SacI site located adjacent to the 5' LTR (data not shown). We are presently studying the structure of these deleted proviruses in order to understand how their defectiveness relates to downstream transcription of c-*myc*.

B. Human Leukemias and Lymphomas

Activation of c-*myc* by promoter insertion in B cell lymphomas is the first example of tumorigenesis associated with a highly elevated expression of a cellular oncogene. Recently we have begun to look at oncogene expression in human tumors. We have undertaken an analysis of *myc* gene expression in human leukemias and lymphomas. Preliminary data from this analysis are presented here.

Our choice of the *myc* gene and our selection of the type of human tumor to analyze were based on the following factors: (1) the results obtained in our animal model system; (2) the possibility of obtaining relatively pure tumor cell populations from leukemic peripheral blood samples (Greaves *et al.*, 1980); (3) the fact that different precursor cell populations can be characterized by conventional staining techniques and also by using specific monoclonal antibodies (cell sorter analysis) (Haynes, 1981); and (4) the observation that several types of human lymphomas and acute and chronic leukemias are associated with nonrandom chromosome abnormalities (Rowley, 1980).

Since cellular oncogenes appear to be highly conserved in vertebrate genomes throughout evolution, we expected to find a human endogenous oncogene analogous to the c-*myc* gene present in chicken cells. Preliminary evidence indicates that this is in fact the case. We have recently isolated, from a human recombinant DNA library, a clone containing sequences homologous to a portion of the viral *myc* gene (B. G. Neel, unpublished observations).

We have, therefore, analyzed human c-*myc* gene expression using three different probes: (1) the chicken c-*myc* gene, which has been cloned from two B cell lymphomas (clones BN1 and CR1, from tumors 7 and 10, respectively). In addition to the cellular *myc* sequences, these clones also contain a portion of the right viral LTR; (2) the v-*myc* gene, which has been cloned from MC29 virus transformed quail cells by T. Papas and collaborators (Lautenberger *et al.*, 1981); (3) HM-10, a clone containing at least a portion of the human c-*myc* gene. The three probes give identical results in "dot blot" experiments in which serial twofold dilutions of cellular RNAs were spotted into nitrocellulose paper and hybridized to radiolabeled probe (Thomas, 1980).

DNA and RNA samples were prepared from patients and normal donors. A representative result is shown in Fig. 4. In this case, total nucleic acids from peripheral blood leukocytes from a normal individual have been extracted, DNA and RNA separated in CsCl gradients, and "dot blots" prepared and hybridized with the v-*myc* probe. It is clear that the signal in the total nucleic acids (lane A) is due to the presence of DNA, since the DNA fraction (lane C) is positive whereas the RNA fraction (lane B) is negative. This result was expected, since the human genome contains a gene which is homologous to v-*myc*.

It is also evident that transcripts of the human c-*myc* gene are almost completely absent from the RNA of normal leukocytes (the film was exposed for two weeks). Figure 5 shows a similar hybridization with eight other samples of RNA extracted from leukocytes from eight normal individuals. Transcripts of the human c-*myc* gene seem to be completely undetectable in these samples (the largest amount of RNA analyzed was 1 μg). On the other hand, the same probes give a strong signal when hybrid-

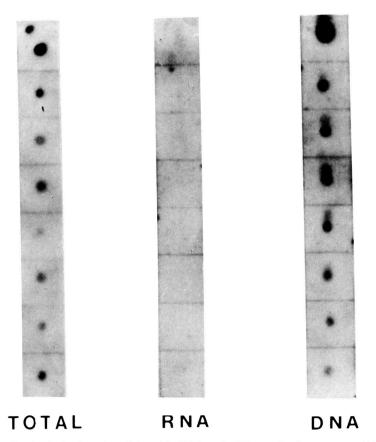

TOTAL   RNA   DNA

Fig. 4. Analysis of total nucleic acids, RNA, and DNA samples from a normal blood donor. "Dot blot" analysis has been performed as described by Thomas (1980). The amount of nucleic acid in the uppermost sample was always 1 μg and serial twofold dilutions were then spotted into the paper. The probe utilized was the v-*myc* clone kindly provided by T. Papas (Lautenberger *et al.*, 1981).

ized with total RNA extracted from tumor samples (leukemias, lymphomas), as shown in Fig. 6. Six out of ten samples analyzed were positive (lowest RNA levels still showing a positive signal range between 5 and 50 ng). The positive samples consist of one out of four samples from chronic lymphatic leukemias, two out of three from non-Hodgkin's lymphomas, and three out of three from acute lymphatic leukemias.

For one of the ALL samples (#3), we have performed two additional controls. In order to rule out the possibility that expression of c-*myc* was a polymorphic phenotype occurring in certain families and not linked to the disease, we have analyzed RNA samples extracted from peripheral blood leukocytes from the family of #3. The controls of Fig. 5, numbers 5

NORMAL

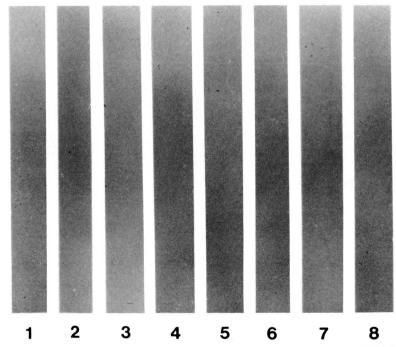

Fig. 5. Analysis of *myc* RNA expression in peripheral blood leukocytes (PBL) from normal donors. The samples were blotted and hybridized as described in Fig. 4. The amount of RNA in the uppermost sample was 0.5 μg. Samples 5 to 8 correspond to the family of ALL #3 (see Fig. 6).

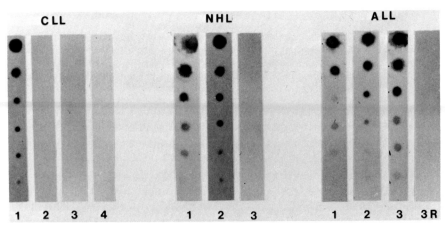

Fig. 6. Analysis of c-*myc* expression in total RNA from different leukemias and lymphomas. "Dot blot" analysis was performed as described in Fig. 4. The uppermost sample was in every case 1 μg of RNA. The hybridizing probe was v-*myc* as described in Fig. 5. Samples ALL #3 and ALL #3R correspond to the same ALL patient at diagnosis and after chemotherapy and remission, respectively.

to 8, clearly show that both parents plus two brothers of the ALL patient do not express high levels of *myc* transcripts. Furthermore, an RNA sample extracted from the same ALL patient after remission induced by chemotherapy also shows that the hybridization signal is now totally absent (Fig. 6, samples ALL #3 and #3R). Presumably, leukemia cells have been eliminated from the peripheral blood in the course of chemotherapy and only a residual population of normal leukocytes remains (white cell counts dropped from 75×10^6 per mm^3 down to 3×10^6 per mm^3).

III. Discussion

We have recently shown that in B cell lymphomas induced by ALV, the expression of an endogenous oncogene, c-*myc*, is highly enhanced (30- to 100-fold) by the integration of the ALV provirus next to the c-*myc* gene. This new mechanism of oncogenesis has been termed promoter insertion, since the ALV provirus supplies a new promoter for transcription of the adjacent cellular sequences (Neel *et al.*, 1981; Hayward *et al.*, 1981; Astrin *et al.*, in preparation). In this chapter, we have reported some studies on the ALV integration sites and the structure of the proviruses integrated next to c-*myc* in the chicken lymphomas. We have also described preliminary results on the expression of a similar oncogene, the human c-*myc* gene, in human lymphomas and leukemias.

Endogenous oncogene expression has recently been associated with both *in vivo* tumorigenesis (Hayward *et al.*, 1981; Astrin *et al.*, in preparation; Payne *et al.*, 1981) and with the capability for unlimited proliferation *in vitro* (Scolnick *et al.*, 1981). Furthermore, the presence of a viral promoter (the MuLV LTR) has also been associated with an enhanced efficiency of malignant transformation after transfection of the endogenous oncogene c-*mos* into NIH-3T3 cells. On the other hand, Cooper and Neiman (1981) have recently reported that although they find promoter insertion and c-*myc* activation in B cell lymphomas, neither ALV nor chicken c-*myc* sequences are present in NIH-3T3 cells transformed by transfection with DNA from the tumors. These results seem to indicate that ALV integration next to c-*myc* does not play an essential role in the transformation of NIH-3T3 cells by transfection. However, NIH-3T3 cells can be transformed by transfection with MC29 transformed cell DNA and MC29 virus can be rescued from the transfected clones (Copeland and Cooper, 1980). A possible interpretation of the above observations is that the NIH-3T3 transfection assay detects a secondary event either related or unrelated to ALV integration next to c-*myc*. For example, NIH-3T3 cells might be at a different stage in a multistep process leading to neoplastic transformation and for this reason they would require a different genetic event in order to be transformed. In this respect, it is interesting to note that we have detected transcripts of the endogenous c-*myc* gene in NIH-3T3 cells (unpublished results).

In the case of the human peripheral blood leukocytes (PBL), our preliminary results indicate that the expression of the human c-*myc* gene is also enhanced severalfold in some of the (human) leukemias and lymphomas, as compared to the expression in PBL from normal blood donors. We have not calculated the exact copy number of the *myc* RNA transcripts present in normal versus leukemic PBL. However, by comparing similar amounts of RNAs on "dot blots," the elevation in some of the leukemic samples seems to be at least 20-fold. In control experiments, we have shown that small amounts of DNA contamination can impair our analysis. However, RNA purification through CsCl gradients effectively eliminates all DNA contamination.

There are at least three possible explanations for the elevated expression of c-*myc* sequences in human leukemias and lymphomas: (1) c-*myc* expression may be associated with a particular phenotype, being expressed only in certain lineages and/or stages of differentiation, but it may be completely unrelated to the onset and maintenance of the neoplastic state; (2) c-*myc* activation may be associated with cell proliferation, but may not itself be the trigger to neoplastic transformation; (3) c-*myc* activation may actually be the trigger to neoplastic transformation; that is, the oncogenic event may be activation of the *myc* gene, which in turn causes cell transformation.

While it is difficult to completely rule out the possibilities indicated in point (1), there is some evidence indicating that they are unlikely. So far, we have detected c-*myc* expression in different leukemias and lymphomas which appear to possess unrelated differentiation markers. For example, we have seen *myc* expression in B, T, and null cell leukemias as well as in non-Hodgkin's lymphomas. It seems unlikely, although not impossible, that the same differentiation specific marker is present in distant or unrelated cell types. It is known that other sequences are expressed only in leukemias or are induced after viral transformation. For example, Gianni *et al.* (1978) have observed an enhancement of globin sequence expression in certain human leukemias. Certainly, the oncogene we are studying is quite different from globin genes, since its homologue in the avian species has been shown to be responsible for induction not only of acute leukemias, but also of solid tumors, like carcinomas and sarcomas (Beard, 1980). Moreover, Ramsay *et al.* (1980) have recently shown that mutants of MC29 defective for transformation of macrophages are mutated in the *myc* portion of the viral genome, thus showing that the v-*myc* gene is actually responsible for macrophage transformation *in vitro*. Thus it seems possible that the elevated expression of the *myc* gene in leukemic cells and lymphomas is related directly to the transformed state of the cells. Whether the oncogenic event is actually activation of the *myc* gene remains to be determined.

References

Astrin, S. M., Rovigatti, U. R., Rogler, C. E., Skalka, A. M., Neel, B. G., and Hayward, W. S. Viral oncogenesis by promoter insertion: Avian leukosis virus DNA is integrated next to the cellular *myc* gene in 83% of virally induced lymphomas. (in preparation).

Beard, J. W. (1980). Biology of avian oncornoviruses. *In* "Viral Oncology" (G. Klein, ed.) pp. 55–87, Raven, New York.

Cooper, G. M., and Neiman, P. E. (1981). Two distinct candidate transforming genes of lymphoid leukosis virus-induced neoplasms. *Nature (London)* **292**, 857–858.

Copeland, N. G., and Cooper, G. M. (1980). Transfection by DNAs of avian erythroblastosis virus and avian myelocytomatosis virus stain MC29. *J. Virol.* **33**, 1199–1202.

Fishinger, P. J. (1979). Type C RNA transforming viruses. *In* "Molecular Biology of RNA Tumor Viruses" (J. P. Stephenson, ed.) pp. 163–198, Academic Press, New York.

Gianni, A. M., Della Fevera, R., Polli, E., Merisio, I., Giglioni, B., Corri, P., and Ottolenghi, S. (1978). Globin RNA sequences in human leukemic peripheral blood. *Nature (London)* **274**, 610–612.

Greaves, M. F., Hebeshaw, J. A., and Stansfeld, A. G. (1980). Lymphoproliferative disorders. *In* "Atlas of Blood Cells' Function and Pathology" (D. Zucker-Franklin, M. F. Greaves, C. E. Grossi, and A. M. Marmont, eds.) pp. 409–524, Ermes Ed., Milano.

Haynes, B. F. (1981). Human T lymphocyte antigens as defined by monoclonal antibodies. *Immunol. Rev.* **57**: 127–160.

Hayward, W. S., Neel, B. G., and Astrin, S. M. (1981). Activation of a cellular *onc* gene by promoter insertion in ALV-induced lymphoid leukosis. *Nature (London)* **290**, 475–480.

Klein, G. (1981). The role of gene dosage and genetic transpositions in carcinogenesis. *Nature (London)* **294**, 313–318.

Lautenberger, J. A., Schulz, R. A., Geron, C. F., Tsichlis, P. N., and Papas, T. S. (1981). Molecular cloning of avian myelocytomatosis virus (MC29) transforming sequences. *Proc. Natl. Acad. Sci. U.S.A.* **78**, 1518–1522.

Neel, B. G., Hayward, W. S., Robinson, H. L, Fang, J., and Astrin, S. M. (1981). Avian leukosis virus-induced tumors have common proviral integration sites and synthesize discrete new RNAs: Oncogenesis by promoter insertion. *Cell* **23**, 323–344.

Payne, G. S., Courtneidge, S. A., Crittenden, L. B., Fadly, A. M., Bishop, J. M., and Varmus, H. E. (1981). Analysis of avian leukosis virus DNA and RNA in bursal tumors: Viral gene expression is not required for maintenance of the tumor state. *Cell* **23**, 311–322.

Purchase, H. G., and Burmester, B. R. (1978). Neoplastic Diseases: Leukosis/Sarcoma group. *In* "Diseases of Poultry" (M. S. Hofstad, B. W. Calnek, C. Helmboldt, W. M. Reid, and H. W. Yoder, Jr., eds.) pp. 502–568, Iowa State Univ. Press, Ames, Iowa.

Ramsay, G., Graf, T., and Hayman, M. J. (1980). Mutants of avian myelocytomatosis virus with smaller *gag* gene-related proteins have an altered transforming ability. *Nature (London)* **288**, 170–172.

Rowley, J. D. (1980). Chromosome abnormalities in human leukemia. *Annu. Rev. Genet.* **14,** 17–39.

Scolnick, E. M., Weeks, M. O., Shih, T. Y., Ruscetti, S. K., and Dexter, T. M. (1981). Markedly elevated levels of an endogenous *sarc* protein in a hemopoietic precursor cell line. *Mol. Cell. Biol.* **1,** 66–74.

Thomas, P. S. (1980). Hybridization of denatured RNA and small DNA fragments transferred to nitrocellulose. *Proc. Natl. Acad. Sci. U.S.A.* **77,** 5201-5205.

Weiss, R. A., Teich, N. M., Varmus, H., and Coffin, J. M., eds. (1982). RNA Tumor Viruses. Cold Spring Harbor Lab, Cold Spring Harbor, New York (in press).

21

Mutated Developmental Genes: Cause for Malignancy in *Drosophila*

ELISABETH GATEFF

I. Introduction

The fruit fly *Drosophila melanogaster* shows that mutated developmental genes are causally involved in the induction of malignant and benign tumors (Gateff, 1978a,b,c; 1982a). These genes are instrumental in basic developmental processes such as the control of cell division rates, morphogenetic events, and pattern formation. The affected cells, which are incapable of differentiating, retain their capacity to divide, and thus, give rise to malignant or benign tumors.

Twenty-five such genes have been studied. These are distributed over the entire genome and affect tissues and cells in the embryo, the larva, and the adult. The affected tissues and cells are the neuroblasts, the blood cells and other not yet identified cell types in the embryo, the neuroblasts, the imaginal disc cells and the primordial blood cells in the larva, and the gonial cells in the adult. With the exception of the nonlethal gonial cell tumors, all other tumors are lethal at specific developmental stages. Furthermore, most genes are recessive and are chemically induced (Gateff, 1978a; 1982a). Some of the mutants, however, are spontaneous and occur also in natural populations (see, for example, Golubovsky, 1978; Golubovsky and Sokolova, 1973).

The interference of *Drosophila* tumor genes with differentiation and development points strongly to the possibility that cancer, in general, may be causally related to genetic changes that prevent cell differentiation. The achievements of two fields of research have recently provided support for this notion: (1) retroviral oncogenes (Bishop, 1982) and (2) transfection experiments with DNA from normal and tumorous cells (for review see Weinberg, 1981).

It is well substantiated by now that retroviral oncogenes (*v-onc*) originated from cellular genes (Scolnick *et al.*, 1973; Stehelin *et al.*, 1976a,b; Frankel and Fischinger, 1976; Hanafusa *et al.*, 1977; Spector *et al.*, 1978; Andersson *et al.*, 1979; Sheiness and Bishop, 1979). Evidence is swiftly accumulating which shows that on the genomes of a variety of vertebrate species *c-onc* sequences exist (Stehelin *et al.*, 1976a,b; Spector *et al.*, 1978; for review see Bishop, 1982). Recent reports show even homologies of *v-oncs* with human DNA sequences (Roussel *et al.*, 1979; Spector *et al.*, 1978; Goff *et al.*, 1980; Wong-Staal *et al.*, 1981; Dalla Favera *et al.*, 1981; Murray *et al.*, 1981). Furthermore, Shilo and Weinberg (1981b) also found homologous sequences on the *Drosophila* genome to five oncogenes.

Proteins related to the *v-src* gene product, the $pp60^{src}$ of avian sarcoma virus, have been isolated from a variety of vertebrates (Oppermann *et al.*, 1979; Karess *et al.*, 1979; Collett *et al.*, 1979; Barnekow *et al.*, 1982).

Finally, transfection studies show that the genomes of a variety of vertebrate species may contain putative transforming genes (for review see Weinberg, 1981).

All the above evidence, paired with the knowledge concerning the genetics of human tumors (Knudson, 1978; Knudson and Meadows, 1978) and the tumors of *Xiphophorus* fish hybrids (Anders and Anders, 1978), strongly suggests the causal involvement of genetic factors in the origin of cancer in general.

This chapter deals with the *Drosophila* mutants developing malignant or benign neoplasms in particular tissues and at particular developmental times.

II. The *Drosophila* Tumor Mutants

During the past 6 years three reviews have appeared that discuss the *Drosophila* tumor mutants in detail (Gateff, 1978a,b,c,). A fourth review has recently been submitted (Gateff, 1982b). For this reason, I will briefly describe the different mutants and will concentrate on their discussion in the light of recent achievements in molecular biology.

A. Embryonic Lethal Tumor Mutants

Among the known embryonic mutants, two have been found that develop malignant growth. These are the $Df(1)Notch^8$ (N^8) and the temperature-sensitive (ts) mutant $shibire^{ts1}$ (shi^{ts1}) (Table I).

In the case of the shi^{ts1} mutant, an exposure of 4 to 6 hours to the restrictive temperature between the 3.5 and 14 hours of embryonic life causes disorganized, lethal growth. The growth is autonomous, since implantation of pieces of embryos into wild-type adult hosts gives rise to transplantable malignant tumors comparable to the *in situ* primaries (MacMorris-Swanson and Poodry, 1981). The neoplastically transformed cell type(s) have not yet been identified.

The above tumor mutant shows that between 3.5 and 14 hours of embryonic life, the shi^{ts1} wild-type allele is active and becomes irreversibly damaged when exposed to the restrictive temperature for up to 6 hours during the temperature-sensitive period. These observations allow the conclusion that the shi^{ts1} wild-type gene product must carry important information for the normal differentiation of the embryonic pattern. The cells lacking this information express tumorous growth.

The second mutant, $Df(1)N^8$ (N^8), represents a small deficiency in which the differentiation of the ventral ectoderm is impaired. In the wild-type the ventral region differentiates ectoderm and neuroblasts, while in N^8 exclusively neuroblasts are produced, which differentiate further into neurons (Poulson, 1945). Autonomous tumorous growth ensues when the anterior portions of older N^8 embryos are implanted into the body cavity of wild-type female flies (Gateff and Schneiderman, 1974). The tumorous growth was transplanted for 14 further transfer generations *in vivo* before being discontinued, and showed, in addition to neuroblasts, blood cells growing in a malignant fashion. Thus, the N^8 tumor represents a mixed tumor, consisting of cells belonging to two germ layers, i.e., the ectoderm and the mesoderm.

TABLE I

Drosophila melanogaster Mutants Showing Malignant and Benign Neoplasms[a]

Designation of neoplasm	Tumor mutants on chromosome No.		
	I	II	III
Embryonic tumors	*Df(1)Notch*[1], 1–3.0[1]; shibire[ts1], 1–52.2[2]	—	—
Malignant neuroblastoma	Lethal(1)2,[b,c]; lethal(1)2269[b,c]	14 Alleles of lethal(2) giant larvae; Df(2) lgl net, 2–00[9]; lethal(2)1542[b,c]	Lethal(3)giant larvae[b,c]; lethal(3)brain tumors[ts1b,c]
Intermediate imaginal disc neoplasm with compact lethal mode of growth	Lethal(1)2,[b,c]; lethal(1)2269[b,c]; lethal(1)disc large-1, 1–36[3c]; lethal(1)benign wing imaginal disc neoplasm, 1–34[c]; lethal(1)1pr-2, 1–36.2[4c]; shibire[ts1], 1–522.2[2]	14 Alleles of lethal(2) giant larvae (two of them ts[19]; Df(2) lgl net, 2–00[9], lethal(2)giant disc,[11]; lethal(2)1542[b,c]	Lethal(3)giant larvae,[b,c]; lethal(3)brain tumor[ts1b, c]
Intermediate imaginal disc neoplasm with invasive, lethal mode of growth	Lethal(1)disc large-1, 1–36[3c]; lethal(1)benign imaginal disc neoplasm, 1–34[c]; lethal(1)disc. large-2, 1–24.9[c]	—	—

	Lethal(1)malignant blood	Lethal(2)malignant blood neoplasm[b,c]	Lethal(3)malignant blood
Malignant blood cell neoplasm	Lethal(1)malignant blood neoplasm, 1–39[c], tumorous-lethal, 1–34.5[5c]		neoplasm-1, between h-th[c]; lethal(3)malignant blood cell neoplasm-2[b,c]
Benign gonial cell neoplasm	2 Alleles of female sterile(1) 231, in Df B138L–B170R[6]; female sterile(1)1621, 1–11.7[7]; fused, 1–59.5[8] (10 alleles)	Benign(2) gonial cell neoplasm, between 13.0 and 48.5[c]; female sterile(2) of Bridges, 2–5[12]; 5 alleles of narrow, 2–83[13]	—

[a] References: [1]Mohr, 1919; Gateff and Schneiderman, 1974; [2]Grigliatti et al., 1973; MacMorris-Swanson and Poodry, 1981; Williams, 1981; [3]Kiss et al., 1978; [4]Stewart et al., 1972; [5]Corwin and Hanratty, 1976; [6]Gans et al., 1975; King, 1979; [7]Gollin and King, 1981; [8]King et al., 1957; [9]1(2)gl alleles and Of(2) lgl net Golubovsky and Sokolova, 1973; Gateff et al., 1977; [10]Hanratt, personal communication; [11]Bryant and Schubiger, 1971; [12]Koch and King, 1964; [13]King and Bodenstein, 1965.

[b] Not located.

[c] The remaining mutants were isolated by Gateff, 1978a,b,c.

B. Larval Lethal Tumor Mutants

In the larva three types of tumors were encountered: (1) neuroblasto-mas, derived from the adult optic neuroblasts and ganglion-mother cells in the adult optic centers of the larval brain, (2) imaginal disc tumors, and (3) hematopoietic tumors (Table I).

1. Larval Lethal Mutants Developing Malignant Neuroblastoma

Seven independent, nonallelic mutated genes cause malignant neuro-blastoma (Table I). Among the many genes instrumental in the morpho-genesis of the adult optic centers, these seven genes seem to be involved in a most basic way in the differentiation of the optic neuroblasts into ganglion-mother cells and further into adult optic neurons.

Characteristic for all these mutants are extremely enlarged brain hemi-spheres, the enlargement being due to the malignant neoplastic growth of the adult optic neuroblasts and the ganglion-mother cells (Gateff, 1978a,b,c; 1982a).

In the wild type, the adult optic neuroblasts divide unequally and give rise to new optic neuroblasts and ganglion-mother cells. The ganglion-mother cells, in turn, divide an unknown number of times and differenti-ate finally into adult optic neurons. For the development of the wild-type nervous system consult Kankel et al. (1980).

Mutant optic neuroblasts and ganglion-mother cells, in contrast, fail to differentiate and continue to divide. The tumorous neuroblasts and gangli-on-mother cells invade the larval portions of the brain hemispheres and cause a complete loss of the original brain morphology.

The malignant mode of growth of the optic neurogenic cells is ex-pressed autonomously after implantation of small pieces of mutant brain into the body cavity of a wild-type fly. In histological preparations one can witness an enormous growth and invasion of the malignant cells into the ovaries, the gut, and the thoracic musculature. The autonomous growth of the neurogenic cells causes, finally, the death of the adult host. The tumorous neuroblasts and ganglion-mother cells can be transplanted for many transfer generations.

Two ts alleles at the l(2)gl locus have been isolated (Hanratty and Adler, personal communication). The time of gene activity responsible for the development of neuroblastomas was determined in transplantation ex-periments by Gateff and Schneiderman (1969, 1974) around the middle of embryonic life. Similar results were obtained by Sokolova and Golu-bovsky (1978) in heteroallelic combinations of ts l(2)gl alleles.

A lethal giant larvae locus has also been reported in another Drosophi-la species D. hydei (Srdic and Gloor, personal communication; Srdic and

Frei, 1980), which indicates that this gene may cause similar tumors also in other Dipteran species.

Another *ts* mutant, *lethal (3) brain tumor* [ts] *(l(3)bt[ts])*, was recently isolated on chromosome 3 (Gateff, 1982b). At the restrictive temperature (29°C), in the adult optic centers a neuroblastoma develops and the imaginal discs show tumorous growth. The time of gene activity responsible for the development of brain and imaginal disc tumors falls during the first part of embryonic life (Fig. 1; E. Gateff, unpublished). During this time, at the restrictive temperature, the gene product is synthesized, but its function is impaired, probably due to steric changes of the gene product. A second phase of gene activity associated with abnormalities of the imaginal discs was found during larval life, and a third one was detected during oogenesis, in the developing adult, where tumorous egg chambers are produced which lead to sterility (see below).

As in the last mutant, in most of the other mutants developing neuroblastomas, the imaginal discs also show tumorous growth. Their description follows in the next section.

2. Larval Lethal Mutants Developing Imaginal Disc Tumors

The imaginal discs are the primordia of the adult integument. They are disc-shaped and exhibit a folded epithelium in which the cells are arranged in monolayers. The imaginal discs originate in the embryo from nests of 10 to 50 cells. During larval life the small nests of cells grow and consist shortly before metamorphosis of about 30,000 to 50,000 cells. Under the influence of the hormones at metamorphosis and during adult development in the pupa they secrete their prospective adult cuticular patterns, such as the head with the eyes and the antennae, or the thorax with all its appendages. See Poodry (1980) and Bryant (1978) for further information on wild-type imaginal disc development.

Mutant imaginal discs are, instead of disc-shaped and exhibiting a monolayer epithelium, clumped and of highly variable morphology. The tumorous imaginal disc cells are arranged primarily in clustered array (Gateff, 1978a,b,c; 1982a). In some of the mutants they invade the central nervous system and thus cause the destruction of portions of it (Table I).

The above morphological changes are closely associated with the loss of the capacity of the imaginal disc tissue to differentiate when implanted into a ready-to-pupariate wild-type larva and allowed to complete adult development with the host. Wild-type imaginal discs, in contrast, differentiate under the above conditions into their prospective cuticular patterns.

Moreover, all tumorous imaginal discs exhibit autonomous, lethal

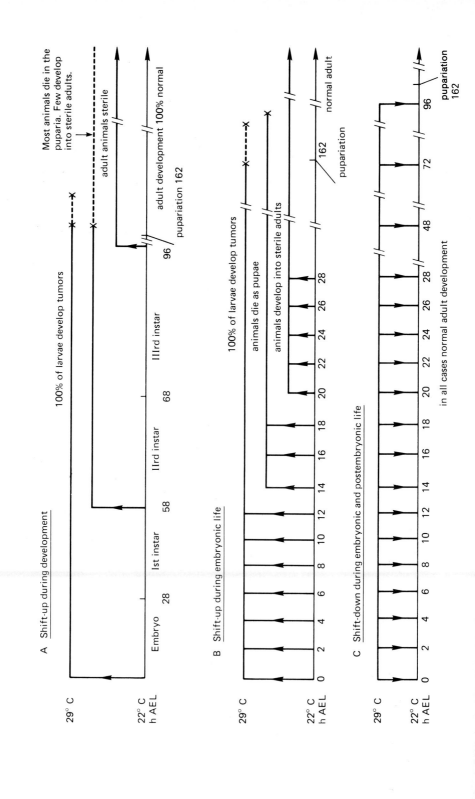

A Shift-up during development

100% of larvae develop tumors

Most animals die in the puparia. Few develop into sterile adults.

adult animals sterile

adult development 100% normal

adult development 162

puparilation 162

29° C

22° C
h AEL

Embryo   Ist instar   IIrd instar   IIIrd instar

28   58   68   96

B Shift-up during embryonic life

100% of larvae develop tumors

animals die as pupae

animals develop into sterile adults

normal adult

pupariation

162

29° C

22° C
h AEL

0   2   4   6   8   10   12   14   16   18   20   22   24   26   28

C Shift-down during embryonic and postembryonic life

in all cases normal adult development

pupariation
162

29° C

22° C
h AEL

0   2   4   6   8   10   12   14   16   18   20   22   24   26   28   48   72   96

growth after transplantation into the body cavity of wild-type female flies. Here, they grow fast into compact tumors which can be subcultured *in vivo* for numerous transfer generations. Wild-type imaginal discs, in contrast, never grow in a tumorous, lethal fashion in wild-type adult hosts.

Thus, the imaginal discs of all 12 imaginal disc tumor mutants (Table 1) combine characteristics of truly benign and truly malignant neoplastic growth, e.g., they grow in a compact, noninvasive way after transplantation, but are lethal to their hosts due to their fast autonomous growth.

With the help of the temperature-sensitive $l(2)gl$ allele $l(2)gl^{ts1}$, Hanratty and Gough (1982) determined the time of the $l(2)gl$ gene activity. They found a biphasic temperature sensitivity; one ts period during embryonic, and the other during larval life. The larval ts period affected the differentiation of cuticular structures, while the embryonic ts period was apparently connected with tumorous development of the imaginal discs. It was further found that the $l(2)gl^+$ function is required throughout embryonic life, up until the early third larvae instar for the normal development of the wing imaginal disc. This corresponds well with the findings of Gateff and Schneiderman (1969, 1974) who determined in transplantation experiments the time of gene activity responsible for imaginal disc tumor development around the middle of embryonic life.

In the new autosomal, recessive-lethal mutant $l(3)bt^{ts1}$, the ts period for imaginal disc as well as for brain tumor development was established during the first half of embryonic life (Fig. 1; Gateff, 1982a; see Section II,B,1). Thus, the wild-type $l(3)bt^{ts1+}$ gene product acts during the early part of embryonic life in the adult neuroblasts and the imaginal disc primordia by initiating a determinative developmental step. At the restrictive temperature the gene product is nonfunctional and thus incapable of inducing the above steps. The cells, devoid of this information, remain undifferentiated and continue to divide in a malignant neoplastic fashion. For tumorous growth to ensue, the animals have to be kept at the restrictive temperature for the rest of embryonic and throughout larval life. Shift-down at any time during development brings about normal differentiation of the adult optic centers in the larval brain and the imaginal discs

Fig. 1. Shift-up (arrow up; A, B) and shift-down (arrow down; C) experiments, performed with the *ts* mutant lethal (3) brain tumor^{ts1} ($l(3)bt^{ts1}$). In the shift-up experiments (A,B) adults were allowed to lay eggs for 2 hours at the permissive temperature (22°C), after which the adults were removed. The eggs/larvae were shifted to the restrictive temperature at the indicated hours after egg laying (h AEL). In the shift-down experiments (C) eggs were collected, as above, at 2-hour intervals at the restrictive temperature, and were brought down to the permissive temperature at various h AEL. (For further details see text.)

(Fig. 1). Thus, the continuous presence of the functional gene product is a prerequisite for normal development to take place.

The previously described embryonic tumor mutant shi^{ts1} (see Section II,A) does not develop tumorous imaginal discs *in situ* at the restrictive temperature. However, after transplantation and subculture of the morphologically normal eye-antennal imaginal discs in the abdomens of wild-type host flies, tumorous growth ensues at the restrictive temperature (Williams, 1981). Wild-type eye-antennal imaginal discs, in contrast, never grow in a tumorous fashion under the above circumstances. After 48 hours in subculture *in vivo* the tumorous growth pattern is irreversibly established, and persists also at the permissive temperature.

The above cases demonstrate that the wild-type alleles of the various tumor mutants possess different modes of action. The elucidation of the molecular events underlying the different mutant phenotypes has already begun with the first attempts to clone the $l(2)gl^+$ gene (O. Schmidt, personal communication).

3. *Larval Lethal Mutants Developing Hematopoietic Tumors*

The hematopoietic organs in the wild-type larva are the so-called "lymph glands." In the hematopoietic organs, located along the dorsal heart vessel, the two blood cell types originate, which are found freely in the hemolymph: (1) the plasmatocytes and (2) the crystal cells (Gateff, 1977; Shrestha and Gateff, 1982a). The plasmatocytes originate from proplasmatocytes and the crystal cells from procrystal cells. Plasmatocytes show two morphological variants, the podocytes and the lamellocytes, which function as phagocytes and in addition are capable of encapsulating and melanizing larger foreign objects. The crystal cells, characterized by crystalline inclusions, are most probably involved in the coagulation of the hemolymph. For more details on the free blood cells in the hemolymph consult Rizki (1957; 1978) and Shrestha and Gateff (1982a).

Table I shows five mutants that develop hematopoietic tumors. In all five cases the neoplastic blood cells are the cell types of the plasmatocyte line. No crystal cell tumors have yet been found.

Characteristic for the five blood tumor mutants are very much enlarged hematopoietic organs and increased blood cell counts (Gateff, 1978a,b,c; Shrestha and Gateff, 1982b; Hanratty and Ryerse, 1981). Furthermore, the tumorous plasmatocytes seem not to be able to recognize "self" from "not self" and, thus, invade the host tissues and cause their partial or complete destruction.

The five blood tumor mutants can be subdivided into two types: The first type shows no impairment of plasmatocyte differentiation, (*l(1)mbn*,

Tum[1]) and the second mutant type exhibits a tumor which consists largely of immature plasmatocytes (*l(2)mbn, l(3)mbn-1, l(3)mbn-2;* Table I). Thus, in the first two mutants, plasmato-, podo-, and lamellocytes can be observed in large amounts in the hematopoietic organs. In contrast, in the wild-type hematopoietic organs, differentiated cell types belonging to the plasmatocyte line can rarely be observed. It appears that in these mutants, the demand for plasmatocytes in the hemolymph and their supply by the hematopoietic organs is abnormally regulated. Characteristic for the mutant plasmatocytes and their morphological variants the podo- and lamellocytes is the increased amount of primary and secondary lysosomes when compared to their wild-type counterparts. This stands in close relation to their increased phagocytic activity (Shrestha and Gateff, 1982b). Small pieces of mutant hematopoietic organs, implanted into the body cavity of wild-type flies, grow in an autonomous malignant fashion.

The remaining three mutant alleles seem to impair the differentiation of the cells of the plasmatocyte line (Shrestha, 1979; Shrestha and Gateff, 1982b). This causes the accumulation of large amounts of immature plasmatocyte-like cells in the hemolymph. A small percentage of cells, nevertheless, engages in an abnormal differentiation process which yields giant plasmato-, podo-, and lamellocytes. In these cells one finds enormous amounts of primary and secondary lysosomes (Shrestha, 1979; Shrestha and Gateff, 1982b). These cells also show increased phagocytic activity. Giant lamellocytes sometimes accumulate and melanize into small melanotic masses.

C. Mutants Developing Germ-Line Tumors in the Adult

The first cells set aside in the embryo are the pole cells, the precursors of the male and female germ cells. After the migration of the pole cells into the gonads during gastrulation, they remain quiescent for quite some time before they divide and transform into primary spermatogonia or oogonia in the second part of larval life. During adult development and in the adult, primary spermatogonia and oogonia differentiate into sperms (Lindsley and Tokuyasu, 1980) and eggs (Mahowald and Kambysellis, 1980).

Many hundreds of genes affect either male or female germ cell differentiation. Mutations in such genes affect differentially only female or male germ cell differentiation. In contrast only a small number of genes is active in both the female and male germ cells.

Tumor mutants belonging to either of the two classes have been found. Five ovarian tumor mutants, studied extensively by King and collaborators, affect only the female sex (King, 1970; King et al., 1978; King and Buckles, 1980; Gollin and King, 1981; Table I). In all these mutants cyst formation is interrupted.

In the wild-type germarium oogonia divide and give rise to cystoblasts which in turn become cystocytes. The progeny of each cystocyte, resulting from four consecutive incomplete mitoses, remain connected with a complex canal system and form a cyst of 16 cystocytes. The cyst becomes enveloped by follicle cells. Within the follicle one of the 16 cystocytes develops into the oocyte and the remaining 15 differentiate into nurse cells.

In the above mutants, cyst formation is interrupted at either the early or late cystocyte divisions resulting in tumorous follicles in which, in addition to numerous single cystocytes, groups of two and more can also be observed.

The *ts* mutant $l(3)bt^{ts1}$, discussed above in connection with the occurrence of brain and imaginal disc tumors (see Sections II,B,1 and 2), also develops tumorous egg chambers. In such egg chambers, one finds cystocytes in addition to many smaller cells. The mutant has not yet been studied histologically, but it appears to belong to the above mutant type, since the male sex is not affected. (For reviews on these mutants see Gateff, 1978a,b,c; 1982a.)

An interesting germ-line tumor mutant belonging to the rare type, affecting both sexes, is the recently discovered mutant *benign gonial cell neoplasm (bgcn)* (Gateff, 1982b). The *bgcn* ovary is filled entirely with single cells which appear to be cystoblasts. These cells are engaged in continuous cell divisions. No trace of differentiation into cystocytes and cyst formation can be observed. The tumorous mode of growth is autonomous also after transplantation of mutant ovarioles into wild-type female flies. Mutant ovaries of third instar larvae implanted into wild-type larvae of comparable age also behave autonomously, indicating that the $bgcn^+$ allele must act some time between pole cell formation and the beginning of the third larval instar.

In the *bgcn* male testis, similarly, large clusters of primary spermatocytes can be observed which never differentiate into secondary spermatocytes or any of the postmeiotic spermatid stages.

All germ-line tumors are benign, i.e., they do not cause the death of the host.

III. Viruses in *Drosophila* Tumor Cells

Two viruses have been found in tumorous blood cell lines cultured *in vitro*: (1) a reovirus designated as F_B (Gateff *et al.*, 1980; Haars *et al.*, 1979) and (2) the *Drosophila* C virus (DCV), a picornavirus (Plus *et al.*, 1975). In addition, in fine structure preparations of all tumorous cells the so-called virus-like particles (*vlp*) have been found mainly in the nucleus (for review see Gateff, 1978a). They show a single envelope and have a diameter of 36 nm.

The above two viruses are certainly not causally related to the tumors, since they are frequently found in natural and laboratory populations of *Drosophila*. The nature of the *vlp*s, on the other hand, is still not known. Two recent papers, one by Heine *et al.* (1980) and the other by Flavell and Ish-Horovicz (1981) give some reasons for speculations that *vlp*s may be a retroviral entity. Heine *et al.* (1980) found in a subcellular fraction, which was associated with reverse transcriptase activity and a high molecular weight, polyadenylated RNA, particles of 40 nm in diameter, which comes close to the 36 nm of *vlp*s measured by Akai *et al.* (1967) in tumors of *Drosophila*.

The second paper, by Flavell and Ish-Horovicz (1981), correlated one of the moderately repetitive gene families, the *copia* gene family (for review, see Spradling and Rubin, 1981) with covalently closed, circular DNA containing either one or two direct terminal repeats. This circular DNA resembles closely integrated proviruses of vertebrate retroviruses. However, until more data are available on this subject, nothing more than speculations can be forwarded (see Gateff, 1982a, for further discussion).

IV. Retroviral Cellular Oncogenes and Transfection Studies: Relationships to the *Drosophila* Genes Causing Tumors

Even though genetic factors have been considered in many systems (Knudson, 1978; Knudson and Meadows, 1978; Lynch, 1976; Anders and Anders, 1978; Gateff, 1978a,b,c; Ponder, 1980; Arrighi *et al.*, 1981), a unifying concept was missing.

Recent molecular and genetic studies with retroviral oncogenes have directed attention to distinct cellular genomic sequences causally associated with the transformed malignant state of particular cell types. Molecular hybridization studies of more than 15 different isolates of retroviral oncogenes to the genomes of a variety of species provided compelling evidence for the hypothesis that oncogenes may be transduced cellular genes (for review, see Bishop, 1982). Cellular genomic sequences corresponding to viral oncogenes (*v-onc*) were shown to possess a high degree of evolutionary conservation. For the best studied oncogene, the *src* gene of Rous sarcoma virus (RSV), complete conservation was found in all tested avian species (Spector *et al.*, 1978). In the case of other vertebrates the homology diminished with the evolutionary distance between the species (Stehelin *et al.*, 1976a,b; Hanafusa *et al.*, 1977; Spector *et al.*, 1978; Wang *et al.*, 1980; Oskarsson *et al.*, 1980).

In the human genome, Dalla Favera *et al.* (1981) found a single constant locus homologous to the transforming *v-sis* gene of simian sarcoma virus. In the spontaneous melanomas, occurring with high frequency in fish hybrids among *Xiphophorus maculatus* and *Xiphophorus helleri* (Anders and Anders, 1978), endogenous *pp60^{src}* expression was detected (Barnekow *et al.*, 1982). Moreover, Schwab (1981) reported *v-src* homologous sequences on the genome of the above fish hybrids and could obtain transformation of NIH 3T3 mouse cell *in vitro* by transfecting with *src* genomic DNA. Barnekow (1982) measured *pp60^{c-src}* kinase activity in various metazoan animals. She found the cellular *src* product in sponges, in the nervous system of cockroaches, Amphioxus, western brook lamprey, cat shark, black striped cichlid and codfish, but failed to detect it in protozoa and plants. In *Drosophila*, Shilo and Weinberg (1981b) found genomic sequences homologous to *v-abl*, *v-src*, *v-ras*, *v-myc* and *v-fes*.

The conclusion from all the above studies is that the genomes of animals contain *v-onc* homologous sequences, which during evolution have become viral entities by transduction. Maybe in the future, one or the other of the here described *Drosophila* genes, causing tumors, will prove homologous to some *v-onc* gene. In *in vitro* cultured blood cells derived from the *l(2)mbn* blood tumor mutants, A. Barnekow (personal communication) showed *pp60^{c-src}* protein kinase activity, which may indicate that the above mutant cellular gene may be homologous to *v-src*. Further studies will, however, be needed in order to ascertain this possibility.

The function of the *c-onc* genes in the cell is at present not known. However, studies by Graf *et al.* (1980) suggested that the various *c-onc* genes may play a role in the differentiation of particular cell types. They showed that oncogenes exhibit target cell specificity in their capacity to transform cells *in vivo* as well as *in vitro*. The various avian (acute) leukemia viruses replicate and produce transforming proteins in nontarget cells. However, these cells do not transform as a result of the viral infection. It is assumed that in target cells the viral gene product inhibits the action of the corresponding cellular protein, whose function may be to induce a particular state of differentiation. Thus, cellular differentiation is prevented by the competitive inhibition of the cellular protein by the viral product.

In *Drosophila* it is already well established that the genes causing malignant or benign tumors function autonomously in specific cell types and they are regarded as involved in cell-specific differentiation steps (Gateff, 1978a,b,c; 1982a). In this respect similarities between the *Drosophila* genes, involved in tumor induction, and viral oncogenes are apparent.

However, this may not be a general principle since Chen *et al.* (1981) found that the feline sarcoma virus (FeSV) also transforms cells from embryonal layers other than the mesoderm which is usually its target. Thus, different pathways of malignant neoplastic transformation will have to be considered.

The *Drosophila* system shows that a particular tumor phenotype can be induced by a number of nonallelic mutated genes. For instance, six independent mutated genes cause malignant neuroblastomas. This implies that during development, in the neuroblasts, a number of genes are instrumental in directing fundamental differentiation steps.

With different *v-src* genes the situation seems to be analogous. The *src* genes of the Fuginami sarcoma virus and RSV both cause sarcomas in chicken fibroblasts despite their differing sequence composition, and thus different gene products (for review see Bishop, 1982).

Of the 25 *Drosophila* mutants listed in Table I, in three cases the mode of action of the gene is known. These are the mutants N^8, $l(2)gl$, and $l(3)lt^{ts1}$. In these three mutants the tumorous condition results from the absence of a functional gene product. In the case of N^8 and the $Df(2)lgl$ *net* the gene deficient state exhibits the most extreme tumor phenotype. The $l(3)bt^{ts1}$ mutant is comparable to the above two mutants, since even though the product is made it is nonfunctional at the restrictive temperature, which practically equals the absence of the gene product (see Sections II,C,1 and 2).

Retroviral oncogenes, on the other hand, show that the transformed state and its maintenance in a fibroblast, for instance, depend on the constant presence of a highly elevated functional gene product (as reviewed by Bishop, 1982).

Although the slow transforming RNA tumor viruses do not possess an oncogene, they can cause malignant neoplastic transformation of cells. Viruses, such as the avian and the murine leukemia viruses activate a cellular gene by integration of the provirus adjacent to the cellular gene. The transcription of the gene begins at the proviral promoter which results in an enhanced gene expression and transformation (Neel *et al.*, 1981; Hayward *et al.*, 1981).

Since most cancers are not of viral origin, it was important to establish whether the *c-oncs* or other genes on the genomes from virus negative cells are capable of transforming. This approach was taken by a number of investigators who transfected *NIH 3T3* mouse cells *in vitro* with DNA from normal and tumorous cells from mice, chickens and humans (Andersson *et al.*, 1979; Cooper *et al.*, 1980; Shih *et al.*, 1979, 1981; Cooper and Neiman, 1980; Krontiris and Cooper, 1981; Shilo and Weinberg, 1981a; Lane *et al.*, 1981; Murray *et al.*, 1981; for review see Weinberg, 1981).

All the above studies showed an elevated transformation frequency in the *in vitro* transfection-focus assay. Moreover, these studies suggest that tissue-specific cellular genes may become abnormally regulated through DNA shearing (Cooper and Neiman, 1980). During shearing the regulatory sequences of a particular cellular transforming gene may be removed, causing an aberrant gene expression and thus malignant neoplastic transformation. The transfected DNA, furthermore, may cause mutations in cellular transforming genes.

The mutagenic effect of exogenous DNA is well established in *Drosophila* (Gershenson, 1980). More importantly, the transfection with foreign DNA showed a high degree of specificity of the mutagenic effect. In contrast to mutagens, which induce at random mutations at many loci, exogenous DNA mutated only very few specific loci (Gershenson, 1980).

In conclusion, 25 loci on the *Drosophila* genome are presently known to cause benign and malignant tumors in specific embryonic, larval and adult cells (Table I). The wild-type alleles of these genes control at particular times particular differentiation steps in specific cell types. In cancer induction we will have to consider different modes of abnormal genomic expression, such as gene mutation or abnormal gene regulation. It may become evident in the future that in addition to the family of *c-oncs* homologous to *v-oncs*, other gene families instrumental in malignant neoplastic transformation may also exist. I can well conceive that genes involved in the differentiation of *Drosophila* neuroblasts, gonial cells, or blood cells may function also in mouse, rat or human neuroblasts, gonial cells, or blood cells. Cloned *Drosophila* tumor genes may hybridize to different animal genomes and, thus, may serve as probes for the identification of genes involved in differentiation and malignant transformation of particular cell types in other animals and humans.

Acknowledgments

This research was supported by the Deutsche Forschungsgemeinschaft SFB46. The skilled technical assistance of D. Willer and I. Brillowski is gratefully acknowledged. I am also grateful to Prof. K. Sandes for providing the research facilities.

References

Akai, H., Gateff, E., Davis, L. E., and Schneiderman, H. A. (1967). *Science (Washington, D.C.)* **157**, 810–813.
Anders, A., and Anders, F. (1978). *Biochim. Biophys. Acta* **516**, 61–95.
Andersson, P., Goldfarb, M. P., and Weinberg, R. A. (1979). *Cell* **16**, 63–75.

Arrighi, F. E., Rao, P. N., and Stubblefield, E. (eds.). (1981). "Genes, Chromosomes, and Neoplasia." Raven, New York.

Barnekow, A. (1982). *Cancer Res.* (submitted).

Barnekow, A., Schartl. M., Anders, F., and Bauer, H. (1982). Submitted to *Cancer Res.*

Bishop, J. M.(1982). *In* "RNA Tumor Viruses," Cold Spring Harbor Laboratory, Cold Spring Harbor, New York (in press).

Bryant, P. J. (1978). *In* "The Genetics and Biology of *Drosophila*" (M. Ashburner and T. R. F. Wright, eds.), Vol. 2c, pp. 230–325. Academic Press, New York.

Bryant, P. J., and Schubiger, G. (1971). *Dev. Biol.* **24**, 233–363.

Chen, A. P., Essex, M., Shadduck, J. A., Niederkorn, J. Y., and Albert, D. (1981). *Proc. Natl. Acad. Sci. U.S.A.* **78**, 3915–3919.

Collett, M. S., Erikson, E., Purchio, A. F., Brugge, J. S., and Erikson, R. L. (1979). *Proc. Natl. Acad. Sci. U.S.A.* **76**, 3159–3163.

Cooper, G. M., and Neiman, P. E. (1980). *Nature (London)* **287**, 656–659.

Cooper, G. M., Okenquist, S., and Silverman, L. (1980). *Nature (London)* **248**, 418–422.

Corwin, H. O., and Hanratty, W. P. (1976). *Mol. Gen. Genet.* **14**, 345–347.

Dalla Favera, R., Gelman, E. P., Gallo, R. C., and Wong-Staal, F. (1981). *Nature (London)* **292**, 31–35.

Flavell, A. J., and Ish-Horowicz, D. (1981). *Nature (London)* **292**, 591–595.

Frankel, A. D., and Fischinger, P. J. (1976). *Proc. Natl. Acad. Sci. U.S.A.* **73**, 3705–3709.

Gans, M., Audit, C., and Masson, M. (1975). *Genetics* **81**, 683–704.

Gateff, E. (1977). *Ann. Parasitol. Hum. Comp.* **52**, 81–83.

Gateff, E. (1978a). *In* "The Genetics and Biology of Drosophila" (M. Ashburner and T. R. F. Wright, eds.), Vol. 2b, pp. 181–275. Academic Press, London.

Gateff, E. (1978b). *Science (Washington, D.C.)* **200**, 1448–1459.

Gateff, E. (1978c). *Biol. Rev.* **53**, 123–168.

Gateff, E. (1982a). *In* "Advances in Cancer Research" (S. Weinhouse and G. Klein, eds.), Vol. 37. Academic Press, New York.

Gateff, E. (1982b). *Cell Differ.* (in press).

Gateff, E., and Schneiderman, H. A. (1969). *Natl. Cancer Inst. Monogr.* **31**, 365–397.

Gateff, E., and Schneiderman, H. A. (1974). *Wilhelm Roux' Arch. Entwicklungsmech. Org.* **176**, 23–65.

Gateff, E., Gissman, L., Shrestha, R., Plus, N., Pfister, H., Schroder, J., and zur Hausen, H. (1980). *In* "Invertebrate Systems *in vitro*" (E. Kurstak, K. Maramorosch, and A. Dubendorfer, eds.), pp. 517–533. Elsevier North-Holland Biomedical Press, Amsterdam.

Gershenson, S. M. (1980). *In* "Well-being of Mankind and Genetics, Proceedings of the XIV International Congress of Genetics" (M. E. Vartanian, ed.), Vol. I, Book two, pp. 96–115. MIR Publishers, Moscow.

Goff, S. P., Gilboa, E., Sitte, O. N., and Baltimore, D. (1980). *Cell,* **22**, 777–786.

Gollin, M. S., and King, R. C. (1981). *Dev. Genet.* **2**, 203–218.

Golubovsky, M. D. (1978). *Drosophila Inform. Serv.* **53**, 179.

Golubovsky, M. D., and Sokolova, K. (1973). *Drosophila Inform. Serv.* **50**, 124.

Graf, T., Beng, H., and Hayman, M. J. (1980). *Proc. Natl. Acad. Sci. U.S.A.* **77**, 389–393.

Grigliatti, T. A., Hall, L., Rosenbluth, R., and Suzuki, D. T. (1973). *Mol. Gen. Genet.* **120**, 107–114.

Haars, R., Zentgraf, H., Gateff, E., and Bautz, F. A. (1979). *Virologie* **101**, 124–130.

Hanafusa, H., Halpern, C. C., Buchhagen, D. L., and Kawai, S. (1977). *J. Exp. Med.* **146**, 1735–1747.

Hanratty, W. P., and Gough, T. L. (1982). *Genet. Res.* (submitted).

Hanratty, W. P., and Ryerse, J. S. (1981). *Dev. Biol.* **83**, 238.

Hayward, W. S., Neel, B. G., and Astrin, S. M. (1981). *Nature (London)* **290**, 475–480.

Heine, C. W., Kelly, D. C., and Avery, R. J. (1980). *J. Gen. Virol.* **49**, 385–395.

Kankel, D. R., Ferrus, A., Garren, S. H., Harte, P. J., and Lewis, P. E. (1980). *In* "The Genetics and Biology of Drosophila" (M. Ashburner and T. R. F. Wright, eds.), Vol. 2d, pp. 295–363. Academic Press, New York.

Karess, R. E., Hayward, W. S., and Hanafusa, H. (1979). *Proc. Natl. Acad. Sci. U.S.A.* **76**, 3154–3158.

King, R. C. (1970). *In* "Ovarian Development in Drosophila Melanogaster," pp. 33–98. Academic Press, New York.

King, R. C. (1979). *Int. J. Insect Morphol. Embryol.* **8**, 297–309.

King, R. C., and Bodenstein, D. (1965). *Z. Naturforsch.* **20**, 292–297.

King, R. C., and Buckles, B. D. (1980). *Drosophila Inform. Serv.* **55**, 74–75.

King, R. C., Burnett, R. G., and Staley, N. A. (1957). *Growth* **21**, 239–261.

King, R. C., Bahn, M., Horowitz, R., and Rarramendi, P. (1978). *Int. J. Insect Morphol. Embryol.* **7**, 359–378.

Kiss, I., Scabad, J., and Major, J. (1978). *Mol. Gen. Genet.* **164**, 77–83.

Knudson, A. G. (1978). *In* "Tumors of Early Life in Man and Animals" (L. Severi, ed.), pp. 765–775. Perugia Quadrenn. Int. Conf. Cancer, Monteluce, Italy.

Knudson, A. G. and Meadows, A. T. (1978). *In* "Cell Differentiation and Neoplasia" (F. Grady, ed.), pp. 88–92. Raven, New York.

Koch, E. A. and King, R. C. (1964). *Growth* **28**, 325–369.

Krontiris, T. G. and Cooper, G. M. (1981). *Proc. Natl. Acad. Sci. U.S.A.* **78**, 1181–1184.

Lane, M.-A., Sainten, A., and Cooper, G. M. (1981). Submitted to *Proc. Natl. Acad. Sci. U.S.A.*

Lindsley, D. L. and Tokuyasu, K. T. (1980). *In* "The Genetics and Biology of *Drosophila*" (M. Ashburner and T. R. F. Wright, eds.), Vol. 2d, pp. 226–287. Academic Press, New York.

Lynch, H. T., ed. (1976). "Cancer Genetics." Thomas, Springfield, Illinois.

MacMorris-Swanson, M., and Poodry, C. A. (1981). *Dev. Biol.* **84**, 465–470.

Mahowald, A. P., and Kambysellis, P. (1980). *In* "The Genetics and Biology of *Drosophila*," (M. Ashburner and T. R. F. Wright, eds.), Vol. 2d, pp. 141–209. Academic Press, New York.

Mohr, O. L. (1919). *Genetics,* **4**, 275–282.

Murray, M. J., Shilo, B. Z., Shih, C., Cowing, D., Hsu, H. W., Neel, B. G., Hayward, W. S., Robinson, H. L., Fang, J. M., and Astrin, S. M. (1981). *Cell* **23**, 323–334.

Oskarsson, M., McClements, W. L., Blair, D. G., Maizel, J. V., and VandeWoude, G. F. (1980). *Science (Washington, D.C.)* **207**, 1222–1224.

Oppermann, H., Levinson, A. D., Varmus, H. E., Levintow, L., and Bishop, J. M. (1979). *Proc. Natl. Acad. Sci. U.S.A.* **76**, 1804–1808.

Plus, N., Croizier, G., Jousset, F. X., and David, J. (1975). *Ann. Microbiol. (Paris)* **126**, 107–117.

Ponder, B. A. J. (1980). *Biochim. Biophys. Acta* **605**, 369–410.

Poodry, C. A. (1980). *In* "The Genetics and Biology of *Drosophila*" (M. Ashburner and T. R. F. Wright, eds.), Vol. 2d, pp. 407–432. Academic Press, New York.

Poulson, D. F. (1945). *Am. Nat.* **79**, 340–363.

Rizki, M. T. M. (1957). *J. Morphol.* **100**, 437–458.

Rizki, M. T. M. (1978). *In* "The Genetics and Biology of Drosophila" (M. Ashburner and T. R. F. Wright, eds.), Vol. 26, pp. 397–448. Academic Press, New York.

Roussel, M., Saule, S., Lagrou, C., Rommens, C., Beug, H., Graf, T., and Stehelin, D. (1979). *Nature (London)* **281**, 452–455.

Schwab, M. (1981). *Cong. Int. Soc. Dev. Biol. 9th,* Basel, Switzerland (Abstr.).

Scolnick, E. M., Rands, E., Williams, D., and Parks, W. P. (1973). *J. Virol.* **12,** 458–463.

Sheiness, D. K., and Bishop, J. M. (1979). *J. Virol.* **31,** 514–521.

Shih, C., Shilo, B. Z., Goldfarb, M. P., Dannenberg, A., and Weinberg, R. A. (1979) *Proc. Natl. Acad. Sci. U.S.A.* **76,** 5714–5718.

Shih, C., Padhy, L. C., Murray, M., and Weinberg, R. A. (1981). *Nature (London)* **290,** 261–264.

Shilo, B.-Z., and Weinberg, R. A. (1981a). *Nature (London)* **289,** 607–609.

Shilo, B.-Z. and Weinberg, R. A. (1981b). *Proc. Natl. Acad. Sci. U.S.A.* **75,** 6789–6792.

Shrestha, R. (1979). Ph.D. Thesis, Fakultat fur Biologie, Albert-Ludwigs-Universitat, Freiburg, Federal Republic of Germany.

Shrestha, R., and Gateff, E. (1982a). *Dev. Growth Differ.* **24,** 65–82.

Shrestha, R., and Gateff, E. (1982b). *Dev. Growth Differ.* **24,** 83–98.

Sokolova, K., and Golubovsky, M. D. (1978). *Drosophila Inform. Serv.* **53,** 195–196.

Spector, D. H., Varmus, H. E., and Bishop, J. M. (1978). *Proc. Natl. Acad. Sci. U.S.A.* **75,** 4102–4106.

Spradling, A. C. and Rubin, G. M. (1981). *In* "Annual Review of Genetics" (H. L. Roman, A. Campbell, and L. M. Sandler, eds.), Vol. 15, pp. 219–264. Annual Reviews Inc., Palo Alto, California.

Srdic, Z., and Frei, H. (1980). *Differentiation* **17,** 187–192.

Stehelin, D., Guntaka, R. V., Varmus, H. E., and Bishop, J. M. (1976a). *J. Mol. Biol.* **101,** 349–365.

Stehelin, D., Varmus, H. E., Bishop, J. M., and Vogt, P. K. (1976b). *Nature (London)* **260,** 170–173.

Stewart, M., Murphy, C., and Fristrom, J. (1972). *Dev. Biol.* **27,** 71–83.

Wang, L. H., Snyder, P., Hanafusa, T., and Hanafusa, H. (1980). *J. Virol.* **35,** 52–64.

Weinberg, R. A. (1981). *Biochim. Biophys. Acta* **651,** 25–35.

Williams, J. M. (1981). *Drosophila Inform. Serv.* **56,** 158–161.

Wong-Staal, F., Dalla Favera, R., Franchini, G., Gelmann, E. P., and Gallo, R. C. (1981). *Science* **213,** 226–228.

22

Genetic Instability in Cancer Cells: Relationship to Tumor Cell Heterogeneity

PETER C. NOWELL

I. Introduction

It is the thesis of this chapter that genetic instability in neoplastic cell populations provides one basis for the heterogeneity that is characteristically observed in tumors regardless of what parameter is measured. Further, I would like to suggest that genetic instability underlies a very important aspect of heterogeneity, the sequential appearance within the neoplasm of subpopulations with increasingly malignant characteristics.

It has long been recognized that there is a tendency for many tumors, over time, to become progressively more aggressive in their behavior, although the time course may be quite variable. The stepwise nature of this clinical and biological phenomenon of "tumor progression" was recognized by Foulds (1975), and others suggested that it might reflect sequential appearance within the tumor of increasingly genetically altered subpopulations (Makino, 1956; DeGrouchy and DeNava, 1968). It was further postulated that this "clonal evolution" (Cairns, 1975; Nowell, 1976; Klein, 1979) might result from enhanced genetic lability within the tumor cell population, which increased the probability of genetic errors (often recognizable cytogenetically), and their subsequent selection.

I would like to review briefly the evidence that tumor cell populations are indeed more genetically unstable than comparable normal cells, and that such instability may contribute significantly to the generation of increasingly altered subpopulations within the tumor, recognized as both heterogeneity and clonal evolution. I will also suggest some implications that these findings may have for the control of human cancer. It is important to stress, however, that this discussion is concerned with only one basis for the heterogeneity typically observed in many tumors, and is not intended to exclude the contribution of other phenomena discussed at length elsewhere in this volume.

II. Evidence for Increased Genetic Lability of Tumor Cell Populations

When tumors are examined histologically, one is often struck by the presence of obvious mitotic abnormalities. In fact, such observations led workers such as Von Hansemann (1890) and Boveri (1914) to the earliest theories concerning an important role of chromosomal alterations in the development of cancer. Such histological studies also suggest that the genetic instability represented by mitotic abnormalities may become more pronounced as a neoplasm evolves. In advanced malignancies, a wide variety of mitotic variants are commonly observed with each cell generation, as compared to relatively few in early benign lesions (Oksala and Therman, 1974).

Experimental data indicating that tumor cell populations are more genetically labile than comparable normal cells are being reported with increased frequency. Although the results are not completely uniform, there is evidence, both *in vivo* and *in vitro*, that neoplastic cells are more susceptible to chromosome breakage, nondisjunction and ploidy changes, sister chromatid exchange (SCE), and other genetic alterations than comparable normal cells (Weiner *et al.*, 1974; Sokova *et al.*,1976; Danes, 1978; Otter *et al.*, 1978; Parshad *et al.*, 1979; Shiraishi and Sandberg, 1979). For instance, Nichols (1982) has demonstrated that some SV40-transformed cell lines showed increased mutation rates as compared to controls, and Sager (Chapter 25) has observed a similar phenomenon with tumorigenic versus nontumorigenic Chinese hamster cell lines. There are even limited experimental data indicating that this enhanced mutability increases with tumor progression, as discussed by Fidler in Chapter 9.

An observation directly relevant to human neoplasia has recently been reported by Fialkow *et al.* (1981). They studied chromosome abnormalities in EBV-transformed B lymphoblastoid cell lines established from the blood of normal donors as well as from an individual with Philadelphia chromosome-positive chronic granulocytic leukemia (CGL). Lines established from normal donors were generally karyotypically normal during the first year *in vitro*. In contrast, cytogenetic changes were detected after only 15–45 days in culture in 8 of the 47 B cell lines established from the patient. Moreover, the aberrations were not found at random but were detected only in cells from lines that were considered part of the neoplastic clone based on the fact that they were all of the same glucose-6-phosphate dehydrogenase (G6PD) phenotype. The authors suggested that the genetically labile B lymphocytes arose from the same aberrant marrow stem cell as the Ph-positive leukemia. In this view, the genetically unstable neoplasm arose first, and then, as the result of its lability, a cell with the Philadelphia chromosome was generated, producing a subline with greater selective growth advantage and ultimate appearance of clinical leukemia.

Taken together, the still limited studies on the genetic instability of neoplastic cells suggest that there is indeed a greater frequency of mitotic errors and other genetic changes in many neoplastic cell populations. The results further indicate that the high level of mitotic activity in some tumors only partially accounts for this difference, and that, in addition, each cell division carries an increased risk for genetic variation. More data are clearly needed, however, to determine how consistently this is the case, and the relationship of such lability to tumor progression and tumor heterogeneity. The next section is a discussion of this latter question.

III. Contribution of Genetic Instability to Tumor Progression and Tumor Heterogeneity

Cytogenetic, biochemical, and immunological data support the view that most tumors are of unicellular origin (Harnden, 1977; Fialkow, 1979; Nowell, 1981) and thus are "clones" in the sense of being derived from a single altered cell. As previously indicated, a number of workers (Makino, 1956; DeGrouchy and DeNava, 1968; Cairns, 1975; Nowell, 1976; Klein, 1979) have suggested that the clinical and biological events described as "tumor progression" represent the effects of genetic instability in the neoplastic clone, and the sequential selection of variant subpopulations produced as a result of that genetic lability. In this concept of "clonal evolution," most variants arising in the tumor cell population are considered not to survive; but those few mutants that have a selective growth advantage expand to become predominant subpopulations within the neoplasm and demonstrate the characteristics that we recognize as tumor progression. The continued presence of multiple subpopulations within the tumor provides the basis for the heterogeneity which is typically observed.

Most of the data that support these concepts have been derived from chromosome studies (and this may have caused excessive emphasis on the role of cytogenetic abnormalities, as compared to submicroscopic alterations, in discussing the types of genetic change involved in this process). In general, most neoplasms show visible chromosome changes (as discussed by Sandberg, Chapter 23), and advanced malignancies show more extensive cytogenetic aberrations than earlier stages of neoplasia (Rowley, 1980a; Nowell, 1981). It has rarely been possible, however, to do sequential studies of the same tumor and so determine whether biological progression of the neoplasm to more "malignant" characteristics was associated with the emergence of new predominant subpopulations of tumor cells having additional genetic alterations, recognizable cytogenetically.

A. Clonal Evolution and Tumor Progression

Fortunately, such serial studies have been done in certain of the human hematopoietic tumors, as well as in a few experimental malignancies in animals. Interestingly, the best documented data in man are the findings in chronic granulocytic leukemia (CGL), which has already been mentioned. In this disorder, characteristically, both the early and late stages of the disease, as recognized clinically, are accompanied by chromosomal abnormalities. The early stage of CGL is typically a benign disorder characterized by a relatively slowly expanding neoplastic clone consisting mostly of differentiated myeloid elements. At this time, the neoplastic cells nearly always contain the Philadelphia chromosome (a translocation from the long arm of chromosome 22, usually to the long arm of chromosome 9) as the only cytogenetic change. After several years, the clinical picture often changes dramatically. The well differentiated cells are replaced by a rapidly expanding population of undifferentiated myeloblasts, crowding the blood and bone marrow, and leading to the death of the patient in so-called "blast crisis."

In this accelerated phase, a subpopulation of cells with karyotypic abnormalities in addition to the Philadelphia (Ph) chromosome often becomes predominant. These additional changes are not consistent from case to case, but frequently involve one one or more of several specific alterations (a second Ph, iso 17q, trisomy 8) (Rowley, 1980b; Sandberg, Chapter 23). It is thus possible to speculate that tumor progression in CGL results from further mutation in a cell of the original clone, often recognizable cytogenetically, allowing a more aggressive subpopulation to develop and overwhelm the patient. As already noted, the initial appearance of the Philadelphia chromosome may itself represent a similar example of sequential genetic change in a genetically unstable neoplastic population originally chromosomally normal (Fialkow et al., 1981).

As yet, the specific genes and gene products involved in these stages are not known, but one could postulate that the second cytogenetic abnormality within the CGL clone might further alter membrane receptors for local growth regulators so that nearly all the cells with the additional chromosome change remain as blasts, with very few undergoing terminal differentiation. This would lead to a rapid expansion of the stem cell pool and the clinical picture of the blast crisis. With the increasing evidence that techniques of modern molecular genetics may be capable of identifying and characterizing specific cancer genes and their products within the cells of human tumors, as well as in other species, direct evidence relevant to such hypotheses may be forthcoming in the not too distant future (Murray et al., 1981; Astrin, Chapter 20).

Similar sequential patterns of karyotypic alteration associated with clinical progression have been reported in other human leukemic and preleukemic disorders (Rowley, 1980a; Nowell, 1982), but many cases do not follow the protracted time course necessary for repeated investigations. We have recently studied over a 5-year period a patient with the rare T cell variant of chronic lymphocytic leukemia (CLL) whose tumor cells showed evidence of cytogenetic evolution in parallel with changes in the biological and clinical characteristics of her disease (Nowell et al., 1981). She first developed a pseudodiploid subpopulation with two characteristic chromosome markers (3q+ and 14q+) and associated loss of some T cell properties. She then progressed to poorly differentiated lymphoma (Richter's syndrome) with extensive chromosome changes in addition to the 3q+ and 14q+ in the cells of the solid tumor. It is interesting that in this single patient there was cytogenetic evidence of clonal evolution producing, first, biological changes in the cells without clinical significance, and, finally, extensive alterations in growth characteristics which proved fatal. Furthermore, the sequential cytogenetic changes in her cells apparently reflected genetic instability inherent within the neoplastic population, as previously discussed for CGL, as the patient had received no mutagenic therapy and there was no history of exposure to chromosome-damaging agents in the home or workplace (Mitelman *et al.*, 1979).

Some chromosomal data have also been obtained in experimental animals which support the concept of sequential genetic changes and clonal evolution underlying tumor progression. In a number of primary sarcomas induced in rats and mice by the Rous virus, the karyotype was initially normal (Mark, 1969; Mitelman, 1971). Serial biopsies of individual tumors as they gradually acquired more malignant properties, including increased growth rate and reduced collagen production, revealed the sequential appearance of new subpopulations identified cytogentically, overgrowing and replacing the original diploid tumor cells. In the studies of Rous sarcomas in rats, involving both primary lesions and transplantable tumors derived from them, chromosome banding data have indicated a relatively consistent pattern of stepwise karyotypic change, with first the addition of chromosome 7, then 13, and then 12 (Mitelman, 1971; Levan and Mitelman, 1976). These further cytogenetic alterations apparently provided additional selective growth advantages over earlier tumor cells, both diploid and aneuploid, and Isaacs (Chapter 7) describes a similar phenomenon in another rat tumor.

B. Coexisting Subpopulations and Tumor Heterogeneity

In both the human and animal studies, the chromosome data have frequently also indicated the continuing coexistence of multiple subpopulations within the tumor during these evolutionary stages (Mark, 1969; Mitelman, 1971; Nowell, 1981; Rowley, 1980b; Sandberg, Chapter 23). This is well documented in CGL, when, as noted above, one or more subpopulations with cytogentic changes in addition to the Philadelphia chromosome frequently appear in association with the accelerated phase of the disease (Rowley, 1980b). These new subclones may have cytochemical and membrane characteristics that differ from the original neoplastic cells, and a similar basis for heterogeneity has been recognized in human acute leukemia as well (Rowley, 1980a; Nadler, Chapter 4). Thus, we have observed a patient with CGL who, in the late stages of the disease, had two populations of immature neoplastic cells in the peripheral blood, one with myeloid characteristics and the other with lymphoid markers. Their relative frequency, when correlated with cytogenetic data, indicated that the myeloid cells had 46 chromosomes (with one Ph chromosome) and that the lymphoid elements were an evolved subline of the same neoplasm with 50 chromosomes (including two Ph's) (Hutchinson *et al.*, 1981). We have also recently studied a child with acute leukemia whose neoplastic cells appeared to constitute several subpopulations, one with only T cell markers; one with T, B, and monocytic markers; and terminally, an additional subset with T and B markers. Chromosome studies on this patient indicated again that these were related subclones of the same neoplasm, present in varying proportions at different times during the course of the disease (Hann *et al.*, in press). There are many other reports of cytogenetic evidence for coexisting subclones in a variety of leukemias and solid tumors, ranging from several major subpopulations, as above, to multiple small ones recognized as related only by the presence of a distinctive abnormal marker chromosome in all metaphases (Nowell, 1981; Rowley, 1980a; Sandberg, Chapter 23; Nowell *et al.*, 1982; Balaban *et al*, 1982).

These various findings indicate that, through cytogenetic techniques, genetically aberrant subpopulations have been identified in many neoplasms, apparently reflecting underlying genetic instability, and associated with both tumor progression and heterogeneity. In the next section I will discuss some of the possible mechanisms that might account for this apparent increase in genetic lability and the resultant heterogeneity and evolution within the tumor.

IV. Possible Mechanisms for Increased Genetic Instability in Tumor Cells

Table I summarizes a variety of mechanisms that could account for the apparent increased mutability of tumor cell populations, providing a basis for clonal evolution and some aspects of tumor heterogeneity. The categories listed in Table I are by no means mutually exclusive, and at various stages of tumor development and in different neoplasms, different mechanisms could operate. Each of the categories will be discussed briefly.

A. Inherited Defects

In a small segment of the population, increased genetic lability in neoplastic cells may not result from an acquired alteration, but rather reflect

TABLE I

Possible Mechanisms of Genetic Instability in Tumor Cell Populations

---

A. Inherited defects
   1. "Chromosome breakage" syndromes
   2. Subclinical gene defects
   3. Constitutional chromosome abnormalities
B. Acquired defects
   1. Gene mutations
      a. DNA repair
      b. DNA replication
      c. Mitotic apparatus
   2. Chromosome alterations
      a. Aneuploidy
      b. Translocations and "transposable elements"
      c. SCE; HSR and DMs
C. Extracellular factors
   1. Viruses
   2. Radiation and mutagenic chemicals
   3. Nutritional deficiencies

---

an inherited gene defect present in all cells of the body. Of particular interest are the so-call "chromosome breakage syndromes," such as Bloom's syndrome (BS), Fanconi's anemia (FA), ataxia telangiectasia (AT), and xeroderma pigmentosum (XP) (German, 1977; Hecht and McCaw, 1977; Setlow, 1978). These individuals apparently have an inherited defect in DNA repair, or in some other aspect of DNA "housekeeping," although the details have not been completely worked out in all instances. As an oversimplified generalization, it can be suggested that the genetic instability resulting from the inherited gene defect leads to persistent chromosome aberrations, cytogenetically abnormal clones, and ultimately the increased incidence of neoplasia which characterizes these syndromes.

It is possible that inherited gene defects with similar effects may be present in individuals without recognizable clinical syndromes. There have been children described, for instance, with unexplained familial disorders of blood formation who do not fit one of the recognized chromosome breakage diseases (Li et al., 1978; Nowell, 1977). These children may demonstrate cytogenetically abnormal clones among circulating lymphocytes or in the bone marrow, and some ultimately progress to leukemia. It has not yet been demonstrated that such patients carry a gene defect influencing karyotypic stability, but the parallels with known chromosome breakage syndromes suggest that some of these unexplained disorders may represent "subclinical" inherited defects in DNA housekeeping.

It has also been recognized that individuals with constitutional chromosome abnormalities, and particularly Down's syndrome, show evidence of increased susceptibility to cytogenetic damage and rearrangement when exposed to clastogenic agents *in vitro* (Seabright, 1976). It is not clear whether the specific chromosomal alteration in the patient's cells has, itself, a destabilizing effect, or whether both the constitutional abnormality and the increased fragility reflect an inherited defect in chromosomal stability analogous to that discussed in the preceding paragraphs. In at least some families, the latter possibility seems supported by the presence of different constitutional chromosome alterations in family members as well as a general familial increase in cancer incidence (Law *et al.*, 1977; Miller *et al.*, 1961).

B. Acquired Defects

For the vast majority of patients with cancer, it is assumed that there is no constitutional abnormality in genetic stability, and that the increased lability within the neoplastic clone is the result of an acquired alteration. Many kinds of acquired defects have been suggested by various workers, with some supporting evidence in studies of different tumors.

Single gene mutations of various types could destabilize the genome. Such "mutator" genes might result in abnormalities in DNA repair similar to those in the "chromosome breakage syndromes" or other defects in repair mechanisms. Alternatively, such a gene might involve the DNA synthetic apparatus, resulting, for instance, in more error-prone pathways being utilized within the tumor cells and hence increasing the probability for subsequent mutations. The product of a mutator gene might even involve the mitotic apparatus itself, resulting, for example, in defective polymerization of microtubules, instability of the mitotic spindle, and an increased probability of nondisjunction and other chromosomal rearrangements. Although these various possibilities have not been widely explored, there are, in fact, limited data indicating the action of each of these various types of mutator genes in certain neoplastic cell populations (Cairns, 1975; Heston, 1977; Loeb *et al.*, 1975; Chan and Becker, 1979).

In addition to these specific mutations, one can postulate that *chromosomal alterations*, once established within the tumor cell population, may themselves contribute to the continuing, and perhaps increasing, genetic instability within the neoplastic cells. Aneuploidy, for instance, could result from one of the mutagenic mutations suggested in the preceding paragraphs, and so might appear during evolution of the tumor. Once present, it could readily contribute to the production of further genetic errors. Aneuploid cells are more susceptible than normal to further chromosomal rearrangements (Högstedt and Mitelman, 1981) and, as already noted, may also be more easily damaged by clastogenic agents (Seabright, 1976).

Even balanced translocations in a cell may increase the probability of mitotic errors; and recently the related phenomenon of "transposable elements," originally described in maize, has been reintroduced as a possible important consideration in mammalian neoplasia. In this concept, certain DNA segments may move about within the genome and exert various kinds of destabilizing effects on other segments, adjacent to their sites of insertion. This phenomenon is discussed in detail by Sager (Chapter 25).

Several additional types of chromosomal alterations, recognizable in tumor cells, might also increase genetic instability in the neoplastic clone as well as having specific direct effects in terms of alterations in gene products. It has been postulated, for instance, that abnormal sister chromatid exchanges might play a significant role in tumor development by generating homozygosity of critical recessive genes (Passarge and Bartram, 1976); and so, if a somatic alteration in the neoplastic cells produced increased SCE within the population, the probability of further significant genetic changes would also be enhanced. Similarly, the phenomenon of homogeneous staining regions (HSR) and related double minutes (DMs) could have a dual effect. The HSR, as observed in various tumors, apparently represents an area of gene amplification within a chromosome, and the increased gene product from this site could have an important role in the growth of certain neoplasms. If, as has been suggested, the HSR can break down into separate DMs which are ultimately lost from the cell, the HSR could also contribute to genetic instability in the system (Balaban-Malenbaum and Gilbert, 1978). This topic also is considered at length elsewhere (George and Powers, Chapter 24).

A number of kinds of acquired specific mutations and chromosomal alterations may thus underlie the observed genetic lability in different tumor cell populations, operating through various forms of gene duplication, deletion, position effects, and imbalance. It should be recognized that different types of genetic change could occur at different times during tumor development, even within the same neoplasm. I have already noted that chromosomal alterations might result from a gene mutation acquired earlier, and then, in turn, contribute to a cascade of increasing instability.

I have also pointed out in the earlier discussion of the studies by Fialkow et al. (1981) in CGL, that in some instances the acquired mutagenic mutation might actually occur before a cell acquires a sufficient selective growth advantage to generate a recognizable neoplastic clone. This has also been observed in connection with chemical carcinogenesis in the rat liver, where most of the earliest nodules arising in the exposed animal subsequently regress spontaneously (Farber and Cameron, 1980), apparently having only a temporary growth advantage within an hepatic microenvironment badly damaged by the cytotoxic effects of the carcinogen. There does appear to be, however, within the proliferating cells of these "preneoplastic" nodules an increased probability of mutation, resulting in the outgrowth from an occasional nodule of a true neoplasm. Clearly, the acquisition of a heritable growth advantage and the acquisition of genetic instability may both be very important early events in tumor development, and the specific conditions of carcinogenesis in a particular individual may determine which occurs first.

C. Extracellular Factors

In additon to these inherited and acquired mechanisms that may underlie genetic instability in different neoplasms, it is also possible that extracellular factors may contribute to the sequential mutational events involved in clonal evolution and the acquisition of heterogeneity. If, for instance, an oncogenic *virus* is the causative agent, its incorporation into the genome of the cell may not only trigger the initial transformation event, but could also have a continuing destabilizing effect on adjacent segments of the host cell genome. Some theories of viral oncogenesis, such as Temin's "provirus" concept (1980), have envisioned viral elements as functioning, in some respects, like the "transposable elements" described above, and such possibilities are considered in Chapter 20. One can also suggest circumstances in which the persistence of intact virus within the tumor could have a continuing direct damaging effect on the genome of host cells (Nichols, 1982).

Similarly, the continued presence of a long-lived carcinogenic chemical or radioisotope in an individual, or repeated doses of such clastogenic materials through occupational or other exposure, could also result in sequential mutations within the tumor (Nowell, 1976). The mutagenic therapeutic agents used in cancer treatment (radiation, chemotherapy) might contribute significantly in this way to later stages of clonal evolution and tumor progression in some patients. It has even been suggested that *nutritional* changes within a neoplasm may play a role in its genetic instability. Deficiencies of single essential amino acids and of oxygen have been shown to increase the frequency of nondisjunction in cell culture. With the reduced circulation in many areas of rapidly growing tumors, such phenomena might well help to explain the many mitotic abnormalities observed in aggressive malignancies (Freed and Schatz, 1969; Oksala and Therman, 1974).

V. Clinical Implications of Genetic Instability in Tumors

The general concept of genetic lability and resultant clonal evolution and heterogeneity within neoplastic cell populations which has just been discussed presents a somewhat discouraging prospect from the standpoint of clinical control of cancer. The hope for many years has been to find a consistent metabolic alteration in tumor cells which could be exploited therapeutically. It seems increasingly likely that if such a common alteration does occur as the first step in many neoplasms, it may initially represent only a relatively minor quantitative change in a critical gene product, with its identification made extremely difficult by the many subsequent evolutionary steps between the initial alteration and the fully developed malignancy as one sees it clinically. These sequential stages are not only multiple, but also, to some degree, random, reflecting the particular environmental pressures that influence the development of each tumor.

Under these circumstances, one may ultimately have to consider each advanced malignancy as an individual therapeutic problem. If so, immunotherapy would seem theoretically the most hopeful approach to specific destruction of residual tumor cells, after the maximum effect of nonspecific modalities such as surgery, radiation, and current chemotherapy. It is clear, however, that our present knowledge is not adequate to allow confident manipulation of the immune system to the benefit of the patient (Siegel and Cohen, 1978).

This approach may ultimately prove useful, but one must still recognize the definite handicap to the therapist which will be imposed by the genetic lability and resultant heterogeneity of the tumor cell populatiom. With variants being produced, and even increasing in frequency with tumor progression, the neoplasm will continue to generate mutant sublines, perhaps resistant to whatever treatment the physician introduces. The same capacity for variation and selection which permitted the evolution of a malignant population from the original aberrant cell also provides the opportunity for the tumor to adapt successfully to the inimical environment of therapy to the detriment of the patient. This clinical difficulty has been clearly recognized by several other contributors to this volume (Goldie, Chapter 8; Trope, Chapter 10).

If complete eradication of the tumor cell population, then, seems likely to continue to be a therapeutic problem, one might also consider the potential for reversibility of the neoplastic process, as has been suggested by several authors (Braun, 1969; Mintz, 1978) and discussed in other chapters (Markert, Chapter 15; Pierce, Chapter 16). Is it likely that a "cure" can be produced by providing an environment that forces the tumor cell population to cease unbalanced proliferation and move into a state of controlled differentiation? A few such circumstances have been demonstrated experimentally, both *in vivo* and *in vitro* usually involving tumors with a diploid or near-diploid karyotype and with some characteristics of "embryonic rests" (e.g., neuroblastoma, teratocarcinoma), presumably still somewhat responsive to normal developmental influences (Mintz, 1978; Markert, Chapter 15; Pierce, Chapter 16). This approach may be of interest, particularly for neoplasms with little or no demonstrable chromosome change, such as certain cases of leukemia; but for common human malignancies (lung, colon, breast, etc.), which are typically highly aneuploid, the possibility of generating *in vivo* the conditions necessary to force normal patterns of differentiation in these neoplastic populations seems much less likely. The predominant sublines in these tumors have been selected through many steps for proliferative capacity and lack of response to growth controls. However, even in these tumors with major chromosomal abnormalities, banding studies often indicate that the components of the normal genome are still present, although rearranged, and their potential reversibility to normal growth characteristics cannot be categorically excluded. Certainly, these lines of investigation should be continued, as well as increased efforts to understand and control the mechanisms of genetic instability which permit early benign diploid tumors to evolve through multiple subpopulations into the highly aneuploid and heterogeneous malignancies which are the typical clinical presentation of human cancer.

VI. Summary

1. Considerable evidence now exists that tumor cell populations are, to some degree, more genetically unstable than comparable normal cells. This lability might result from inherited gene defects, acquired activation of "mutator" genes, chromosomal rearrangements, or continued effects of clastogenic agents in the tumor environment.

2. There is also increasing evidence that most tumors are clones (i.e., unicellular in origin) and that the phenomenon of tumor progression results from acquired genetic changes in the original clone, which allow sequential appearance and selection of more aggressive subpopulations.

3. Many aspects of tumor heterogeneity apparently reflect continued coexistence within the neoplastic clone of multiple subpopulations with differing selective growth advantages under different conditions within the host.

4. These concepts of genetic instability and associated clonal evolution are discouraging from a clinical standpoint, since each advanced human

malignancy may be heterogeneous and highly individual genetically and biologically when first seen by the physician. Each patient's cancer may thus require individual specific therapy, and even this may be thwarted by the emergence of genetically variant sublines resistant to treatment.

References

Balaban-Malenbaum, G., and Gilbert, F. (1978). *Science (Washington, D. C.)* **198**, 739–742.

Balaban, G. Herlyn, M., Guerry, D., and Nowell, P. (1982). *Proc. Am. Assoc. Cancer Res.* **23**, 34.

Boveri, T. (1914). *In* "Zur Frage der Entstehung maligner Tumoren." Fischer Jena.

Braun, A. C. (1969). "The Cancer Problem," Columbia Univ. Press, New York.

Cairns, J. (1975). *Nature (London)* **255**, 197–200.

Chan, J., and Becher, F. (1979). *Proc. Natl. Acad. Sci. U.S.A.* **76**, 814–818.

Danes, B. S. (1978). *Cancer* **41**, 2330–2334.

DeGrouchy, J., and De Nava, C. (1968). *Ann. Intern. Med.* **69**, 381–391.

Farber, E., and Cameron, C. (1980). *Adv. Cancer. Res.* **31**, 125–225.

Fialkow, P. (1979). *Annu. Rev. Med.* **30**, 135–143.

Fialkow, P., Martin, P., Najfeld, V., Penfold, G., Jacobson, R., and Hansen, J. (1981). *Blood* **58**, 158–163.

Foulds, L. (1975). "Neoplastic Development, " Vol. 2. Academic Press, New York.

Freed, J. J., and Schatz, S.A. (1969). *Exp. Cell Res.* **53**, 393–398.

German, J. (1977). *In* "Human Genetics" (S. Armendares, and R. Lisker, eds.), pp. 64–68. Excerpta Medica, Amsterdam.

Hann, H.-W., Nowell, P., Koch, P., Minowada, J., Leitmeyer, J., and August, C. *J. Natl. Cancer Inst.* (in press).

Harnden, D. (1977). *In* "Human Genetics" (S. Armendares, and R. Lisker, eds.), 355–366. Excerpta Medica, Amsterdam.

Hecht, F., and McCaw, B. (1977). *Prog. Cancer Res. Ther.* **3**, 105–123.

Heston, L. (1977). *Science (Washington, D.C.)* **196**, 322–323.

Högstedt, B., and Mitelman, F. (1981). *Hereditas* **95**, 165–167.

Hutchinson, R., Rosenstock, J., Nowell, P., and Finan, J. (1981). *Med. Pediatr. Oncol.* **9**, 467.

Klein, G. (1979). *Proc. Natl. Acad. Sci. U.S.A.* **76**, 2442–2446.

Law, I. P., Hollinshead, A. C., Whang-Peng, J., Dean, J. H., Oldham, R. K., Herberman, R. B., and Rhode, M. C. (1977). *Cancer* **39**, 1229–1236.

Levan, G., and Mitelman, F. (1976). *Hereditas* **84**, 1–14.

Li, F. P., Potter, N. U., Buchanan, G. R., Vawter, G., Whang-Peng, J., and Rosen, R. B. (1978). *Am. J. Med.* **65**, 933–939.

Loeb, L., Battula, N., Springgate, C., and Seal, G. (1975). *In* "Fundamental Aspects of Malignancy," pp. 243–256. Springer-Verlag, Berlin and New York.

Makino, S. (1956). *Ann. N.Y. Acad. Sci.* **64**, 818–823.

Mark, J. (1969). *Eur. J. Cancer* **5**, 307–318.

Miller, O. J., Breg, W. R., Schmickel, R. D., and Tretter, W. (1961). *Lancet* **2**, 78–79.

Mintz, B. (1978). *Annu. Symp. Fundam. Cancer Res. Proc.* **30**, 27–53.

Mitelman, F. (1971). *Hereditas* **69**, 155–162.

Mitelman, F., Nilsson, P., Brandt, L., Alimena, G., Montuoro, A., and Dallapiccolo, B. (1979). *Lancet* **2**, 1195–1197.

Murray, M., Shilo, B., Shih, C., Cowing, D., Hsu, H., and Weinberg, R. (1981). *Cell* **25**, 355–361.

Nichols, W. (1982) *In* "Chromosome Breakage and Neoplasia" (J. German, ed.), Wiley, New York (in press).

Nowell, P. (1976). *Science (Washington, D.C.)* **194**, 23–28.

Nowell, P. (1977). *Am. J. Pathol.* **89**, 459–476.

Nowell, P. (1982). *In* "Cancer: A Comprehensive Treatise" (F. Becker, ed.), Vol. 1, 2nd ed., pp. 3–46. Plenum, New York.

Nowell, P., Finan, J., Glover, D., and Guerry, D. (1981). *Blood* **58**, 183–186.

Nowell, P., Finan, J., and Vonderheid, E. (1982). *J. Invest. Dermatol.* **78**, 69–75.

Oksala, T., and Therman, E. (1974). *In* "Chromosomes and Cancer" (J. German, ed.), pp. 239–263. Wiley, New York.

Otter, M., Palmer, C., and Baehner, R. (1978). *Proc. Am. Assoc. Cancer Res.* **19**, 202.

Parshad, R., Sanford, K. K., Tarone, R. E., Jones, G. M., and Baeck, A. E. (1979). *Cancer Res.* **39**, 929–933.

Passarge, E., and Bartram, C. (1976). *In* "Birth Defects," 177–180 Original Article Series, The National Foundation, New York.

Rowley, J. D. (1980a) *Cancer Genet. Cytogenet.* **2**, 175–198.

Rowley, J. D. (1980b) *Clin. Haematol.* **9**, 55–86.

Seabright, M. (1976). *Chromosomes Today* **5**, 293–297.

Setlow, R. (1978). *Nature (London)* **271**, 713–717.

Shiraishi, Y., and Sandberg, A. A. (1979). *J. Natl. Cancer Inst.* **62**, 27–33.

Siegel, B., and Cohen, S. (1978). *Fed. Proc. Fed. Am. Soc. Exp. Biol.* **37**, 2212–2214.

Sokova, O., Volgareva, G., and Pogosiantz, H. (1976). *Genetika* **12**, 156–159.

Temin, H. (1980). *Cell* **21**, 599–600.

Von Hansemann, D. (1890). *Virchows Arch. Pathol. Anat. Physiol.* **119**, 298–307.

Weiner, F., Dalianis, T., Klein, G., and Harris, H. (1974). *J. Natl. Cancer Inst.* **52**, 1779–1785.

23

Chromosomal Changes in Human Cancers: Specificity and Heterogeneity

Avery A. Sandberg

TUMOR CELL HETEROGENEITY
Copyright © 1982 by Academic Press, Inc.
All rights of reproduction in any form reserved.
ISBN 0-12-531520-1

367

Even though the title of this symposium is "Tumor Cell Heterogeneity: Origins and Implications," and certainly heterogeneity characterizes the karyotypic* findings in the cells of human cancer and leukemia (Sandberg 1980),† advances in cancer cytogenetics and the acquisition of a large body of data in various human leukemias and cancers have afforded the opportunity for (1) correlations with a number of clinical, histological, and prognostic parameters, which have revealed specific karyotypic changes in some states, (2) application of the cytogenetic findings in the planning of therapy, (3) the unraveling of possible causative agents in leukemia, and (4) an understanding of the biology of some human leukemias and tumors. In this chapter an attempt will be made to present a concise historical background to chromosome studies in human cancer and leukemia during the last 25 years; and then to discuss the chromosome findings as they relate to a number of areas of human neoplasia, including, in particular, causation of cancer and heterogeneity of the karyotypic aspects of tumors and their cells.

Meaning and order in new scientific endeavors require time for the acquisition of sufficient data and their correlation with appropriate parameters and the refinement of techniques necessary for more sophisticated approaches to problems. Chromosome studies in human cancer and leukemia are no exception. Thus, even though the most specific and characteristic karyotypic anomaly in human neoplasia described to date, i.e., the Philadelphia (Ph¹) (Fig. 1) chromosome in chronic myelocytic leukemia (CML) (Nowell and Hungerford 1960), was found within 4 years after the correct number of chromosomes in human somatic cells was established (Tjio and Levan 1956) and methodologies developed for cytogenetic examination of a variety of human cells and tissues, it has taken another two decades to unravel some of the more subtle, complex, and less common karyotypic characteristics of certain leukemias and tumors; this was primarily due to the necessity of developing and utilizing techniques that reveal more of chromosomal structures than afforded by previously used less refined methods. Once karyotypic data were obtained, it did not take long to correlate these with a number of parameters, thus revealing some rather interesting and intriguing promulgations and/or conclusions.

---

*The terms "karyotypic," "chromosomal," and "cytogenetic" will be used interchangeably in this chapter.

†The number of references has been kept to a minimum in order to conserve space. However, the reader will find more detailed information and a large list of references (more than 4000) on the subjects presented in the book by the author entitled, "The Chromosomes in Human Cancer and Leukemia," Elsevier North-Holland, New York, 1980.

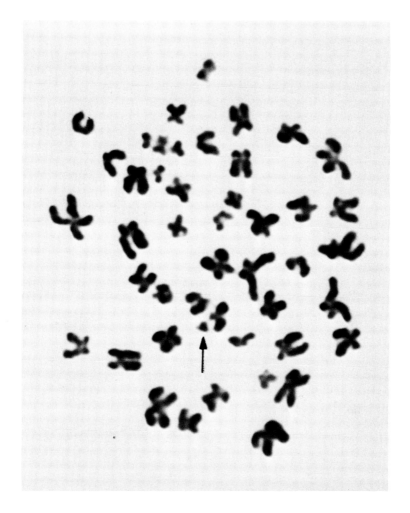

Fig. 1. Bone marrow metaphase containing a Ph¹ chromosome (arrow), shown to date to be the most common and characteristic cytogenetic finding in human neoplasia, in this case chronic myelocytic leukemia (CML). The somewhat fuzzy appearance of the chromatids is not unusual and can be observed in a significant number of cases of leukemia or cancer. Without banding it was difficult to identify the exact origin of the Ph¹, which ultimately was shown with banding to be due to a translocation between chromosomes 9 and 22 in the preponderant number of cases of CML. The origin of Ph¹ is invariably due to deletion of one chromosome 22.

I. Historical Background to Cytogenetic Studies in Human Cancer and Leukemia

The short historical background to the study of chromosomal changes in human neoplasia reflects the fact that advances in the cytogenetics of human cancer, as is true of most scientific disciplines, are at the mercy of methodological advances (Wake *et al.*, 1981). When the latter occur, progress is made almost immediately in expanding our knowledge and the characterization of new syndromes associated with chromosomal changes and their significance in human cancer and leukemia (Sandberg, 1981b; Sandberg and Wake, 1981).

The era of chromosome analysis in human neoplasia can be arbitrarily divided into three periods: before 1960, the period of 1960–1970, and that of 1970 to the present.

A. Period before 1960

In addition to the Ph[1], a number of cytogenetic laboratories examined and established the chromosome constitutions of various human cancers (primarily in effusion material), and in bone marrow cells of various leu-

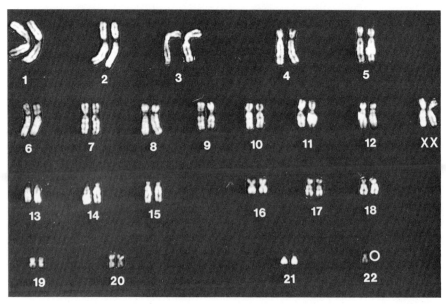

Fig. 2. Karyotype of a meningioma consisting of 45 chromosomes, the missing chromosome being a 22, a finding characterizing a significant number of meningiomas.

kemias. It became apparent that cancerous tissues almost invariably have chromosome changes, numerical and/or morphological, though it was often difficult (see below) to be certain of the identification of the abnormal (marker) chromosomes and not infrequently even of normal chromosomes in such preparations. Nevertheless, it was during this period that the presence of readily recognizable, ranging from minor to remarkable, karyotypic changes were described in various cancers and leukemias (Sandberg, 1980). Except for the Ph¹, however, this era failed to yield other specific or characteristic chromosome changes in human neoplasia.

B. Period of 1960–1970

During this period the information was greatly expanded. It was established that almost all human cancers have chromosomal changes, ranging from subtle ones to greatly increased chromosome numbers with and without a large number of abnormal marker chromosomes (Fig. 2). In a

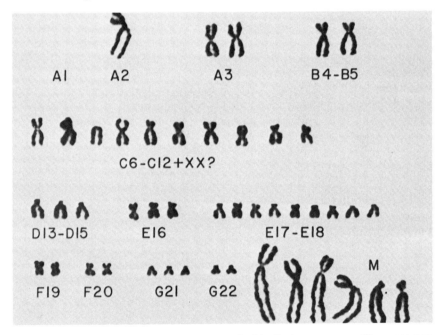

Fig. 3. Unbanded karyotype of a tumor cell with 45 chromosomes. Chromosomes are missing in groups A, A2, C, and D. Extra chromosomes appear to be present in groups E and G. The six marker chromosomes shown in the right lower corner could not be identified rigorously as to their origin. Undoubtedly, the genesis of some of these markers could have been established with banding techniques. In this particular cell the markers are larger in size than any of the normal chromosomes.

few conditions nonrandom and in some specific karyotypic changes were described, which were later confirmed and elaborated on by banding techniques in the 1970s. Thus, for example, monosomy 22 in meningioma (Fig. 3) (Zang and Singer 1967), missing or extra chromosomes in group C in some cases of acute myeloblastic leukemia (AML), and chromosomal changes in disorders with high risk of cancer (Bloom's syndrome, ataxia telangiectasia, Fanconi's anemia, and others) were established; again these were critically analyzed when banding techniques became available. The preponderant number of observations made during this period have withstood the test of time with banding techniques. Even though the latter did lead to a greatly increased number of nonrandom karyotypic changes being recognized in human leukemia, few mistakes (at least serious ones) in the analysis of chromosome findings in human cancer and leukemia were made by cytogeneticists prior to 1970.

C. 1970 to Present

The introduction of banding techniques (Figs. 4–6), starting with Q banding in 1970, led to the recognition of subtle karyotypic changes in human neoplasia by revealing subchromosomal structure. Thus, about 350 bands were arbitrarily defined in the human chromosomes (the 22 autosomes and X and Y sex chromosomes). Recent advances with high resolution banding have yielded about 1500 bands (Yunis, 1980); the possibility exists that conditions previously thought to be associated with normal (diploid) karyotypes may be proved to have subtle changes only recognized with such high resolution banding. However, to date, except for revealing more details about already established karyotypic changes, high resolution banding has not revealed any new cytogenetic syndromes in human neoplasia. Undoubtedly, further refinements in various techniques will reveal even more subband structures with the number of recognizable bands exceeding 3000–4000.

It was also during this period that a sufficient body of cytogenetic information became available in human leukemias suitable for correlations with various prognostic, cytological and clinical parameters. This resulted in the cytogenetic definition of a number of subgroups of leukemias with very similar cytology, response to therapy, and prognosis. Examples are shown in Tables I and II. In Table I are presented the salient features of a subgroup of acute myeloblastic leukemia (AML) associated with t(8;21)(q22;q22), and characterized by common histological and clinical aspects. In Table II are shown prognostic parameters characterizing cytologically recognizable subgroups of acute lymphoblastic leukemia (ALL).

During the 1970s the introduction of methods for demonstrating sister chromatid exchanges (SCE) led not only to the recognition and study of this phenomenon in normal and abnormal states, but also the application of SCE as a sensitive test for mutagenic and/or carcinogenic agents and environments. The application of this approach in the future, particularly in the area of public health, will undoubtedly find much use.

Most importantly, the seemingly confusing body of cytogenetic data in human cancers was shown to contain within it definite nonrandom or specific chromosomal changes characterizing certain states (Tables III–VI). Undoubtedly, future studies, probably based on even more refined techniques, will continue to reveal more conditions characterized by specific chromosome changes, as well as more details about those already established, thus affording means of sorting out the seeming heterogeneity of some of the chromosome findings in human neoplasia.

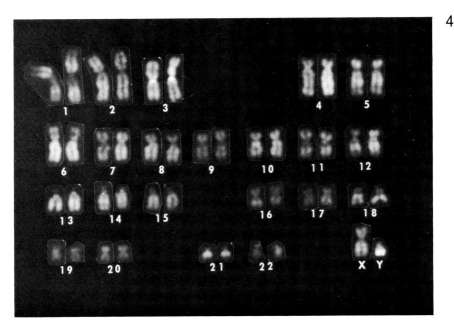

4

Figs. 4–6. Three normal karyotypes obtained with three different banding techniques: Q (Fig. 4), R (Fig. 5), and C (Fig. 6). Each one of these banding techniques reveals different characteristics of the chromosomes. For example, the Q banding technique (Fig. 4) reveals the various bands which afford the cytogeneticist the opportunity to identify each chromosome rigorously, with the long arms of the Y chromosome fluorescing very brightly. The R banding technique (Fig. 5) is a useful one for establishing translocations, since it favors the staining and recognition of telomeric (end regions) areas of the chromosomes. The C banding technique (Fig. 6) is one that reveals paracentric heterochromatin and is also useful in recognizing translocations, particularly those containing more than one centromere. (See p. 374.)

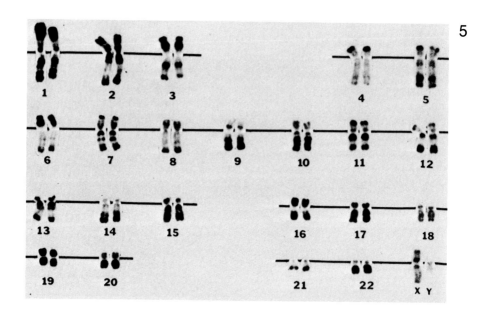

5

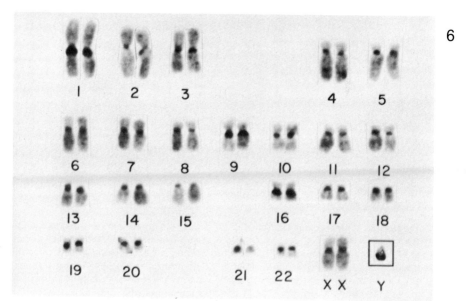

6

Figs. 5 and 6

TABLE I

AML with 8;21 Translocation[a]

---

1. M2 of Fab classification
2. Relatively good prognosis
3. Auer bodies present
4. Missing sex chromosome common
5. Additional karyotypic changes affect disease negatively

---

[a] See Second International Workshop on Chromosomes in Human Leukemia (1980) for further details.

TABLE II

Median Survivals in ALL as Related to Karyotypic Changes[a]

Chromosome findings	Approximate median survival (months)
t(8;14)	5
t(4;11)	8–10
t(9;22)(Ph[1]+)	12
Pseudodiploid	>24
6q −	>36
Hyperdiploid	>36
Diploid	>36

[a] Based on reports of the Third International Workshop on Chromosomes in Leukemia (1981).

TABLE III

Nonrandom Translocations Characterizing Human Leukemias and Cancers

Translocation	Condition in which found
t(9;22)(q34;q11)	CML, acute leukemias (AML, ALL)
t(8;21)(q22;q22)	AML (M2)
t(4;11)(q21;q23)	ALL
t(8;14)(q23;q32)	ALL (L3), Burkitt's lymphoma, other lymphomas
t(15;17)(q24;q21)	APL (M3)
t(11;C)(q21–23;C)	ANLL
(C = #6, #9, #10, #17)	
t(3;8)(p25;q21)	Mixed tumor of parotid
t(6;14)(q21;q24)	Serous cystadenocarcinoma of ovary
t(9;11)(p21;q23)	Acute monoblastic leukemia (M5)

TABLE IV

Nonrandom Morphological Chromosome Changes in Human Cancer and Leukemia

Chromosome involved	Condition in which found
1p−	Malignant melanoma
1p−(p34)	Neuroblastoma
1q+	Breast cancer
3p−	Small cell cancer of lung
5q−	Refractory anemia; ANLL (EL and AML)
6q−	Lymphoma, ALL
7q−	ANLL (EL and AML)
11q−	ANLL (AMoL and AMMoL)
12q−	Complicating acute leukemia
14q+	Lymphoma, ALL, CLL
14q+(q32)	Adult T cell leukemia
i(17q)	CML (BP)
20q−	PV
21q−	Thrombocythemia?
22q−	CML, meningioma
1p−,i(1q)	Endometrial cancer
3p−,3q−,5q−,7q−	Complicating leukemia

TABLE V

Nonrandomness of Missing or Extra Chromosomes in Human Cancer and Leukemia

Chromosome involved	Condition in which found
−5	ANLL (EL and AML), complicating acute leukemia
−7	ANLL (EL and AML), complicating acute leukemia
+8	ANLL, CML (BP)
+12	Hematological conditions, especially CLL
+21	ALL
−22	Meningioma
±3, −5, −7, ±12, ±17	Complicating leukemia

TABLE VI

Common Chromosome Translocations in Lymphoma

Lymphomas (non-Burkitt's)
t(1;14)(q23;q32)
t(8;14)(q22;q32)
t(10;14)(q24;q32)
t(11;14)(q13;q32)
t(14;14)(q24;q32)
t(14;18)(q32;q21)
t(Y;14)(q12;q24?)

Burkitt's lymphoma
t(2;8)(p12;q23)
t(8;14)(q23;q32)
t(8;22)(q24;q11−13)

II. Chromosomal Heterogeneity in Human Tumors

Tumor cell heterogeneity probably has its basis in the diversity of the chromosome changes observed in cancer cells and in the genomes of the human population. Though it is possible that the former reflect in a large measure the remarkable diversity of the latter, it is possible that the interaction between these two parameters (karyotype of the tumor and genome of the host) may account, to a large extent, for tumor cell heterogeneity. Some of the salient features of the chromosome heterogeneity among tumors will be outlined.

A. Heterogeneity between Tumors of Different Sites and Histology

Though they lack the specificity akin to that of nonrandom or specific karyotypic changes the modal chromosome number and the distribution of such numbers in various cancers show differences among tumors of different sites. For example, cancer of the uterus is more likely to have a

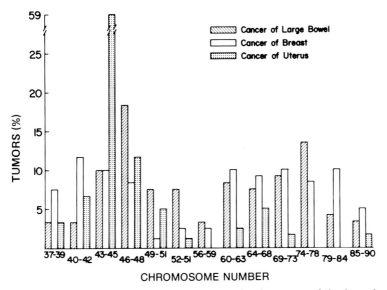

Fig. 7. Distribution of modal chromosome number in cancer of the large bowel, breast and uterus. The most common modal number in cancer of the uterus is in the near-diploid range (43–45 chromosomes), with a few of the tumors having a modal chromosome number in the triploid range. On the other hand, cancer of the large bowel or breast, though having some tumors with a modal chromosome number in the diploid range, are predominantly hyperdiploid or near-triploid.

modal chromosome number in the hypodiploid range (43–45 chromosomes) than cancer of the breast or large bowel (Fig. 7). The latter two tumors also have a significant percentage of cases with a near-triploid modal number, which is not true of cancer of the uterus. This type of heterogeneity may be reflected in (or reflect) the biology of the tumor and the site of its origin. To date, the mechanisms responsible for the wide range of the modal chromosome numbers in tumors, i.e., those of one site being near-diploid and those of another site near-triploid or near-tetraploid, remain unknown, though they may be related to variability in the abnormalities of the mitotic process in cancer cells (Oksala and Therman, 1974). These may possibly reflect different causative factors and/or the host's genetic variability in the various tumors.

Even in tumors of different sites but with the same modal chromosome number, the distribution and/or morphological features of the chromosomes will differ profoundly. Most importantly, certain specific translocations, morphological changes in specific chromosomes and other non-random anomalies may characterize tumors of a specific site and histology, for example, small cell cancer of the lung (Whang-Peng et al., 1982), ovarian serous cystadenocarcinoma (Wake et al., 1980), mixed tumor of the parotid gland (Mark et al., 1980), and meningioma (Zang and Singer, 1967). Thus, there is a basic heterogeneity of the chromosome constitutions among tumors of different sites. In time, it is possible that each specific tumor will be shown to have a consistent, characteristic, and specific karyotypic change. Such a change may possibly be related to the etiology of each tumor.

B. Chromosomal Heterogeneity between Tumors of the Same Site

Having stated that tumors at different sites or in different organs show a diversity in their chromosomal constitution, it must not be assumed that tumors originating at a similar site (or organ) have identical or similar karyotypes (Fig. 8). Even when such tumors have a consistent and basic karyotypic anomaly (e.g., a translocation between chromosomes 6 and 14 in cystadenocarcinoma of the ovary), the total cytogenetic picture will differ from tumor to tumor in the additional (secondary?) karyotypic changes associated with the specific anomaly (Figs. 9–14). Tumors of the lung differ in their chromosome constitution, e.g., small cell cancers have a 3p– anomaly, which does not characterize adenocarcinoma or epidermoid cancer of the lung. Thus, it is possible that tumors of very similar histology may have a basic and consistent karyotypic change, which, as mentioned previously, may be related to the causation of the tumor, with the secondary and additional chromosomal changes being sufficiently diverse so that no two tumors of the same site and histology appear to have identical karyotypes. Whether these diverse secondary changes reflect the basic genetic variability among human beings and, thus, paradoxically constitute a phenotypic phenomenon of this variability among patients and/or whether these secondary changes are related to external phenomena affecting the tumor after its development is an area that requires much more work and information.

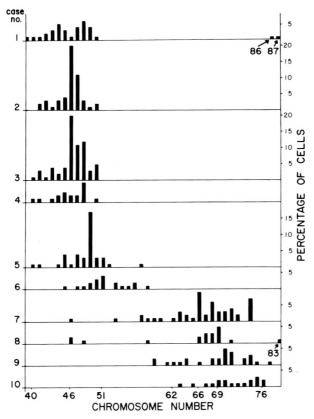

Fig. 8. Distribution of chromosome number in 10 cases of colon cancer, showing that five of the tumors had chromosome numbers in the diploid range and the other five in the triploid range. In addition, the distribution of the chromosome numbers, including the modal ones, differs from one tumor to another.

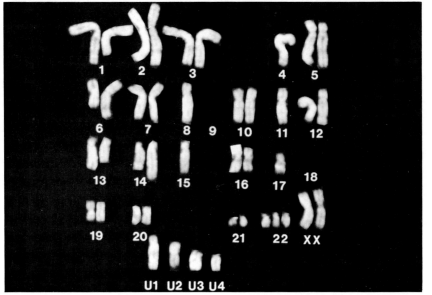

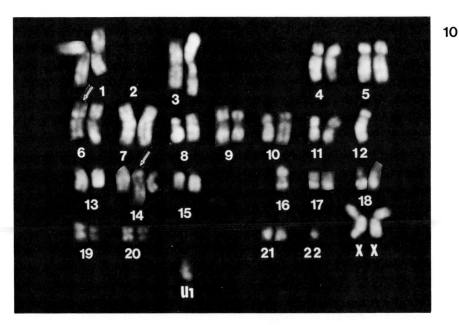

10

Figs. 9–14. In these figures are shown six karyotypes, each originating from a different serous cystadenocarcinoma of the ovary. In each case the specific karyotypic change, i.e., t(6;14), is present with the secondary changes being quite different in each of the tumors. Thus, the karyotypes shown in Figs. 9–11 are near-diploid and, yet, each one of them differs considerably from the other. These three karyotypes are remarkably different from those shown in Figs. 12–14 which have a much higher chro-

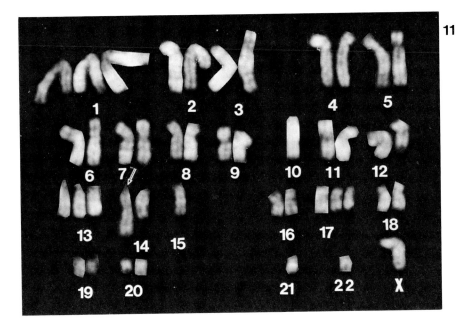

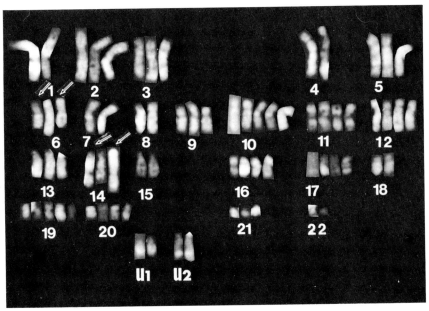

mosome number than those shown in Figs. 9–11 and containing varying numbers of markers. Thus, these six karyotypes demonstrate the remarkable karyotypic heterogeneity that may exist in tumors of the same site and histology, though, as indicated, they are all characterized by a specific chromosomal change consisting of a translocation between chromosomes 6 and 14. (See p. 382.)

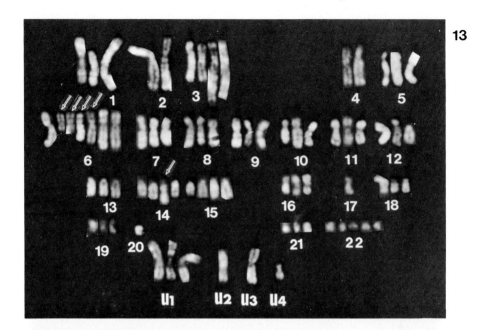

13

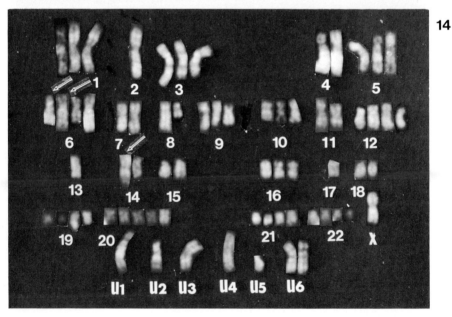

14

Figs. 13 and 14

C. Chromosomal Heterogeneity among Cells of Individual Tumors

Within the same tumor, even when all of the cells are characterized by a specific karyotypic anomaly, e.g., t(6;14) in ovarian serous cystadenocarcinoma or the Ph^1 in CML, chromosomal variability may exist between the cells of each tumor (Figs. 15 and 16). Such variability may involve only a small percentage of the cells and/or be characterized by minor karyotypic changes or affect a preponderant number of the cells, with remarkable variations in the karyotypic changes. With the progression of the tumor and/or recurrence some changes in the karyotype of the modal cells may occur but these are usually a variation on the theme of the original chromosomal abnormality. Thus, chromosomal instability and

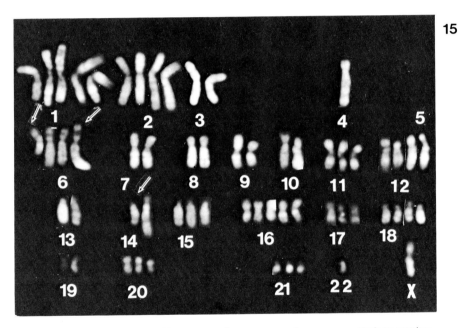

15

Figs. 15 and 16. Q-banded karyotypes from a case of a serous cystadenocarcinoma of the ovary showing the type of heterogeneity which may exist in a single tumor. Though each cell contains the specific chromosomal change consisting of a translocation between chromosomes 6 and 14, other changes characterize the cells. Thus, the cell shown in Fig. 15 contains a marker (M1) as well as extra or missing chromosomes constituting a karyotypic makeup remarkably different from that of the cell shown in Fig. 16; it must be remembered that these two cells originated from the same tumor and reflect the type of chromosomal heterogeneity which may characterize a single tumor. However, the basic chromosomal change, i.e., t(6;14), is evident in both cells, as it was in all the cells of this particular tumor. (See p. 384.)

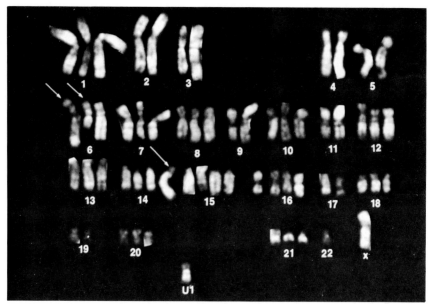

16

Fig. 16

heterogeneity may not necessarily be *de novo* phenomena in cancer cells, but a continuous process of karyotypic selection from preexisting cells present in a tumor population. It should be pointed out that generally chromosomal heterogeneity between tumors, even when characterized by nonspecific karyotypic changes, is much wider than within the cells of a single tumor. In the latter, though the cells may show a wide range of chromosome numbers and a variety of karyotypes, the chromosomal changes have a common theme, a central cytogenetic motif. Thus, the widest heterogeneity in chromosomal changes exists between tumors of different sites or histology; the least exists within the cells of a single tumor.

Single tumor heterogeneity may indicate biological heterogeneity, particularly if the genotype is reflected in the phenotype. If a tumor starts from a single cell, then the heterogeneity may indicate progression and divergence from the original tumor. However, a common theme must then pervade the tumor cell population, this theme probably being responsible for the cancerous behavior of the original cell and its products. On the other hand, the secondary chromosome changes may play a role in such parameters as metastatic spread, resistance to chemotherapy and/ or radiation and other clinical aspects of the tumors. For example, there may exist within a tumor a subpopulation of cells with secondary karyotypic changes sufficiently divergent from the rest of the cell population to render them resistant to chemotherapy, with these cells ultimately characterizing recurrence or progression of the tumor when the sensitive cells have been ablated with therapy.

III. Characteristics of Karyotypic Findings in Human Tumors

The characteristics of the chromosomes in human neoplasia to be described below may not necessarily be found in every case. However, they occur with a sufficiently high frequency to deserve emphasis. The abnormalities to be described are seen more frequently in so-called solid tumors than in the leukemias and, hence, this section has addressed itself primarily to tumors, though examples from the leukemias will be called on whenever a cogent point has to be made.

A. Some Physical Characteristics of Tumor Chromosomes

Before discussing some of the other karyotypic changes in human tumors, a finding that characterizes most of the solid tumors and some of the leukemias should be stressed. This finding consists of the fuzzy and ill-defined appearance of the chromosomes in a substantial number of cancers and leukemias. What is perplexing about this appearance of the chromosomes is that apparently similar leukemias and tumors may not show this fuzzy appearance, the cause of which, to date, has not been elucidated. This fuzzy and ill-defined appearance of the chromosomes presents a major obstacle in their banding and, thus, has prevented the detailed analysis of a significant number of tumors and leukemias. Though some evidence exists that this fuzziness is probably not related to the DNA and some of the proteins of chromosomes, no cogent evidence exists for or against this contention. Thus, the fuzziness of the chromosomes may not only have important basic and theoretical implications in the biology of human cancer and leukemia, but also practical reflections in the difficulty with which such chromosomes can be analyzed, particularly with banding techniques.

B. Aneuploidy in Human Tumors

One of the interesting characteristics of the distribution of the chromosome number in human neoplastic cells, in contrast to observations in normal cells, is the wide spread of the chromosome number (Fig. 17).

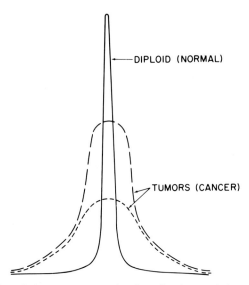

Fig. 17. Distribution of chromosome number in cells of normal tissues (diploid) and in primary and metastatic tumors (long hatches, primary, short hatches, metastatic). As can be seen, in normal tissue the mode of 46 is rather sharp with only a few cells having missing or extra chromosomes. On the other hand, in cancerous tissue there is a wide distribution of the chromosome number with a considerable number of cells having numbers over a wide range below and above the modal number. In metastatic tumors the cells belonging to the chromosome modal number may constitute a small percentage of the total cell population.

Thus, in normal tissue more than 90% of the cells have the modal chromosome number, i.e., 46 chromosomes, whereas in tumors it is not unusual to find only a small proportion of the cancer cells in the modal range with a wide distribution occurring about the mode. Obviously, this indicates tremendous heterogeneity among the cancer cell population, which is even more noticeable in metastatic tumors, particularly effusions. In addition, metastatic lesions generally tend to have a much higher chromosome number (Fig. 18) and contain more marker chromosomes than do the original tumors, possibly indicative that the cells that tend to metastasize are also more cytogenetically advanced, as far as their chromosomal aberrations are concerned.

For all practical purposes all human cancers are aneuploid. This in large measure reflects in all probability the advanced biological state at which such tumors are seen, for in the case of the leukemias diploidy has been encountered in a significant number of cases, this possibly being related to the earlier stages at which such diseases are diagnosed. However, in a recent publication it was demonstrated that in acute nonlymphoblastic leukemia, which until recently was thought to be characterized by diploidy

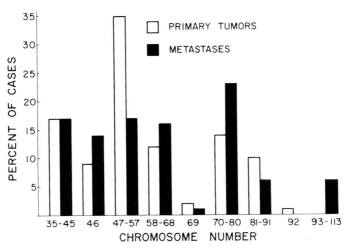

Fig. 18. Modal chromosome number in primary and metastatic tumors. Generally, the metastatic tumors tend to have higher modal chromosome numbers than the primary lesions, with some of the metastatic tissues having modal chromosome numbers above the tetraploid.

in about half the cases, chromosomally abnormal clones may be found with a newly developed technique (Yunis *et al.*, 1981). This finding may indicate that even in some leukemias, diploidy may be a rather rare phenomenon. Thus, for all practical purposes it can be stated that human neoplastic cells are characterized by chromosomal abnormalities, however insignificant or subtle they may be, and, hence, the finding of any chromosomal abnormalities in cells points to the malignant nature of such cells. The chromosome number in human neoplastic cells vary from low to near-haploid, as seen in some cases with lymphoblastic leukemia, to extremely high counts (more than 100 or 200 per cell) (Sandberg, 1980). Extremely aberrant cells with hundreds of chromosomes have been described, though these are patently very rare in human cancer.

The significance of tumors which have modal chromosome numbers in the near-diploid range versus those whose numbers are in the triploid or tetraploid ranges remains to be determined. Some evidence exists that there may be some relation between the modal chromosome number and sensitivity, for example, to irradiation. Furthermore, in some tumors a bimodal distribution may be evident, with one peak being in the near-diploid range and another one in the near-tetraploid or near-triploid range. In all probability the latter ranges were generated from cells in the near-diploid range; once the chromosome numbers are established, it is possible that differences may exist in the characteristics of the cancer cells which depend on the modal chromosome number.

C. Basic Karyotypic Theme of Human Tumors

When human tumors are examined, generally it can be shown that certain karyotypic changes characterize a preponderant number of cells, even though as indicated previously there may be heterogeneity in the cells regarding the number of such changes. Thus, for example, when a number of marker chromosomes characterizes a tumor, these can be observed either in all the cells or in only a portion of the cells with a combination of any of the markers being present in other cells. However, the nature of the markers observed in all the cells will be very similar and indicates the common origin of such cells.

The preponderant number of human tumors have abnormal chromosomes (markers) whose genesis in some cases can be established. In fact, in certain conditions, such as mixed tumor of the parotid gland, ovarian cystadenocarcinoma and others, these markers have been shown to be due to specific translocations, present in almost every tumor, which share a common origin and histology (Figs. 19 and 20). As mentioned above, when tumors recur, either at the primary site or as metastases, the karyotypic picture may vary somewhat from that observed originally, though examination will reveal that the chromosome constitution merely repre-

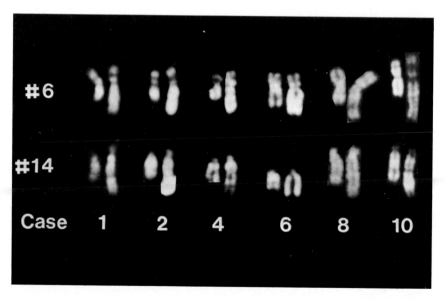

Fig. 19. Translocation between chromosomes 6 and 14 characterizing serous ovarian cystadenocarcinoma. The translocation leads to shortening of chromosome 6 and elongation of one of the chromosome 14, as shown in six different tumors in this figure.

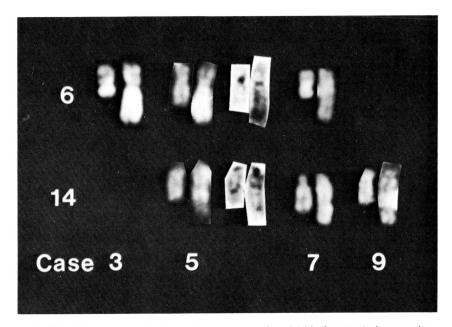

Fig. 20. Translocation between chromosomes 6 and 14 in four cystadenocarcinomas showing some of the progressions which may occur. Thus, in Case 3 the shortened chromosome 6 was present, whereas 14 was lost. Cases 5, 6 and 7 show the translocation between chromosomes 6 and 14, leading to shortening of one chromosome 6 and elongation of a chromosome 14. In Case 9 another variation is shown in which loss of chromosome 6 occurred, whereas the 14q+ was retained. These cases demonstrate what may happen following the specific translocation in cystadenocarcinoma, i.e., in some cases the evidence of a translocation is clear from the presence of abnormal chromosomes 6 and 14, whereas in other cases loss of one of the chromosomes involved in the translocations may occur.

sents a variation on a theme already observed in the original tumor. Thus, the genesis of a new karyotype in human neoplastic cells is extremely rare if it ever occurs at all. It appears that therapy given to patients with cancer or leukemia, be it chemotherapy or various forms of radiation, usually does not change the basic karyotype of the neoplastic cells, though in some cases such agents may lead to the appearance of a second malignancy, particularly acute leukemia, in which case the cells will usually have the karyotypic changes usually observed in such secondary malignancy. In other words, the karyotype of the original tumor appears not to be affected by such therapy; the second malignancy may reflect the effects of the therapy given and demonstrate a karyotype compatible with that seen in secondary malignancy, such as that in acute myeloblastic leukemia.

D. Marker (Abnormal) Chromosomes in Human Tumors

As mentioned above, markers are very commonly present in human tumors, including the leukemias. The origin of these markers may carry some specificity in that it may possibly constitute the original karyotypic change related to the etiology of the neoplasia; or, the markers may reflect secondary events. Often, the origin of markers may be rather difficult to discern. Again, the difficulty in deciphering the origin of such markers can frequently be ascribed to the fuzzy and ill-defined appearance of the chromosomes. The number of marker chromosomes in a human tumor may vary from one to several dozen (Sandberg, 1980). The significance of marker chromosomes in relation to the biology of the tumors has received some attention. For example, the presence of a marker chromosome in bladder tumors of a noninvasive nature usually indicates a high probability of recurrence, whereas the absence of marker chromosomes indicates a high probability of recurrence not taking place (Falor and Ward, 1978; Sandberg, 1977, 1981a). Generally, the more markers in a tumor the more likely the tumor is to behave in a very aggressive fashion, particularly regarding invasiveness and/or metastatic spread. Thus, it would appear that the presence of marker chromosomes indicates a rather advanced biological stage of tumor development characterized by progression.

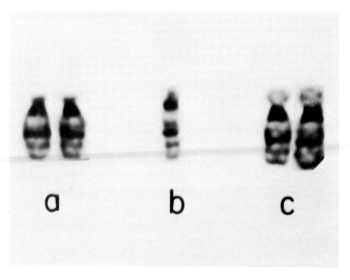

Fig. 21. Three markers (a, b, and c) of identical morphology characterizing three different tumors of different sites. The one shown in (a) was from a breast cancer, the one in (b) from cystadenocarcinoma of the ovary, and the one in (c) from an ovarian cancer.

Identical marker chromosomes may be present in tumors of different origin and histology (Fig. 21), possibly indicating that some of the markers are a secondary phenomenon and do not have the same significance as others, which may be associated with the causation of the tumor. Much remains to be done in this area before the significance of identical markers in different tumors has been deciphered. Undoubtedly, the accumulation of many more data in the future will shed considerable light on the problem of markers and their significance in tumor behavior. In some tumors, the presence of marker chromosomes may indicate resistance to various forms of therapy, whereas in others it points in the opposite direction, i.e., tumors with marker chromosomes being more sensitive to certain forms of therapy than those without or with fewer markers. In any case, the problem of marker chromosomes remains an intriguing one, for obviously it is not only related to the possible causation of the tumors but also to their biological behavior.

E. Specific Changes in Human Tumors

Certain human tumors are characterized by specific chromosomal changes including translocations (Tables II–V). In my opinion these primary changes, which characterize specific groups of tumors, are possibly related to their causation and may reflect their common origin. For example, in the case of acute nonlymphocytic leukemia, certain chromosome changes (–5, –7) are thought to reflect possible exposure to toxic agents (petroleum products, chemical solvents, insecticides, and pesticides), which may, in fact, be implicated in the causation of the leukemias (Mitelman et al., 1981). Similar approaches should be taken in all other human neoplasms, with the chromosomal changes possibly indicating those groups of tumors which may have a common etiology.

In all probability, as a sufficient number of various tumors is examined, each specific group of tumors will all be shown to have specific chromosome changes. Thus, detailed banding analysis, the refinement of existing techniques and the acquisition of more data have clarified some of the rather complex pictures of the chromosome constitutions in human tumors existing prior to 1970. As techniques for the analysis of the chromosomes in human tumors become more refined, specific changes will undoubtedly be shown to characterize specific tumors. The specificity of such changes will not only be useful in the diagnosis and classification of such tumors, and possibly in establishing their common cause, but also of practical value in clinical and therapeutic parameters as well.

F. Heterogeneity of Karyotypic Changes (in Addition to Specific Ones) in Human Tumors

Chromosomal heterogeneity characterizes most of the human tumors (Figs. 22 and 23). In leukemia, however, homogeneity of the karyotypic changes may exist for considerable periods of time, such as the Ph[1] in CML, t(8;21) in AML and t(15;17) in APL, without any additional changes developing until the disease progresses clinically (Sandberg, 1980). This progression may be accompanied by secondary chromosomal changes, in addition to the primary ones. Chromosome heterogeneity is particularly common in solid tumors, undoubtedly reflecting the advanced stage of the tumors; thus, in addition to the specific karyotypic changes, secondary changes are usually observed, accounting for the remarkable chromosome heterogeneity which may be observed in a single

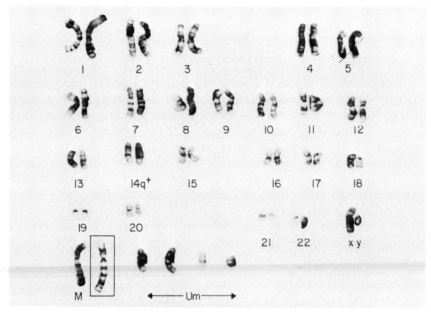

Figs. 22 and 23. Two karyotypes from lymphomas of similar histology, the one in Fig. 22 containing a 14q+ chromosome, an anomaly seen in a substantial number of lymphomas, as well as an identified marker chromosome and four unidentified marker chromosomes. The karyotype with a large number of chromosomes shown in Fig. 23 contains three markers (M_1–M_3) whose origin was identified and 18 markers whose genesis could not be established. Thus, these two karyotypes demonstrate, again, the heterogeneity which may characterize tumors of similar histology, possibly pointing to heterogeneity in causation.

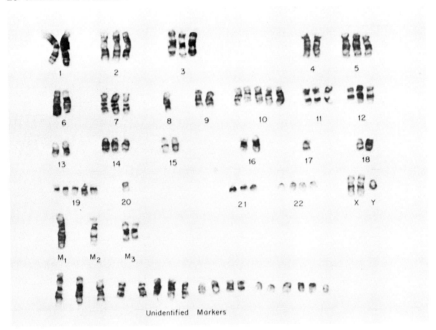

Fig. 23

group of tumors. A good example of that is the heterogeneity observed in ovarian serous cystadenocarcinoma (Figs. 9–14). We have found that almost all of these tumors have evidence for a specific translocation between chromosomes 6 and 14, but are otherwise characterized by remarkable heterogeneity of the chromosomal changes (Wake *et al.*, 1980). Whether these secondary changes reflect the heterogeneity of the genomes among the patients with this tumor, or are related to factors exogenous to the genome, is at the moment unknown. Undoubtedly, these secondary karyotypic changes must play a role in the biology of the tumor, as reflected in its behavior, particularly spread, metastatic ability, and response to therapy. Thus, the secondary chromosomal changes in human tumors represent a challenge to cytogeneticists and oncologists, for these changes probably carry important information which will be deciphered when a sufficient number of tumors has been examined cytogenetically and the findings related to detailed clinical and therapeutic data. It would appear that the primary chromosomal change may be related to the causative aspects of the tumors and that the secondary changes play an important role in the biologic behavior of the tumors. Such chromosomal heterogeneity among tumors undoubtedly is reflected in the heterogeneity of the various aspects of the tumors, including histology, immunology, enzymology, and others.

G. Karyotypic Changes Are Irreversibly Imprinted on Tumors

When a karyotypic change is found in a tumor, this change will persist for the life of such a tumor. This does not mean that additional changes may not occur, but these will usually occur "on top" of existing ones. It is very doubtful whether the karyotypic changes observed in tumors can be reversed, for no evidence exists to date that any form of therapy is capable of modifying the tumor karyotype in the direction of normality. Thus, the karyotypic changes appear to be irreversibly imprinted on the cancer cell, though undoubtedly variations may occur within established karyotypes reflecting in some tumors "phenotypic" manifestations related to the behavior of the cancer cells.

The origin of the heterogeneity of chromosomal changes within a single tumor are still obscure, though irregularities of the mitotic apparatus and related events in cancer cells have been documented (Oksala and Therman, 1974) and may realistically account for some of the changes observed, particularly variations in the chromosome number among the cells of a single tumor.

A moot point is that related to the appearance of cells with chromosomal changes in addition to those present on first examination. Some evidence exists that such cells are already present in the earliest stages of tumor development, but that their number remains quite small; then cells with additional chromosomal changes become apparent only when they gain proliferative advantages over the cells containing fewer chromosomal changes. On the other hand, there is also some evidence that as progression of the tumor occurs, the genesis of cells with additional chromosomal changes becomes evident. At present, this controversy cannot be resolved and further studies consisting primarily of establishing the karyotypes on a large number of cells in early tumor development and following tumor progression with karyotypic analysis should yield some important answers.

Generally, the appearance of chromosomal changes in addition to the specific ones means biological progression of the tumor. For example, in AML cases with t(8;21), the appearance of additional chromosomal changes usually means progression of the acute leukemia, resistance to therapy and short survival (Table I). In CML, the appearance of karyotypic changes in addition to the Ph[1] usually heralds or is associated with the appearance of the blastic phase of the disease (Sandberg, 1980); this blastic phase is similar to acute leukemia, is often resistant to therapy, and is characterized by short survival. Thus, the secondary changes both in leukemia and cancer appear to dictate the biology of the tumor, whereas the primary changes possibly reflect causative parameters.

IV. Significance of Chromosome Changes in Human Cancer

A. Primary Changes

The data on the chromosome changes in human cancer and leukemia obtained to date indicate that in all probability specific human neoplastic conditions are characterized by specific karyotypic anomalies, with such anomalies possibly being related to the etiology of the disease. As shown in Tables III–VI, it is evident that with time, more and more conditions will be shown to be characterized by specific cytogenetic abnormalities. Since such abnormalities are present in the preponderant number of tu-

TABLE VII

Some Applications of Chromosome Findings in Human Cancer and Leukemia, Citing Examples for Each

1. Etiology and causation of human cancer and leukemia
   - (a) Monosomy 5 and 7 in secondary leukemias and Ph[1] in CML
   - (b) Specific karyotypic changes in cancers, e.g., meningioma, serous cystadenocarcinoma of ovary, small cell cancer of lung, etc.
2. Diagnosis and classification (between and within diseases)
   - (a) Ph[1] chromosome in CML
   - (b) t(8;21) subgroup of AML
   - (c) Translocations involving #8 in Burkitt's lymphoma
3. Prognosis and response to therapy
   - (a) Chromosome findings and survival in ANLL
   - (b) Significance of marker chromosomes in bladder cancer recurrence and prognosis
   - (c) Prognosis in Ph[1]-positive leukemia vs. Ph[1]-negative leukemia
4. Disease characterization
   - (a) Translocations in lymphoma
   - (b) NN, AN, and AA characterization of AML
   - (c) MIKA and MAKA groups of ANLL
5. Constitutional and congenital chromosome changes and neoplasia
   - (a) Chromosome breakage syndromes
   - (b) Familial or congenital karyotypic changes associated with high risk of cancer
   - (c) Polymorphism of heterochromatin and cancer susceptibility
6. Chromosome changes and studies in relation to carcinogenesis
   - (a) SCE test
   - (b) Chromosomal changes (breaks, dicentrics, rings, etc.)
   - (c) Consistent karyotypic changes
7. Prevention and public health aspects of cancer and leukemia
   - (a) Monitoring of chromosomal changes and SCE levels
   - (b) Establishment of specific karyotypic changes for specific carcinogens

mors of common site and histology, it can be assumed that they must be related somehow to the causation of the disease.

B. Secondary Changes

The secondary changes may be epiphenomena and/or play an important role in the heterogeneity and variable biology of cancer cells. As indicated previously, these secondary changes probably develop subsequent to the primary chromosomal changes, and, yet, may play a more important role in the behavior and characteristics of cancer cells than do the primary changes. The appearance of cells with secondary changes may be a selective proliferation of cells already existing in the earliest stages of the cancer or these develop *de novo*, a problem that to date has not been solved satisfactorily. The relative heterogeneity of the secondary karyotypic changes in any single tumor may be a reflection of the genotypic heterogeneity and/or due to extraneous factors; again, in this case the significance of one or the other in the genesis of the secondary changes has not been established with certainty. The challenge to cancer cytogeneticists is not only to continue to establish characteristic or nonrandom chromosomal changes in those cancers and leukemias in which this has not been accomplished, but also to address themselves to the nature of the secondary changes and their significance, particularly in the behavior of tumors and leukemia in relation to their aggressiveness, metastatic spread, sensitivity to therapy, and host response (Table VII).

Acknowledgments

The studies performed in the author's laboratory referred to in this chapter were supported in part by a grant (CA-14555) from the National Cancer Institute through the National Bladder Cancer Project.

References

Falor, W. H., and Ward, R. M. (1978). *J. Urol.* **119**, 44–48
Mark, J., Dahlenfors, R., Ekedahl, C., and Stenman, G. (1980). *Cancer Genet. Cytogenet.* **2**, 231–241
Mitelman, F., Nilsson, P. G., Brandt, L., Alimena, G., Gastoldi, R., and Ballapiccola, B. (1981). *Cancer Genet. Cytogenet.* **4**, 197–214.
Nowell, P. C., and Hungerford, D. A. (1960). *Science* **132**, 1497.
Oksala, T., and Therman, E. (1974). *In* "Chromosomes and Cancer" (J. German, ed.), pp. 239–263. Wiley, New York.
Sandberg, A. A. (1977). *Cancer Res.* **37**, 222–229.

Sandberg, A. A. (1980). "The Chromosomes in Human Cancer and Leukemia." Elsevier North-Holland, New York.

Sandberg, A. A. (1981a). *In* "Carcinoma of the Bladder" (J. G. Connolly, ed.), pp. 127–141. Raven Press, New York.

Sandberg, A. A. (1981b). *Int. Adv. Surg. Oncol.* **4**, 311–336.

Sandberg, A. A., and Wake, N. (1981). *In* "Genes, Chromosomes, and Neoplasia" (F. E. Arrighi, P. N. Rao, and E. Stubblefield, eds.), pp. 297–333. Raven Press, New York.

Second International Workshop on Chromosomes in Leukemia. (1980). *Cancer Genet. Cytogenet.* **2**, 89–113.

Third International Workshop on Chromosomes in Leukemia. (1981). *Cancer Genet. Cytogenet.* **4**, 95–142.

Tjio, J. H., and Levan, A. (1956). *Hereditas* **42**, 1–6.

Wake, N., Hreshchyshyn, M. M., Piver, S. M., Matsui, S. I., and Sandberg, A. A. (1980). *Cancer Res.* **40**, 4512–4518.

Wake, N., Slocum, H. K., Rustum, Y. M., Matsui, S., and Sandberg, A. A. (1981). *Cancer Genet. Cytogenet.* **3**, 1–10.

Whang-Peng, J., Bunn, P. A., Jr., Kao-Shan, C. S., Lee, E. C., Carney, D. N., Gazdar, A., and Minna, J. D. (1982). *Cancer Genet. Cytogenet.* (in press.)

Yunis, J. J. (1980). *Cancer Genet. Cytogenet.* **2**, 221–229.

Yunis, J. J., Bloomfield, C. D., and Ensrud, K. (1981). *N. Engl. J. Med.* **305**, 135–139.

Zang, K. D., and Singer, H. (1967). *Nature London* **216**, 84–85.

24

Gene Amplification and Double Minute Chromosomes in Mouse Tumor Cells

DONNA L. GEORGE AND VICKI E. POWERS

I. Introduction

Although nonrandom chromosomal changes have been documented in some malignancies, the nature of the relationship between karyotypic alterations and malignancy remains a fundamental problem in cancer research. Extra-chromosomal nuclear entities termed double minutes (DMs), and distinctively banding, expanded chromosomal segments termed homogeneously staining regions (HSRs) are two intriguing classes of chromosomal abnormality described predominantly in mammalian tumor cells. DMs and/or HSRs have been reported in over 80 human and animal cell tumors of different histological types (Cox *et al.*, 1965; Sandberg *et al.*, 1972; Levan *et al.*, 1977; Barker and Hsu, 1979; Kovacs, 1979; Miller *et al.*, 1979). In human material, they have been described in direct chromosome preparations from some, but not all, tumors of the breast, colon, esophagus, ovary, and pharynx, in neuroblastomas, retinoblastomas, and gliomas, as well as in other tumor cells. Although presently little is known about the molecular composition, mechanism of origin or role of DMs and HSRs in the various tumor cells, they are of interest because of their possible direct relationship to the malignant or differentiated properties of cells in which they are found.

A current hypothesis relating to the origin of these entities proposes that they result from a process of gene amplification, with the amplified sequences represented intrachromosomally as an HSR and extrachromosomally as DMs. This possibility was initially presented for HSRs that arose in a series of methotrexate (MTX)-resistant Chinese hamster cells. Working with these cells, Biedler and Spengler (1976a,b) noted a correlation among the presence and size of HSRs, acquired resistance to high levels of MTX, and overproduction of the target enzyme dihydrofolate reductase (DHFR). Biochemical support for this gene amplification hypothesis followed with the demonstration that increased DHFR activity in some MTX-resistant cells resulted from amplification of DNA sequences containing the DHFR gene (Alt *et al.*, 1978). Amplified copies of the DHFR gene have been localized by *in situ* hybridization to HSRs in some MTX-resistant cells (Nunberg *et al.*, 1978; Dolnick *et al.*, 1979). In other cells, in which high levels of MTX resistance and amplified DHFR genes were lost when the cells were grown in the absence of MTX, the unstably amplified DHFR genes were associated with DMs (Kaufman *et al.*, 1979).

Given the association among DMs, HSRs, and gene amplification in the MTX-resistant cells, we initiated studies to determine if these chromosomal anomalies also result from gene amplification in tumor cells which are not MTX-resistant and in which the HSRs and DMs are stably present under no obvious selection pressure. To test this hypothesis and to compare the structural organization of HSRs and DMs, we have used as a model system two related sublines of a mouse adrenocortical tumor cell line, designated Y1. One of these cell lines (Y1-HSR) contains an HSR-bearing marker chromosome. The other cell line (Y1-DM) contains numerous DMs per cell. In this chapter we will describe studies that support the hypothesis that the DMs and HSRs in the Y1 cells are structurally related, and that these entities result from a process of gene amplification.

II. Double Minutes and Homogeneously Staining Regions in the Y1 Cells

The Y1 clonal cell line was derived from a functional adrenocortical tumor that arose in a male LAF_1 mouse exposed to irradiation in an atomic bomb test (Cohen et al., 1957). Established in culture in 1962, the Y1 cell line has been widely used as a model system for studies on steroid biosynthesis and hormone action. These cells produce steroids constitutively at low levels and at increased levels in response to certain hormones (Stollar et al., 1964; Kowal and Fiedler, 1970).

One subline of Y1 cells that we have analyzed contains a large number of DMs per cell (George and Francke, 1980). In 50 cells analyzed at one passage, the number of DMs varied from 6 to 220 per cell, with an average of 69. A representative metaphase spread of the Y1-DM cell line is shown in Fig. 1A. As seen during mitosis, DMs are small (0.3–0.5 μm diameter), usually paired, Feulgen-positive particles. Unlike typical chromosomes, they show no evidence of centromeric structure and they are distributed randomly to daughter cells at mitosis (Levan and Levan, 1978; Barker and Hsu, 1979). This is probably the reason they vary in number from cell to cell. DMs stain as euchromatin, but sometimes stain much lighter than the

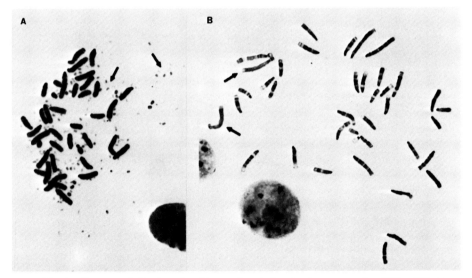

Fig. 1. Representative trypsin–Giemsa banded metaphase spreads of Y1 cell lines. (A)Y1-DM cell line. Arrows point to representative DMs. (B) Y1-HSR cell line. Arrows point to marker chromosome with the HSR. (From George and Powers, 1981. Reprinted with permission of *Cell*, M.I.T. Press.)

other chromosomes of the cell. For this reason, they may be overlooked in some cytological preparations.

Another subline of Y1 cells we have analyzed has a marker chromosome with a large HSR (George and Francke, 1980). HSRs are chromosomal regions that fail to exhibit the differential staining pattern usually obtained with trypsin–Giemsa banding techniques but stain more uniformly (Biedler and Spengler, 1976a). A representative trypsin–Giemsa banded metaphase spread of the Y1-HSR cell line is shown in Fig. 1B. The HSR in these cells is not associated with an identifiable mouse chromosome. Every cell of the Y1-HSR population we have examined contains at least one copy of the HSR-bearing marker chromosome; 4% (4/100) of the cells have two morphologically indistinguishable copies. Based on length measurements of individual chromosomes, we estimate that the HSR comprises 4.2–4.5% of the chromosome complement of these cells. The presence of marker chromosomes shared by the Y1-HSR and the Y1-DM cell lines supports their derivation from a common precursor (George and Francke, 1980).

III. Isolation and Molecular Cloning of DNA from Double Minutes of the Y1 Cells

A. Association between Double Minutes and DNA Amplification

In order to gain some insight into the nature and organization of DNA sequences contained within DMs, we isolated a metaphase chromosome fraction enriched in the DMs of the Y1-DM cell line (George and Powers, 1981). The protocol we used involved the differential centrifugation of a chromosome suspension under conditions that effectively separated DMs from the other metaphase chromosomes of the cell (Barker and Stubblefield, 1979; Blumenthal et al., 1979). DNA obtained from this DM-enriched fraction was digested with the restriction endonuclease EcoRI and cloned in the λ vector Charon 4A. One recombinant, designated Y1dm-1, which was isolated at random from this library, has EcoRI-derived insert fragments 3.8, 3.0, and 2.9 kilobase pairs (kbp) in size (George and Powers, 1981). To determine if sequences complementary to the cloned insert fragments are present in different mouse cell lines and to compare the relative abundance of any such sequences, we isolated DNA from the parental LAF₁ mouse cells. We also isolated DNA from two other mouse cell lines, A9 and 3T3. The C3H-derived A9 cells do not have

DMs or HSRs. The BALB/c-derived, thymidine kinase-deficient 3T3 cells contain a large number of DMs per cell.

When DNA samples from each of these sources were digested with EcoRI and probed by Southern blotting techniques (Southern, 1975) with ^{32}P-labeled DNA from the recombinant Y1dm-1, the results shown in Fig. 2 were obtained. The Y1dm-1 probe hybridized to fragments of similar size in all of the mouse cell lines analyzed. However, the intensity of the hybridization signal was found to be much stronger for DNA from the Y1-DM and Y1-HSR cells than that obtained with equal amounts of DNA from the other sources, including the DM-containing 3T3 cells. This result is consistent with the hypothesis that the cloned sequences in Y1dm-1 are amplified in the genomic DNA of the two Y1 cell lines. We estimate that the Y1dm-1-related sequences are 100–200 times more abundant in the Y1-DM cells than in normal mouse cells (George and Powers, 1981). When cloned DNA fragments from six other recombinants isolated from the Y1 DM–DNA library were analyzed in the same way, similar results were obtained (our unpublished experiments).

B. Structural Relationship between Double Minutes and Homogeneously Staining Regions

It is intriguing that HSRs and DMs are seldom found together in the same cell. A number of cytogenetic analyses have provided indirect evidence that some HSRs and DMs may be functionally and/or structurally related. For example, a human neuroblastoma cell line has been reported to have two populations of cells, one population with an HSR-bearing marker chromosome and another population with DMs (Balaban-Malenbaum and Gilbert, 1977). The loss of DMs with the simultaneous appearance of an HSR has been reported in a human colon carcinoma cell line (Quinn et al., 1979) and in a mouse epithelial tumor cell line (Cowell, 1980). In one study, when cells from an HSR-containing human neuroblastoma cell line were fused to a mouse fibroblast line, the resulting hybrid cells contained varying numbers of DMs but no HSR (Balaban-Malenbaum and Gilbert, 1980).

The absence of specific biochemical or genetic markers for the HSRs and DMs in the above studies prevented a direct determination of the nature of the relationship between these entities in the tumor cells. The availability of cloned probes derived from DMs of the Y1 cells provided a means to approach the problem. Because DNA sequences hybridizing to the recombinant Y1dm-1 are amplified in the Y1-HSR cell line (Fig. 2), we wished to determine if these sequences are located in the HSR of these

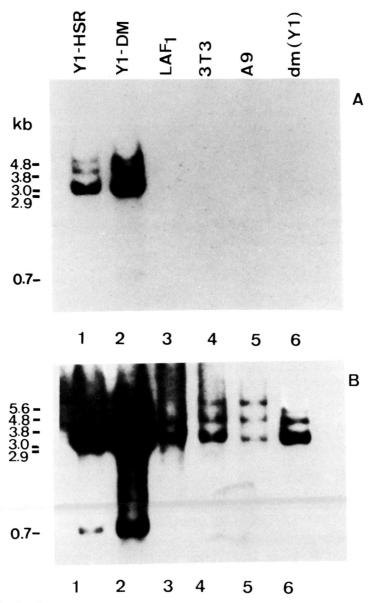

Fig. 2. Southern blot hybridization of ^{32}P-labeled DNA from the recombinant Y1dm-1 to genomic DNA samples. DNA (10 μg) was cleaved with EcoRI, separated by electrophoresis in 0.8% agarose, and transferred to nitrocellulose. Lane 6 contains DNA (<1 μg) from an isolated metphase chromosome fraction enriched in DMs of the Y1-DM cell line. (A) Autoradiogram exposed 16 hours. (B) Autoradiogram exposed 4 days. Band sizes are based on migration of *Hind*III-digested λ DNA.

cells. Therefore, ^{3}H-labeled DNA from Y1dm-1 was used as a probe for *in situ* hybridization (Pardue and Gall, 1975) to metaphase chromosomes of the Y1-HSR cells. The results, illustrated in Fig. 3, showed that the amplified DNA sequences are indeed located within the HSR (George and Powers, 1982a). Thus, the DMs in the Y1-DM cells are structurally related to the HSRs in the Y1-HSR cells.

This conclusion is supported by an additional observation. We have found that a population of cells, derived from the Y1-DM cell line and originally having only DMs, later contained two cell types. Some cells retained DMs. Others in the same culture had lost DMs and gained an HSR-bearing marker chromosome morphologically distinct from that in the original Y1-HSR cell line. From this mixed population we isolated subclones that had either DMs or an HSR, but not both, and DNA was prepared from these subclones. When these DNA samples were analyzed by Southern blot hybridization techniques, the results showed that the cells with an HSR, like the cells with DMs, had retained amplified copies of DNA complementary to the recombinant Y1dm-1 probe (George and Powers, 1982a). Furthermore, the amplified sequences were localized to

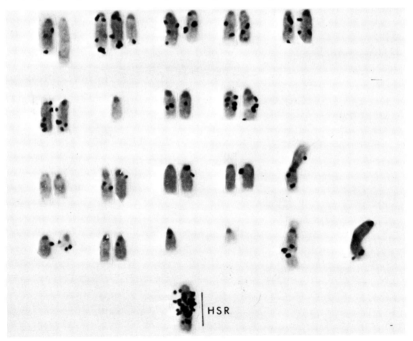

Fig. 3. *In situ* hybridization of ^{3}H-labeled DNA from recombinant Y1dm-1 to metaphase chromosomes of the Y1-HSR cell line. Note accumulation of grains over marker chromosome with the HSR. Exposure time 6 weeks.

the newly arising HSR, as determined by *in situ* hybridization studies. Although these results provide evidence that DMs and HSRs in the Y1 cell lines have DNA sequences in common and under some circumstances one form may give rise to the other, the molecular mechanisms by which this occurs remain unresolved.

IV. Double Minutes and DNA Amplification in 3T3 Cells

To extend our studies on the relationship between DMs and gene amplification, we have utilized a transformed derivative of a 3T3 mouse cell line, discussed in Section III,A. Like the Y1-DM cells, these 3T3 cells contain DMs. In 19 cells analyzed at one passage, the number of DMs varied from 22 to 236, with an average of 130 per cell. However, DNA sequences present in a number of recombinant clones isolated from the Y1 DM–DNA library, which are amplified in the Y1 cells, are not amplified in the 3T3 cells (George and Powers, 1981). Therefore, we initiated experiments to determine if DNA amplification is associated with DMs in the 3T3 cells.

A metaphase chromosome fraction enriched in 3T3 DMs was isolated by a differential centrifugation protocol and a library of DNA fragments from this DM-enriched fraction was cloned in Charon 4A. Of the first five recombinants chosen at random from this library, two were found to contain insert DNA sequences that are amplified in the 3T3 cells. One of these recombinants, designated 3Tdm-7, contains EcoRI-derived insert fragments 2.3, 1.7, and 1.5 kbp in size. When genomic DNA samples from 3T3, Y1-DM, and LAF_1 cells were digested with EcoRI and analyzed on a Southern blot for the presence and relative abundance of sequences complementary to the 3Tdm-7 recombinant, the results shown in Fig. 4 were obtained (George and Powers, 1982b). Hybridization to DNA from the 3T3 cells produced a significantly stronger signal than that obtained with the other cell lines. We estimate that sequences complementary to the 3Tdm-7 recombinant are about 50 times more abundant in the 3T3 cells than in the Y1-DM cells or in genomic DNA from nontransformed NIH/ 3T3 fibroblasts that do not have DMs.

The above results support the hypothesis that DNA sequences in DMs of the 3T3 cells are amplified in these cells. In addition, the data indicate that DMs in the 3T3 cells are not identical in DNA composition to DMs of the Y1 cells. Fragments produced by EcoRI-digestion of cloned sequences in 3Tdm-7, and other recombinants, correspond in size to the fragments to which they hybridize in EcoRI-digested genomic DNA from the different mouse cell lines analyzed (Fig. 4). Similar results have been

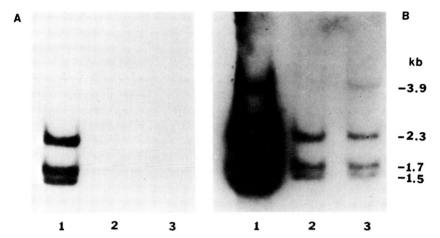

Fig. 4.   Southern blot hybridization of ^{32}P-labeled DNA from recombinant 3Tdm-7 to 10 µg of EcoRI-digested genomic DNA from the following cells: 3T3 (lane 1); Y1-DM (lane 2); normal mouse (LAF₁) fibroblasts (lane 3). (A) Autoradiogram exposed 3 hours. (B) Autoradiogram exposed 3 days. (From George and Powers, 1982b. Reprinted with permission of Cold Spring Harbor Laboratory.)

obtained with other restriction endonucleases (our unpublished observations) and with recombinant clones isolated from the Y1 DM–DNA library (George and Powers, 1981). We conclude, therefore, that these DNA sequences have not undergone any major rearrangement during the amplification process in the 3T3 or the Y1 cells. Also, because we have evidence that the DM-associated DNA from these two mouse cell lines are complementary to DNA sequences present in normal human cells, it should be possible to isolate and characterize such DNA from normal and malignant human material.

V. RNA Complementary to Amplified DNA

An important question relating to the HSRs and DMs in tumor cells concerns whether or not they are transcriptionally active. Experiments in our laboratory have shown that the 3.8 kbp insert in recombinant Y1dm-1 and the 2.3 kbp insert of recombinant 3Tdm-7 are complementary to discrete RNA species in the Y1-DM and the 3T3 cells, respectively. In addition, analysis of cDNA clones constructed from RNA of the Y1-DM cells has provided preliminary evidence that DNA complementary to more than one RNA species is amplified in the Y1-DM cell line (D.L. George and V. E. Powers, unpublished observations). We do not yet know if these RNA transcripts function as messenger RNA or in what way they contribute to the phenotype of these tumor cells. Studies designed to answer these questions are now in progress.

VI. Summary

HSRs and DMs have been described in a variety of mammalian tumor cells, where they appear to be stably present under no obvious selection pressure. We have obtained evidence that these atypical chromosomal structures in two, unrelated, transformed mouse cell lines result from a process of gene amplification. Further, we have found that DMs and HSRs in related Y1 sublines are structurally related, while DMs from the unrealted 3T3 and Y1 cell lines are distinct in DNA composition. Additional studies are necessary to ascertain whether the DMs in these two cell lines, as well as those in other cells, do have some sequences in common.

Modulation in gene number has been documented in both prokaryotes (Perlman and Rownd, 1975; Anderson and Roth, 1977) and eukaryotes. For example, amplification of the DHFR gene has been observed in mammalian cells selected for MTX resistance (Biedler and Spengler, 1976a; Alt *et al.*, 1978); amplification of genetic material coding for the multifunctional protein CAD [carbamyl phosphate synthetase (EC 2.7.2.9), aspartate transcarbamylase (EC 2.1.3.2), dihydroorotase (EC 3.5.2.3)] has been reported in rodent cells selected for resistance to N-(phosphonacetyl)-L-aspartate, a specific inhibitor of aspartate transcarbamylase (Wahl *et al.*, 1979); amplification of the metallothionein-I gene has been seen in cadmium-resistant cells (Beach and Palmiter, 1981). Moreover, detection of DNA amplification has not been limited to situations involving a response to a selective agent. Extrachromosomal amplification of ribosomal RNA genes occurs in amphibian oocytes at a specific stage of development (Brown and Dawid, 1968; Gall, 1968). Also, genes coding for chorion proteins are amplified during oogenesis in *Drosophila melanogaster* (Spradling and Mahowald, 1980). One may speculate, then, that mechanisms of gene amplification may be of general biological significance, having a role in some normal processes of differentiation and development, as well as providing cells with a way to survive adverse environmental conditions.

The mechanism of origin and the function of amplified DNA sequences associated with HSRs and DMs in tumor cells remain to be elucidated. It is important to determine if they function in producing or maintaining malignant transformation, and/or if they are involved in the expression of specific differentiated properties in the tumor cells (Biedler and Spengler, 1976b; Levan *et al.*, 1977). If amplification, or enhanced expression, of otherwise normal cellular genes does play a role in tumorigenesis, the genes involved in different tumors may be specific to a particular cell type or differentiation pathway (Levan *et al.*, 1977; Hayward *et al.*, 1981; Lane *et al.*, 1981; Shilo and Weinberg, 1981). The availability of the DNA libraries derived from DMs of the Y1 and 3T3 cell lines, together with techniques for introducing such DNA into other cells, should promote an understanding of the structural organization and role of these amplified segments in transformed cells. Moreover, HSR- and DM-containing cells should provide workable amounts of what otherwise might be rare cell products for molecular analysis.

Acknowledgment

This work was supported by USPHS Grant CA-29617 from the National Cancer Institute.

References

Alt, F. W., Kellems, R. E., Bertino, J. R., and Schimke, R. T. (1978). *J. Biol. Chem.* **253**, 1357–1370.
Anderson, R. P., and Roth, J. R. (1977). *Annu. Rev. Microbiol.* **31**, 473–505.
Balaban-Malenbaum, G., and Gilbert, F. (1977). *Science (Washington, D.C.)* **198**, 739–741.
Balaban-Malenbaum, G., and Gilbert, F. (1980). *Cytogenet. Cell Genet.* **2**, 339–348.
Barker, P. E., and Hsu, T. C. (1979). *J. Natl. Cancer Inst.* **62**, 257–261.
Barker, P. E., and Stubblefield, E. (1979). *J. Cell Biol.* **83**, 13–16.
Beach, L. R., and Palmiter, R. D. (1981). *Proc. Natl. Acad. Sci. U.S.A.* **78**, 2110–2114.
Biedler, J. L., and Spengler, B. A. (1976a). *Science (Washington, D.C.)* **101**, 185–187.
Biedler, J. L., and Spengler, B. A. (1976b). *J. Natl. Cancer Inst.* **57**, 683–695.
Blumenthal, A. B., Dieden, J. D., Kapp, L. N., and Sidat, J. W. (1979). *J. Cell Biol.* **81**, 255–259.
Brown, D. D., and Dawid, I. B. (1968). *Science (Washington, D.C.)* **160**, 272–280.
Cohen, A. I., Furth, J., and Buffett, R. F. (1957). *Am. J. Pathol.* **33**, 631–651.
Cowell, J. K. (1980). *Cytogenet. Cell Genet.* **27**, 2–7.
Cox, D., Yuncken, C., and Spriggs, A. (1965). *Lancet* **ii**, 55–58.
Dolnick, B. J., Berenson, R. T., Bertino, J. R., Kaufman, R. J., Nunberg, J. H., and Schimke, R. T. (1979). *J. Cell. Biol.* **83**, 394–402.
Gall, J. (1968). *Proc. Natl. Acad. Sci. U.S.A.* **60**, 553–560.
George, D. L., and Francke, U. (1980). *Cytogenet. Cell Genet.* **28**, 217–226.
George, D. L., and Powers, V. E. (1981). *Cell* **24**, 117–123.
George, D. L., and Powers, V. E. (1982a). *Proc. Natl. Acad. Sci. U.S.A.* **79**, 1597–1601.
George, D. L., and Powers, V. E. (1982b). *In* "Gene Amplification" (R. T. Schimke, ed.). *Cold Spring Harbor Lab.*, in press.
Hayward, W. S., Neel, B. G., and Astrin, S. M. (1981). *Nature (London)* **290**, 475–480.

Kaufman, R. J., Brown, P. C., and Schimke, R. T. (1979). *Proc. Natl. Acad. Sci. U.S.A.* **76,** 5669–5673.

Kovacs, G. (1979). *Int. J. Cancer* **23,** 299–301.

Kowal, J., and Fiedler, R. (1970). *Arch. Biochem. Biophys.* **128,** 406–421.

Lane, M. A., Sainten, A., and Cooper, G. M. (1981). *Proc. Natl. Acad. Sci. U.S.A.* **78,** 5185–5189.

Levan, A., and Levan, G. (1978). *Hereditas* **88,** 81–92.

Levan, A., Levan, G., and Mittleman, F. (1977). *Hereditas* **86,** 15–30.

Miller, O. J., Tantravahi, R., Miller, D. A., Yu, L. C., Szabo, P., and Prensky, W. (1979). *Chromosoma* **71,** 183–195.

Nunberg, J. H., Kaufman, R. J., Schimke, R. T., Urlaub G., and Chasin, L. A. (1978). *Proc. Natl. Acad. Sci. U.S.A.* **75,** 5553–5556.

Pardue, M. L., and Gall, J. G. (1975). *In* "Methods in Cell Biology" (D.M. Prescott, ed.), Vol. 10, pp. 1–16. Academic Press, New York.

Perlman, D., and Rownd, R. H. (1975). *J. Bacteriol.* **123,** 1013–1034.

Quinn, L. A., Moore, G. E., Morgan, R. T., and Woods, L. K. (1979). *Cancer Res.* **39,** 4914–4924.

Sandberg, A. A., Sakurai, M., and Holdsworth, R. N. (1972). *Cancer* **29,** 1671–1679.

Shilo, B. -Z., and Weinberg, R. A. (1981). *Nature (London)* **289,** 607–609.

Southern, E. M. (1975). *J. Mol. Biol.* **98,** 503–517.

Spradling, A. C., and Mahowald, A. P. (1980). *Proc. Natl. Acad. Sci. U.S.A.* **77,** 1096–1100.

Stollar, V., Buonassisi, V., and Sato, G. (1964). *Exp. Cell Res.* **35,** 608–616.

Wahl, G. M., Padgett, R. A., and Stark, G. R. (1979). *J. Biol. Chem.* **254,** 8679–8689.

25

The Role of Genomic Rearrangements in Tumor Cell Heterogeneity

RUTH SAGER

I. Introduction

Many lines of evidence have correlated changes at the DNA level with the origin of cancer. The presence of breaks, aneuploidy, and other chromosome changes in tumor cells has been known for a hundred years, but the interpretation of these observations has been another story. Until very recently, the chromosome changes have been mainly viewed as secondary consequences of primary changes occurring elsewhere.

The hypothesis that chromosome changes are causal in the origin of cancer goes back at least to Theodor Boveri (*1*), and was subsequently supported mainly by cytogeneticists. Among oncologists, the Boveri hypothesis went out of fashion as the focus of interest in carcinogenesis shifted to metabolic studies (2,3) and later to viruses (4); and also because a multitude of changes were seen in the chromosomes of tumor cells, changes that were difficult to identify with precision before the development of banding techniques (5,6).

Within the past 10 years or so, a new interest in chromosome changes associated with the origin and progression of cancer has emerged. The emphasis now is on chromosome changes as *causal* events in cancer etiology. Many developments in biological science, some of them ostensibly far removed from cancer research, have contributed to this view. Among the most important has been the recognition that patients with diseases such as Bloom's syndrome, ataxia telangiectasia, xeroderma pigmentosum, and others involving defective DNA repair are also highly cancer-prone (7). Temporal causality has been established in studies of cancer following exposure to ionizing radiation (8), to a variety of chemical agents that damage DNA (9), and to certain viruses that integrate into host chromosomes (10).

Another impressive line of evidence supporting a causal role for chromosome changes in the origin of cancer comes from the discovery that specific nonrandom changes, mainly translocations and deletions, are characteristic of particular forms of cancer: e.g., the 9;22 translocation in chronic myelogenous leukemia (11), the 8;14 translocation in Burkitt's lymphoma (12), the chromosome 22 deletion in meningioma (13), and the interstitial deletion in chromosome 3p in small cell carcinoma of the lung reported at this symposium by Minna (Chapter 2). An up-to-date account of nonrandom chromosome rearrangements associated with cancer has been summarized here by Sandberg (Chapter 22). Other lines of evidence supporting the causality hypothesis, discussed in this symposium, included the progression of chromosome changes seen in prostatic cancer (Chapter 6), the clonal origin of cancer (Chapter 21), and the enhanced expression of endogenous DNA sequences following adjacent integration of retroviral sequences, especially LTRs (Chapter 19).

Changes at the DNA level underlie evolution: *mutation* in the broadest sense, and Darwinian *natural selection*. First, a word about mutations. Ten years ago the exciting news was that carcinogens are mutagenic, and that bacteria could be used to assess the carcinogenic potential of chemicals in the Ames test (14). Bruce Ames' work was a breakthrough, both conceptually and practically, but it also led to narrowing our view of the mutation process in relation to cancer. The Ames test detects nucleotide substitutions and small deletions and consequently attention is focused on this narrow spectrum of changes; but mutations, broadly defined (15) include changes in chromosome number, changes in the arrangement on genes of chromosomes, as well as changes within individual functional sequences. It now appears very likely that the DNA changes leading to cancer involve all these events. At this time, there is no reason to rule out any one of them.

The phenotypic changes seen in cancer are not infinite. A limit to heterogeneity is imposed by the genome. The rearrangements and consequent changes in gene expression that occur in tumor cells do not lead from one differentiation pathway to another. Tumor cells retain some traits diagnostic of their origin. Thus, the genomic rearrangements that are sustained and expressed in cancer cells lie within a narrowly defined sector of development, limited to regions of the genome that are not irreversibly turned off by the normal molecular mechanisms of differentiation.

Natural selection operates on the phenotype, responding to expressed traits whether they are genetic or epigenetic in origin. Natural selection also imposes limits to heterogeneity, since only those cells that are well adapted to their local environment will succeed.

It is my thesis that the same processes that drive evolution, namely *mutation* and *natural selection,* are also the driving forces in carcinogenesis. What is grossly different is the time scale. Evolution occurs over billions of years, whereas cancer occurs within a lifetime. Thus, to understand what causes cancer, we need to understand what mechanisms are responsible for what I call "speeded-up" or *accelerated* evolution.

Natural selection can be speeded up by increasing the stringency of the selective conditions, as in selecting drug-resistant mutants, for example. Some evidence about selection during tumor growth comes from measurements of the rate of tumor growth, the fraction of dividing cells in a tumor, etc. (16). However, the "speed-up" feature that I wish to discuss today concerns mutational events.

II. Transposition as an Evolutionary Mechanism

The modern era in the analysis of genomic rearrangement was ushered in by McClintock's epochal discovery of transposable elements in the corn plant, *Zea mays* (17–22). McClintock established, primarily by genetic methods, that bits of chromosome which she called "controlling elements" could move around in the genome, and that they could induce changes in gene expression, high mutability, chromosome breaks, and rearrangements.

She showed that integration of an element within or close to a gene can either interfere with its expression, or (as in the element called *Spm*) can enhance gene expression. The movement of controlling elements has a random aspect, both in frequency and in location, but also can be regulated to some extent in frequency and in the time during development at which transposition occurs. The transposition event can be visualized, for example, by pigmented spots on kernels arising as the result of movement of a controlling element that had been blocking gene expression by its presence. Depending on gene dosage, the number of spots may vary from few to many, and the size (mirroring the time in development when the rearrangement occurred) from a few cells to a large sector of the kernel. Thus, the process of transposition has both random and regulated features. In addition, regardless of transposition, gene expression also depends on tissue specificity. Pigment synthesis can only be turned on by controlling elements in tissues in which the gene is normally expressed.

Following McClintock's work, transposable elements were identified in bacteria (reviewed in *22*), *Drosophila* (reviewed in *23, 24*), and yeast (*25*). It seems probable that they are present and important in all organisms, though none has yet been clearly identified in mammalian cells. In bacteria (i.e., *E. coli*) transposition accounts for the majority of all spontaneous mutation (*26*). In *Drosophila*, reiterated sequences with inverted repeats at their ends (*24*) such as copia, have very different distributions in the genomes of closely related species (*24,27*) suggesting rapid evolutionary changes. A copia-like element has been identified in a particular mutant at the white locus (*24,28*), further supporting the hypothesis that in *Drosophila* such elements undergo transposition. The genome is estimated to contain about 40 families of these dispersed elements (*24*). A different line of evidence demonstrating the importance of transposable elements in *Drosophila* evolution, comes from the detailed and elaborate studies of mutable genes by M. M. Green and colleagues (*23*). Most recently, the phenomenon of hybrid dysgenesis in *Drosophila*, in which high mutation rates occur in certain hybrid combinations, has been shown to result from transpositional activity (*24,29*).

Thus, transposition is proving to be a highly significant force in evolution. Whether transposition provides the actual mechanism that drives rearrangements in carcinogenesis is not known at this time, but represents a very strong inference.

III. The Origin of Cancer as a Multistage Process

The general hypothesis underlying the ongoing research in my laboratory is summarized in Table I. I have assembled a "most likely scenario," based on the results of many investigators including ourselves. The essen-

TABLE I

Origin of Tumorigenicity: A Multistage Genetic Process

1. Initial DNA damage:
   Induced by radiation, chemicals, viruses or unknown agents
   Leads to:
      Faulty growth control
      Loss of chromosome stability
2. Chromosome breakage and rearrangement:
   Continuing rounds of cell division
   Aberrant transpositions occur leading to genomic rearrangements
   Genetic and phenotypic changes cascade as aberrations continue to arise
3. Selection of successfully growing mutant cells:
   Genomic rearrangements generate new phenotypes
   Selection favors proliferating and well-adapted cells
   Specific phenotypes succeed in different tissues

tial features are (1) the origin of cancer by DNA damage; (2) the further stages dependent not only on continuing rounds of cell division but also on loss of chromosome stability; (3) the occurrence of genomic rearrangements driven by transpositional events; (4) the continuous development of new genotype and phenotypic combinations, which provide the material for natural selection; and (5) the rapid evolution of increasingly better adapted cell types.

On this hypothesis, it is the loss of chromosome stability, leading to rapid and persistent rounds of rearrangement, mediated by transposition, that is the special feature of carcinogenesis. Because of the rate at which these events can occur in destabilized cells, we view it as evolution speeded up.

IV. Experimental Evidence

I wish now to summarize experiments from my laboratory, which I have chosen to illustrate some of the points made in the preceding discussion.

A. Are Rearrangements Causal in the Origin of Tumor Cells?

We approached the problem of causality by a detailed study of the origin of tumor forming ability using CHEF cells which we developed for this purpose (30–34). CHEF cells are Chinese hamster fibroblastic cells of embryonic origin. Two cell lines were initially selected by recloning: CHEF/18 cells which are nontumorigenic; and the CHEF/16 line in which every cell is potentially tumorigenic in the nude mouse as shown by our co-injection procedure (30). Both CHEF/18 and CHEF/16 cell lines are stably diploid in culture (32), but CHEF/16 cells undergo rearrangements during tumor formation (33).

In an intensive study of chemical carcinogenesis with CHEF/18 cells (34), we found that mutants selected for loss of serum growth requirements or of the anchorage requirement for growth remained nontumorigenic in the nude mouse assay with few exceptions. Even low serum, anchorage-free double mutants were non-tumor-forming. Thus, cell culture transformed phenotypes did not correlate with tumorigenicity. The one change that did correlate well with the emergence of tumor-forming ability was the occurrence of chromosome rearrangements as seen in the light microscope (35). Tumor-derived cells from these studies contained heterogeneous chromosome rearrangements but also a high frequency of changes affecting chromosome 3. Remarkably, in a parallel study of chromosome changes occurring during tumor formation by CHEF/16 cells, we again observed a highly nonrandom frequency of changes in chromosome 3, as well as other heterogeneous changes (33).

Taken together, these results suggest an involvement of chromosome 3 in tumorigenicity of Chinese hamster fibroblastic cells. Similar observations were reported some years ago by Bloch-Shachter and Sachs (36). These findings are in line with the many reports of nonrandom rearrangements described in various clinical forms of cancer discussed above. In terms of causality, the association of a gene or chromosomal locus with an altered phenotype, i.e., a disease, has the same implications as in classical genetic mapping, namely that the gene product coded (or regulated) by the particular gene is causally involved in the phenotype. To establish this relationship with translocation junctions or otherwise identified chromosomal regions, one needs to clone out the DNA from the region associated with tumor formation, and test its function by DNA transfer into suitable recipients. Experiments of this type are now within reach.

We already know from published reports (37–39) that DNA extracted from tumor cells can induce 3T3 cells to become tumorigenic. But if carcinogenesis is a multistep process, how can individual DNA sequences carry out this function? One possibility is that prior rearrangements occurring during development of the tumor that was the source of the donor DNA led to coalescence of a single oncogenic sequence. Another possibility is that the recipient 3T3 cells, which are close to tumorigenic (40),

TABLE II

Transfection Experiments with CHEF Cells as Recipients[a]

DNA	Recipient	Foci or colonies per μg DNA per 10^6 cells[b]
Herpes TK-gene	CHEF/16 TK⁻	198[c]
Salmon sperm DNA	LS1-1	0.0005
LS1-1 DNA	LS1-1	<0.005
204-Tu[d]	LS1-1	0.18
EJ[e]	LS1-1	0.59
EJ[e]	CHEF/18	0.15

[a] From Smith et al. (1982).
[b] Background subtracted (control plates taken through experiment with no added DNA).
[c] 1 μg TK clone + 19 μg salmon sperm DNA.
[d] 204-Tu is tumor-derived cell line from CHEF/16.
[e] EJ is human bladder carcinoma cell line.

responded to the tumor-derived donor DNA in a special or indirect way.

We have begun to examine the ability of various DNAs of tumor origin to make CHEF/18 cells tumorigenic in a single transfection step. Since CHEF/18 cells are not spontaneously tumorigenic (34), they are potentially suitable recipients for DNA transfer of tumor forming ability.

CHEF cells are excellent recipients for plasmid DNAs (41). They are also good recipients for genomic DNA, and as shown in Table II, DNA from the human bladder carcinoma cell line EJ induces focus formation in the transformed mutant LS 1-1 and in CHEF/18 cells with yields similar to those reported by other investigators. Our results provide the first evidence that stably diploid, nontumorigenic cells that require chromosome rearrangements in order to become tumorigenic nonetheless can be transformed in a single step by DNA from tumor cells (41). This result supports the hypothesis that the EJ DNA had already undergone prior rearrangements so that it now contains a tumorigenic DNA sequence. Of course, further work is required to establish this hypothesis. I cite this example, although preliminary, because methodologically it represents a sound approach toward analyzing the role of rearrangements in carcinogenesis.

B. An Example of "Speeded-Up Evolution"

We have used the CHEF cell lines to test directly the concept of "speeded-up evolution." One kind of rearrangement that is easy to follow experimentally is the gene amplification that occurs during selection for high levels of resistance to methotrexate (MTX) (*42,43*). We reasoned that tumorigenic and tumor-derived cells should develop MTX resistance faster than stable CHEF cells, assuming that amplification requires genomic rearrangement. We compared three cell lines: CHEF/18 itself; CHEF/16, which is a diploid tumorigenic derivative of CHEF/18;

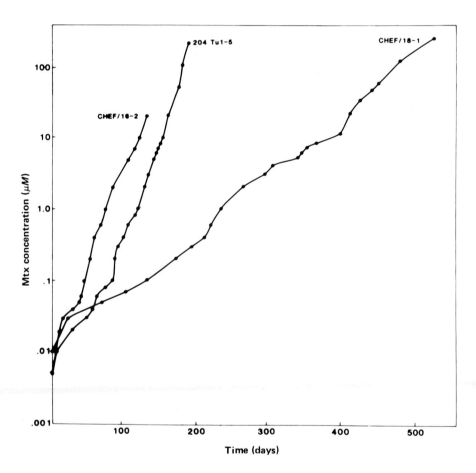

Fig. 1. Time course of development of methotrexate resistance. Nontumorigenic CHEF/18-1 cells, tumorigenic CHEF/16-2 cells, and tumor-derived 204 Tu 1-5 cells were initially resistant to 10 μM MTX. Resistance to increasing concentrations of MTX was selected stepwise, each step represented by a dot. CHEF/16-2 and 204 TU 1-5 developed resistance at four times the rate of CHEF/18-1. (From Sager and Gadi, 1982.)

and 204 Tu, a tumor-derived cell line of CHEF origin. Each cell population was selected by stepwise increases in MTX concentration, starting at 10 n*M*, the sensitivity level of all three strains. The results are shown in Fig. 1. The CHEF/18 cells took four times as long to develop resistance as did the tumorigenic and tumor-derived cells (*44*). This fourfold difference in rate corresponds to a 100-fold difference in resistance at early times in selection and a 1000-fold difference later. The tumorigenic and tumor-derived cell lines increased their resistance at about the same rate. Thus, the tumorigenic and tumor-derived cells both showed speeded up evolution compared to the nontumorigenic CHEF/18 cells. These results strongly support the hypothesis we set out to test, namely, that normal cells (CHEF/18) show a much delayed ability to undergo rearrangement (amplification) either tumor derived cells (204 Tu) which are already rearranged (*33*) or tumorigenic cells (CHEF/16) which are diploid in culture but capable of rapid rearrangement (*33*).

C. Do Changes in DNA Methylation Play a Role in Carcinogenesis?

It seems increasingly likely that changes in DNA methylation (*45,46*) are associated with changes in gene expression. We have examined changes in DNA methylation in various tumor-derived cell lines in the following way. Total cell DNA from a series of tumor cell lines was extracted and cleaved (1) with *Msp*I, which cuts DNA at CCGG and C^mCGG, or (2) with *Hpa*II, which cuts CCGG but not C^mCGG. The digested DNAs were electrophoresed, transferred to paper, and blot hybridized with a set of cDNA probes (*47*). Since we have no specific probes, we used available cDNAs of various genes, two of which β-globin and β-actin, are shown in Figs. 2 and 3. Since all cell lines gave the same pattern with *Msp*I, only the CHEF/18 pattern with *Msp*I is shown here (lane B). The rest of the lanes are DNAs cleaved with *Hpa*II as a measure of comparative methylation at CCGG sites. Lane C is CHEF/18; D and E are azacytidine-treated CHEF/18 cells which have been converted to preadipocytes (*48*). F and G are DNAs from tumors induced by treating CHEF/18 cells with azacytidine (R. Sager, unpublished). H and I are other tumor-derived CHEF cell lines, not from azaC experiments. What is evident is that each of the tumorigenic and tumor-derived cell lines has a unique methylation pattern.

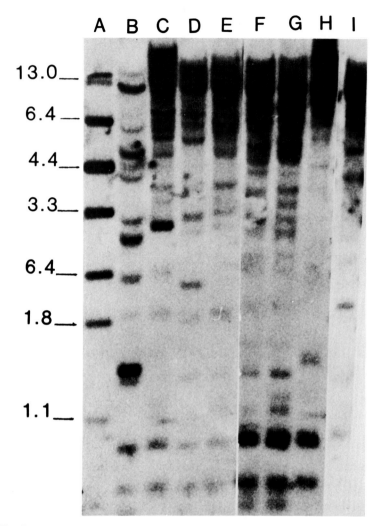

Fig. 2. Methylation patterns of various genomic DNAs blot hybridized to β-actin cDNA. Approximately 10 µg of total cell DNA was digested with *Hpa*II or *Msp*I, electrophoresed on 1% agarose gel at 15 mA for 18 hours at room temperature, and DNA transferred to a nitrocellulose filter by the method of Southern. pA1, A 2000 bp chicken β-actin cDNA cloned in pBR322 [Cleveland *et al.* (1980) Cell 20:95] was labeled with ^{32}P by nick translation and hybridized to the nitrocellulose filter. After washing the filter was exposed to X-ray film at −80°C using an intensifying screen. (A) Molecular weight markers, various digests of approximately 10^{-5} µg pBR322 containing plasmids. (B) CHEF/18, *Msp*I. *Msp*I digests were the same for all cell lines shown. (C–I) *Hpa*II digests. (C) CHEF/18. (D, E) Azacytidine-treated CHEF/18 cells, 708 IV-1 and 708 IV-2. (F, G) Tumor-derived cells from azacytidine-treated CHEF/18 cells, 714dl and 714a3. (H) CHEF/16 ouabain-resistant. (I) tumor-derived cells mutagenized CHEF/18, T30-4. (From Anisowicz and Sager, 1982.)

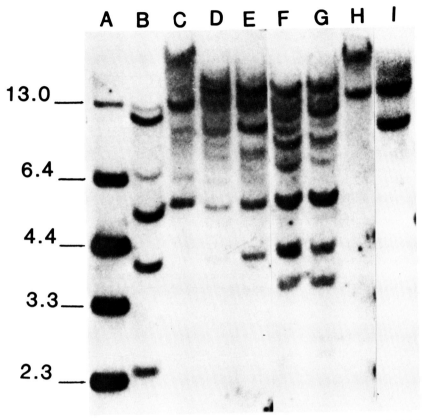

Fig. 3. Methylation patterns of various genomic DNAs blot hybridized to β-globin cDNA. Procedure and DNAs are identical to Fig. 2 except that electrophoresis was on an 0.8% agarose gel and pCRI. βm9, a mouse β-globin cDNA clones in pCRI [Rongeon et al. (1977) Gene 1:229] was labeled with ^{32}P by nick translation and hybridized to the nitrocellulose filter. (From Anisowicz and Sager, 1982.)

V. Concluding Remarks

I propose that normal cells become tumor cells by first undergoing a process leading to genomic destabilization. This instability then leads to the occurrence of continuing cycles of genomic rearrangements, including amplification. These cycles are the motor force of what I have called *speeded-up* or accelerated evolution, and lead to the generation of genomic and phenotypic diversity. Mutations in the broad sense as well as changes in DNA methylation contribute to phenotypic diversity which is acted on by natural selection in tumor formation and progression. A key problem for the future understanding of cancer and for chemotherapy is to find out how the genome becomes destabilized in the first place.

References

1. Boveri, T. (1929). "The Origin of Malignant Tumors." Williams & Wilkins Baltimore, Maryland. (Translated from the German volume of 1914).
2. Greenstein, J. P. (1954). "Biochemistry of Cancer." 2nd edition. Academic Press, New York.
3. Weber, G. (1977). N. *Engl. J. Med.* **296**, 486–493, 541–551.
4. "Tumor Viruses." (1974). *Cold Spring Harbor Symp. Quant. Biol.,* **39**.
5. Yunis, J. J., Sawyer, J. R., and Ball, D. W. (1978). *Chromosoma* **67**, 293–307.
6. Yunis, J. J., Bloomfield, C. D. and Ensrud, K. (1981). *N. Engl. J. Med.* **305**, 135–139.
7. German, J., ed. (1982). "Chromosome Breakage and Neoplasia" (in press).
8. Yuhas, J. M., Tennant, R. W., and Regan, J. D., eds. (1976). "Biology of Radiation Carcinogenesis." Raven, New York.
9. Pullman, B., Ts'o, P. O. P., and Gelboin, H., eds. (1981). "Carcinogenesis: Fundamental Mechanisms and Environmental Effects." Reidel Publ., Hingham, Massachusetts.
10. "Viral Oncogenes." (1980) *Cold Spring Harbor Symp. Quant. Biol.* **44.**
11. Rowley, J. D. (1980). *Cancer Genet. Cytogenet.* **2**, 175–198.
12. Klein, G. (1981). *Nature (London)* **294**, 313–318.
13. Mark, J. (1977). *Adv. Cancer Res.* **24**, 165–222.
14. McCann, J., and Ames, B. B. (1976). *Proc. Natl. Acad. Sci. U.S.A.* **73**, 950–954.
15. Auerbach, C. (1976). "Mutation Research." Wiley, New York.
16. Baserga, R. (1976). "Multiplication and Division in Mammalian Cells." Dekker, New York.
17. McClintock, B. (1951). *Cold Spring Harbor Symp. Quant. Biol.* **16**, 13–47.
18. McClintock, B. (1956). *Cold Spring Harbor Symp. Quant. Biol.* **21**, 197–216.
19. McClintock, B. (1961). *Am. Nat.* **95**, 265–277.
20. McClintock, B. (1965). *Brookhaven Symp. Biol.* **18**, 162–184.
21. McClintock, B. (1978). *Stadler Genet. Symp.* **10**, 25–48.
22. McClintock, B. (1967). *Dev. Biol.* **1**, 84–112.
23. Green, M. M. (1980). *Annu. Rev. Genet.* **14**, 109–120.
24. Spradling, A. C., and Rubin, G. M. (1981). *Annu. Rev. Genet.* **15**, 219–264.
25. Scher, S., and Davis, R. W. (1980). *Science (Washington, D.C.)* **209**, 1380.
26. Arber, W., Humbelin, M., Caspers, P., Reif, H. J., Iida, S., and Meyer, J. (1980). *Cold Spring Harbor Symp. Quant. Biol.* **45**, 38–40.
27. Meselson, M., Dunsmuir, P., Schweber, M., and Bingham, P. (1980). *In* "Genes, Cells and Behavior: A View of Biology Fifty Years Later" (H. Horowitz and E. Hutchings, eds.), pp. 88–92. 50th Anniversary Symp., Calif. Inst. Technol., Pasadena, California.
28. Rasmuson, B., Westerberg, B. M., Rasmuson, A., Gvozdev, V. A., Belyaeva, E. S., and Ilyin, Y. V. (1981). *Cold Spring Harbor Symp. Quant. Biol.* **45**, 545–551.
29. Engels, W. R. (1981). *Cold Spring Harbor Symp. Quant. Biol.* **45**, 561–565.
30. Sager, R., and Kovac, P. (1978). *Somatic Cell Genet.* **4**, 375–392.
31. Sager, R., and Kovac, P. (1979). *Somatic Cell Genet.* **5**, 491–502.
32. Kitchin, R., and Sager, R. (1980). *Somatic Cell Genet.* **6**, 75–87.
33. Kitchin, R., and Sager, R. (1981). *Somatic Cell Genet.* **6**, 615–629.
34. Smith, B. L., and Sager, R. (1982). *Cancer Res.* **42**, 389–396.

35. Kitchin, R., Gadi, I., Smith, B. L., and Sager, R. (1982). *Somatic Cell Genet.* (in press).
36. Bloch-Shachter, N., and Sachs, S. (1977). *J. Cell Physiol.* **93**, 205–212.
37. Shih, C., Padhy, L. C., Murray, M. and Weinberg, R. A. (1981). *Nature (London)* **290**, 261–264.
38. Lane, M., Sainten, A., and Cooper, G. M. (1981). *Proc. Natl. Acad. Sci. U.S.A.* **78**, 5185–5189.
39. Weinberg, R. A. (1981). *Biochim. Biophys. Acta* **651**, 25–35.
40. Kakunaga, T. (1973). *Int. J. Cancer* **12**, 463–473.
41. Smith, B. L., Anisowicz, A., Chodosh, L. A., and Sager, R. (1982). *Proc. Natl. Acad. Sci. U.S.A.* **79**, 1964–1968.
42. Schimke, R. T., Alt, F. W., Kellems, R. E., Kaufman, R. J., and Bertino, J. R. (1977). *Cold Spring Harbor Symp. Quant. Biol.* **42**, 649–657.
43. Dolnick, B. J. (1982). Chapter 11, this volume.
44. Sager, R., and Gadi, I. (1982). (in preparation.)
45. Razin, A., and Riggs, A. D. (1980). *Science (Washington, D.C.)* **210**, 604–610.
46. Ehrlich, M., and Wang, R. Y-H. (1981). *Science (Washington, D.C.)* **212**, 1350–1357.
47. Anisowicz, A., and Sager, R. (1982). (in preparation).
48. Sager, R., and Kovac, P. (1982). *Proc. Natl. Acad. Sci. U.S.A.* **79**, 480–484.

26

The Structure and Function of a Eukaryotic Promoter

STEVEN L. McKNIGHT, MOSES V. CHAO, RAYMOND W.
SWEET, SAUL SILVERSTEIN, AND RICHARD AXEL

I. Introduction

Transcriptional units of eukaryotic cells include precise sites of transcription initiation. Eukaryotic genes are also subject to controlling elements which dictate the frequency of initiation events. Thus, we can anticipate the existence of regulatory DNA sequences that define where along the chromosome transcription is to begin and how frequently this event is to occur. The potential role of specific DNA sequences in regulating the transcription of eukaryotic genes can be examined by testing the function of isolated genes in either soluble transcription systems (*in vitro*) or in appropriate recipient cells (*in vivo*).

The introduction of cloned genes into animal cells offers an opportunity to study the expression of heterologous genes in a transformed host and therefore provides a system in which the functional significance of various features of DNA sequence organization can be examined *in vivo*. In this study, we describe experiments involving the introduction of a viral thymidine kinase (*tk*) gene into *tk⁻* fibroblasts or *Xenopus* oocytes to determine: (1) What sequences are required for accurate and quantitative transcription of this gene? (2) What is the conformation of *tk* regulatory sequences and structural gene sequences when this gene is in the chromosome of a transformed host? (3) What *tk* sequences are essential in modulating the level of *tk* gene expression in response to specific inducers?

II. Results

A. Identifying the Transcriptional Regulatory Sequences of the *tk* Gene

The potential role of specific DNA sequences in regulating the transcription of eukaryotic genes can be examined by testing the function of isolated wild-type or mutant genes in either soluble transcription systems (*in vitro*), or in appropriate recipient cells (*in vivo*). We have used two independent assays to test the functional activity of 5′ deletion mutants of the *tk* gene. Mutants were either tested for the efficiency of transformation of *tk⁻* mouse fibroblasts to the *tk⁺* phenotype or microinjected into *Xenopus laevis* oocyte nuclei. The level of *tk* transcription into microinjected oocytes was measured either by quantitative hybridization mapping or by assaying *tk* enzymatic activity levels. Transformation of cultured mouse fibroblasts will depend on the synthesis of *tk* mRNA. Thus, it is possible to monitor indirectly the effect of specific nucleotide sequences on transcription by determining the transformation efficiency of *tk* deletion mutants.

We first prepared and characterized a systematic series of mutants of the *tk* gene that are truncated in a 5′–3′ direction. The nucleotide sequence encompassing these deletions and surrounding the putative transcription start site is shown in Fig. 1. Deletion mutagenesis experiments began with a plasmid containing 680 nucleotides of DNA flanking the 5′ terminus of the *tk* structural gene and 294 nucleotides of 3′ flanking DNA (McKnight and Gavis, 1980; McKnight, 1980). 5′ deleted molecules were generated by sequential digestion using exonuclease III and S₁. Deletion progressed from a unique Bam HI site 680 nucleotides upstream from the 5′ terminus of the structural gene. Shortened *tk* DNA fragments were ligated to synthetic Bam HI linker molecules and reintroduced into pBR322 vector DNA. The precise endpoints of the 13 5′ deletion mutants chosen for study were determined by DNA sequencing (Maxam and Gilbert, 1980).

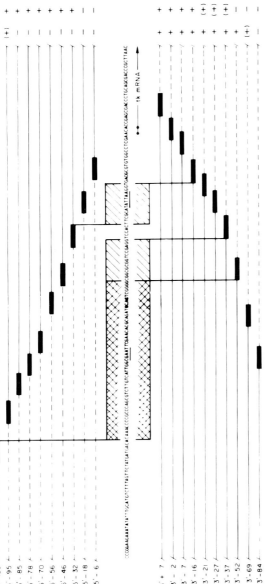

Fig. 1. Schematic diagram showing the boundaries of transcriptional control regions adjacent to the HSV thymidine kinase gene. (Center) The nucleotide sequence of the noncoding strand of the *tk* gene. Underlining: evolutionarily conserved segments. Double-hatched box: extent of quantitative control region. Single-hatched boxes: regions required for accurate transcriptional expression. 5' deletion mutants are shown above the sequence; 3' mutants are shown below. Solid rectangles: positions of synthetic Bam HI linkers. Solid lines: intact *tk* DNA sequences. Dashed lines: pBR322 sequences. (Column A): Whether deletion mutant is expressed quantitatively. Results are derived from transcriptional expression assays in frog oocytes and (for 5' mutants only) in mouse fibroblasts. (Column B): Whether deletion mutant is expressed accurately. Results are derived from transcript mapping assays of RNA synthesized in frog oocytes only. (From McKnight *et al.*, 1981.)

1. *Transformation of tk⁻ Fibroblasts with 5' Deleted tk Genes*

The exposure of *tk⁻* mouse fibroblasts to the HSV *tk* gene results in the generation of numerous *tk⁺* colonies. These transformants integrate and express the donor *tk* DNA. Since transformation to the *tk⁺* phenotype is dependent on the transcription of the donor *tk* gene, the frequency of transformation may serve as an indirect measure of *tk* gene expression.

The "wild-type" *tk* gene, or specific 5' deletion mutants were added to Ltk⁻ cells as a calcium phosphate precipitate (Graham and van der Eb, 1973) in the presence of 20 μg of Ltk⁻ carrier DNA. Following selection in HAT medium for a period of 15 days, surviving (*tk⁺*) colonies were scored: 200 ng of the "wild-type" *tk* gene or deletions that retain 109 or more 5' flanking nucleotides generate equivalent numbers of *tk⁺* transformant colonies; about 500 colonies are obtained per 200 ng donor *tk* DNA per 5 × 10⁵ cells (Fig. 1). Mutants that delete more than 109 5' flanking nucleotides exhibit a marked reduction in transformation efficiency, generating only about 25 *tk⁺* colonies per 200 ng donor DNA. Progressive deletion from position −85 to −6 results in no change in transformation efficiency. Thus, the primary component governing transformation efficiency (and, presumably, transcription) maintains a 5' boundary between 85 and 109 nucleotides from the *tk* gene. This assay detects no other region that influences transformation in either a 3'−5' direction extending to nucleotide −680, or in a 5'−3' direction to nucleotide −6.

2. *Transcription of 5' Deletions of the tk Gene*

The 5' deletion mutants were also assayed for the efficiency and specificity of transcription by microinjection into frog oocyte nuclei: 5-10 ng supercoiled plasmid DNA of each mutant was injected into the nuclei of 100 oocytes (McKnight and Gavis, 1980; Gurdon and Brown, 1978; Kressman *et al.,* 1977). The 5' terminus and relative abundance of the *tk* RNA synthesized in response to microinjection of each deletion mutant were assayed by the S₁ mapping assay (McKnight *et al.,* 1981). Figure 2 shows an autoradiographic exposure of a sequencing gel that was used to size DNA fragments that were protected from S₁ digestion by *tk* mRNA synthesized in oocytes injected with various truncated *tk* genes. From this assay we find that all deletion mutants retaining 109 or more nucleotides of 5' flanking DNA produce *tk* mRNA that protects the same extent of the radiolabeled probe DNA as does authentic *tk* mRNA synthesized either by virus infected cells of DNA transformed cells. Moreover, all such mutants appear to produce a quantity of *tk* mRNA roughly equivalent to the parental *tk* isolate. The 5' deletion mutant that retains only 95 nucleotides of 5' flanking DNA directs the synthesis of roughly 10% the "wild-type" level of specific *tk* mRNA. Mutants that retain between 85 and 32 contiguous 5' flanking nucleotides synthesize about 2%

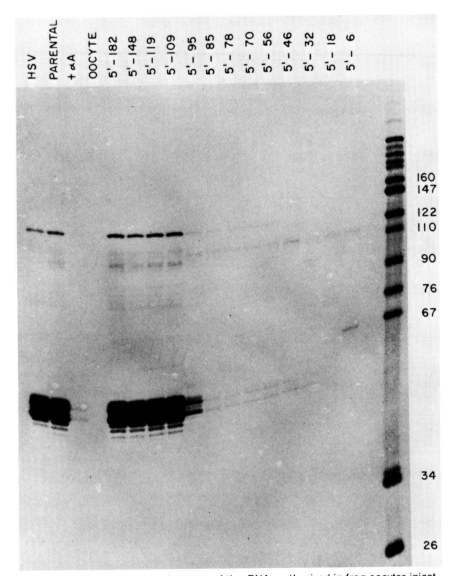

Fig. 2. S₁ nuclease transcript maps of *tk* mRNA synthesized in frog oocytes injected with 5′ deletion mutants. Autoradiographic exposure of a 14% polyacrylamide sequencing gel used to size S₁-resistant *tk* probe DNA. For each experiment, 5 μg RNA
was hybridized with 5 ng radiolabeled *Bgl* II–*Eco*RI probe DNA. RNA –DNA hybrid
molecules were digested with 10 U/m1 S₁ nuclease. (HSV lane) Transcript map of authentic *tk* mRNA. (Parental lane) Transcript map of RNA synthesized in oocytes in response to microinjection of wild-type *ptk 3* (+ αA lane) transcript map of RNA synthesized in oocytes injected with ptk and 1 μg/ml α-amanitin. (Oocyte lane) Transcript map
of RNA prepared from uninjected oocytes. Remaining lanes show transcript maps of
RNA made in oocytes in response to various 5′ deletion mutants. All transcription reac-
tions were assayed in oocytes isolated from a single female frog. Numbers: size of
molecular weight marker DNA fragments (in nucleotides). (From McKnight *et al.*, 1981.)

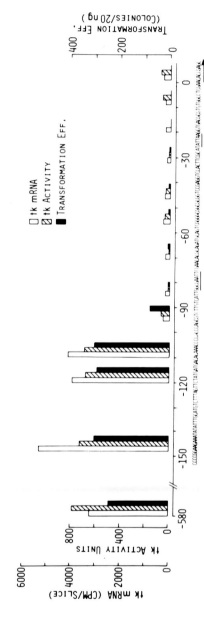

Fig. 3. Transcription efficiency and transcriptional competence of 5′ deletion mutants of the *tk* gene. Transformation efficiency was determined from the number of *tk*⁺ colonies arising from 5 × 10⁵ *tk*⁻ cells exposed to wild-type and various *in vitro* constructed 5′ deletion mutants. *tk* mRNA activity was quantitated from data in Fig. 2. The *tk* activity reflects the level of viral *tk* enzymatic activity synthesized in frog oocytes in response to injection to the various deletion mutants as template. (Data from McKnight *et al.*, 1981.)

the "wild-type" level of specific tk mRNA. Finally, mutants that retain 18 or fewer contiguous 5' flanking nucleotides are incapable of producing *tk* mRNA with the correct 5' terminus. These results are in accord with transformation data (Fig. 3) and precisely define the 5' boundary of a transcriptional control region essential for quantitative expression of the *tk* gene.

3. Transcription of 3' Deleted tk Genes in Oocytes

Analysis of the products of transcription of 3' deletion mutants should allow us to define the 3' boundary of this region, and further permit us to define the components required to specify the site of transcription initiation. The 3' deletion mutants we have prepared maintain a fixed boundary 480 nucleotides upstream from the putative transcription start site of the *tk* gene. The amount of the structural gene and 5' flanking DNA retained by each 3' mutant varies with respect to the extent of deletion progressing in a 3'–5' direction. Mutants are designated according to the 3' end point. For example, a mutant that retains all 480 nucleotides of 5' flanking DNA and only 7 nucleotides of the structural gene is referred to as 3'+7 (see Fig. 1). Exactly the same segment of pBR322 DNA (an internal portion of the plasmid tetracycline gene) is juxtaposed to each deletion end point.

Transcription of 3' deletion mutants was examined after microinjection into frog oocyte nuclei. Since 3' mutants lack most if not all *tk* mRNA coding sequences, we assayed for expression of transcripts complementary to the plasmid tetracycline resistance gene which abuts each deletion end point.

Results with primer extension assays (not shown, see McKnight *et al.*, 1981) show that quantitative transcriptional expression requires sequences that reside 5' to position −52; neither the structural gene nor the 52 nucleotides most proximal to the gene are required to maintain significant levels of transcription. These data precisely define a quantitative transcriptional control region between 52 and 109 nucleotides upstream from the 5' terminus of the *tk* gene. Accurate transcription initiation, however, is only observed for mutants that retain sequences from nucleotide −37 to nucleotide −109. It should be recalled, however, that deletion mutants 3' −21, 3' −27 and 3' −37 synthesize a major transcript bearing an "accurate" 5' terminus along with a low level of transcripts exhibiting heterogeneous 5' termini. Thus, the nucleotide sequence between −16 and −37 seems to enhance the specificity of accurate transcription initiation.

B. Structure of tk Regulatory Sequences in Chromatin

Transformation of the *tk* gene in murine fibroblasts, along with microinjection experiments in the mouse oocyte, clearly delineate the sequences required for accurate and quantitative transcription of the HSV *tk* gene. Only 109 nucleotides of 5′ flanking DNA are required for quantitative expression of *tk* mRNA. Furthermore, the *tk* structural gene is not required to maintain significant levels of transcription. Thus, we have delineated a 100 nucleotide block capable of promoting transcription of virtually any sequence lying proximal to it. We next asked whether this regulatory sequence, when integrated into the chromosome, resides in a unique conformation in association with chromatin proteins.

When mouse Ltk⁻ cells are exposed to a wild-type *tk* gene, transformation to the tk⁺ phenotype results from the integration and expression of a single *tk* gene. A restriction map of one such *tk* transformant, along with the flanking chromosomal DNA, is shown in Fig. 4.

We have designed a series of experiments to examine the accessibility of specific restriction sites within the regulatory region of the *tk* gene. A unique *Eco*RI site exists at position −86, imbedded in the promoter region. A second RI site is present in 3′ flanking DNA, about 1.5 kb from the poly(A) addition site. We have therefore examined the relative accessibility of these two *Eco*RI sites to limited cleavage in intact nuclei. Nuclei were digested with increasing quantities of the enzyme *Eco*RI, deproteinized, and the DNA was then subjected to complete digestion by the enzyme *Sac*I. *Sac*I cuts once within the *tk* structural gene, generating two annealing fragments, 2.8 and 1.8 kb in length. The 5′ 1.8 kb fragment contains the RI site within the promoter region. The 3′ 2.8 kb fragment contains the RI site within 3′ flanking DNA. The relative rate of disappearance of the 5′ and 3′ *Sac*I fragments upon increasing digestion with *Eco*RI therefore provides a measure of the relative accessibility of the two RI sites in chromatin. As observed in Fig. 4, the 5′ Sac fragment is strikingly diminished at an *Eco*RI concentration that leaves the 3′ fragment virtually intact. At higher concentrations of RI, the 3′ fragment begins to disappear, but at rates far slower than those observed for the 5′ fragment. From the relative rates of appearance and disappearance of specific restriction fragments, we estimate that the 5′ RI site within the promoter region is 10 times more accessible to nucleolytic attack than the corresponding site in 3′ flanking DNA.

It should be noted that many nucleases revealed preferred sites of cleavage, even on naked DNA. Control digestions with DNase I or *Eco*RI in a manner described for the experiments with nuclei reveal no such sites of preferential digestion; the 5′ and 3′ *Eco*RI sites in naked DNA are cleaved at equivalent rates. The preferred sites of cleavage suggest that the promoter region in the chromosome is maintained in a unique conformation distinct from structural gene sequences or flanking DNA.

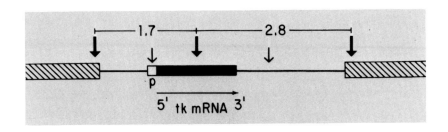

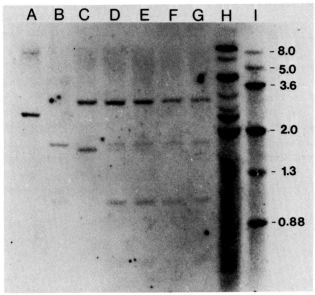

Fig. 4. Accessibility of the *tk* promoter to endonucleolytic attack in chromatin. (A) A restriction map of the *tk* gene integrated into cellular DNA in a transformed cell line, K-2. Crosshatched areas reflect flanking cellular DNA; the extent of the donor fragment integrated is represented by a single line; the darkened area represents the *tk* structural gene; the white box represents the 5' flanking regions which encompass the promoter sequences. Bold arrows denote the sites of cleavage of the enzyme *Sac*I, thin arrows reflect the sites of cleavage for the enzyme *Eco*RI. Note a single *Eco*RI site in the promoter region, and a second site in 3' flanking DNA. (B) 10^7 nuclei derived from the transformant K-2 (the restriction map is shown above) were subjected to digestion with increasing quantities of the enzyme *Eco*RI. Following digestion, the nuclei were deproteinized and the DNA was subjected to complete cleavage with the enzyme *Sac*I. 20 µg of DNA were loaded per lane. Electrophoresis was performed on an agarose slab, transferred to nitrocellulose and hybridized with nick translated ^{32}P-*tk* gene probe. Lane C, 0 *Eco*RI; lane D, 10 units *Eco*RI; lane E, 50 units *Eco*RI; lane F, 100 units *Eco*RI; lane G, 500 units *Eco*RI. Lane A shows a control digestion of purified K-2 DNA with *Eco*RI alone. Lane B shows a digestion of purified K-2 DNA with *Eco*RI plus *Sac*I. Lanes H and I consist of a series of radioactive plasmids cut with a variety of restriction enzymes to provide known size markers.

C. Sequence Elements Responsive to Induction of the *tk* Gene

These experiments define a region close to the *tk* structural gene responsible for maintaining a constitutive level of transcription in the transformed fibroblast for about 5–10 copies of mRNA at steady state. The level of *tk* gene expression can be modulated, however by the expression of a specific herpesvirus encoded protein, VMW-175 (Preston, 1979; Lin and Munyon, 1974; Leiden *et al.*, 1976). Using a discrete set of 5' deletion mutants, we were able to ask whether the sequences responsive to induction reside within the 110 nucleotide promoter region or whether they are distinguishable as a unique subset of sequences either within the structural gene or in flanking DNA.

Initially, clones derived by transformation with the intact "wild-type" *tk* gene were tested to determine whether biochemical transformants maintain the *tk* gene in a form that is responsive to induction by early viral proteins. Transformed cells were infected with the *tk⁻* deletion mutant of HSV-1 (Smiley, 1980). This mutant lacks the 875 base pair *Pst* fragment found within the structural sequences of the DNA that codes for *tk*. The availability of this mutant permits analysis of *tk* activity derived from the integrated transformed *tk* gene without interference from sequences that are derived from the infecting virus. Transformed cells were infected with this *tk⁻* virus to different multiplicities. Poly(A)RNA extracted from infected transformed cells at intervals postinfection was analyzed by Northern blot hybridization analysis (Fig. 5). Comparison of the band intensities obtained following hybridization to RNA isolated from mock infected 6 and 12 hour infected cells reveals a 5- to 10-fold increase in the level of *tk*-specific RNA in response to infection by *tk⁻* virus. We observe a concomitant increase in the level of *tk* during the course of infection. Furthermore, the increase in *tk* activity is dependent on the multiplicity of infection (El Kareh *et al.*, 1981).

These experiments now permit us to ask whether the 109 5' flanking nucleotides essential for transcription are also responsive to induction by infecting herpes proteins. Mutants containing as little as 109 nucleotides are indeed capable of induction to levels roughly equivalent to those observed with mutants retaining over 1 kb of 5' specific information (Table I). Similar results are obtained if the *tk* structural gene is replaced with totally unrelated sequences coding for bacterial genes. These results suggest that the elements controlling constitutive level transcription of the *tk* gene and those elements responsive to inducers of *tk* gene expression are at least partially overlapping and reside quite close to the terminus of the structural gene. This interpretation assumes that the increase in accumulation of *tk* mRNA observed upon induction results from a transcriptional rather than posttranscriptional event.

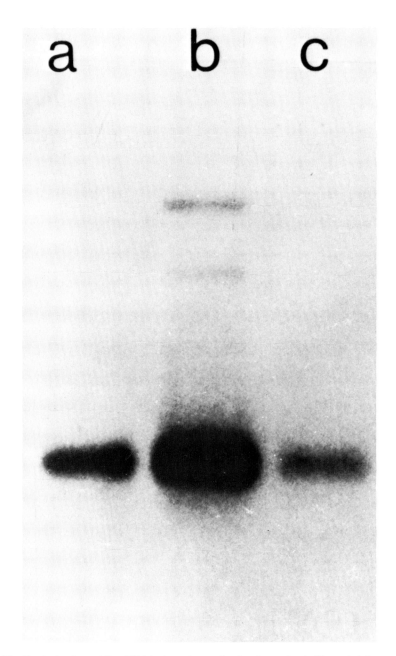

Fig. 5. Induction of *tk* mRNA in transformed cells. 5 µg of poly(A)-containing cytoplasmic RNA was electrophoresed through formaldehyde gels and analyzed by blot hybridization with ³²P-labeled *tk* DNA as probe. RNA from a transformant which has integrated a single copy of the *tk* gene infected with a *tk*⁻ deletion mutant of HSV-1 for 6 (a) or 12 (b) hours or mock infected (c).

TABLE I

Induction of *tk* Activity in Transformed Cells

Mutant[a]	Transformant[b]	*tk* activity[c]		Fold induction
		−	+	
—	Ltk⁻	10	10	0
5′ + 214	1	80	670	8.4
	2	85	400	4.7
	3	90	370	4.1
	4	90	200	2.2
5′ + 149	1	100	520	5.2
	2	70	390	5.5
	3	50	220	4.7
	4	30	70	2.3
5′ +109	1	90	390	4.3
	2	100	420	4.2
	3	40	40	0

[a] Refers to 5′ deletion mutants constructed *in vitro* (see Fig. 1) and used as DNA donor to construct *tk*⁺ cell lines containing a single copy of the *tk* gene.

[b] 1, 2, 3, etc., refer to independent transformants obtained during transfer of specific *tk* deletion mutants.

[c] *tk* activity is expressed as the cpm of [³H]TMP incorporated per μg of cellular protein, either prior to infection (−) or 24 hours postinfection (+) by *tk*⁻ herpesvirus (El Kareh *et al.*, 1981).

III. Discussion

In this study, we have examined the structure and organization of the transcriptional control region of the viral *tk* gene. Two recipient cell types, frog oocytes and mouse fibroblasts, have been used to assay the transcriptional competence of a systematic series of deletion mutants. These results define at least two and perhaps a third region essential for quantitative and accurate transcriptional expression of the HSV *tk* gene. Figure 1 schematically diagrams the results obtained in the present study. One of the functionally important regions we have identified resides between 60 and 100 nucleotides from the structural gene. This region appears to determine the frequency of transcriptional initiation. We therefore refer to this as a quantitative control region. Additional sequences, extending to nucleotide − 37, are required for the quantitative transcriptional control region to accurately promote transcription initiation. Finally, a stoichiometric yield of "accurate" transcripts appears to require 5′ flanking sequences extending from − 109 to − 16. Our results indicate that the quantitative transcriptional control region can act in the absence of sequences that lend absolute accuracy to a reaction. Similarly, the sequences governing accuracy can also function, albeit weakly, in the absence of the quantitative control region. Thus, transcriptional control of the *tk* gene is shown to be effected from two regions that can be physically and functionally distinguished.

One feature of eukaryotic gene promoters which emerges from these data and studies of other genes is the phenomenon of compound or split regulatory signals. Computer assisted sequence comparisons of 5′ flanking DNA have detected two regions of evolutionary conservation: a derivative of the sequence TATAAA commonly observed 25 nucleotides 5′ to the putative start site of transcription and a pentanucleotide homology CCAAT centered roughly 80 nucleotides upstream from the site of initiation. The functional significance of the TATAAA homology was initially demonstrated *in vitro*. Systematic sets of 5′ and 3′ deletion mutants of the adenovirus II (Hu and Manley, 1981), the chicken conalbumin gene (Corden *et al.*, 1980), and the rabbit β-globin gene (Grosveld and Flavell, 1981; Dierks *et al.*, 1981) were tested for transcriptional competence in a cell free assay. These experiments define a control region including the TATAAA element essential for *in vitro* expression of eukaryotic structural genes. The functional significance of this element *in vitro* is strengthened by an elegant single site mutagenesis experiment (Wasylyk *et al.*, 1980).

In vivo expression assays, however, suggest that for SV40 early genes, this component is dispensable (Rio *et al.*, 1980; Myers *et al.*, 1981; Gluzman *et al.*, 1980; Benoist and Chambon, 1981; Ghosh *et al.*, 1981). Our analyses of 3′ mutants of the *tk* gene which delete into or lack this A-T rich sequence exhibit a slight reduction in the specificity of transcription initiation with little effect on the quantity of *tk* RNA synthesized. For SV40 and *tk*, it is apparent that the TATAAA element is not essential for appropriate mRNA expression but may enhance or "focus" the specificity of transcription initiation (Grosschedl and Birnstiel, 1980a; Grosschedl and Birnstiel, 1980b).

In vivo analyses of promoter function have defined sequence elements farther upstream from TATAAA which are essential for efficient levels of transcription. We have defined a transcriptional control region located between 40 and 100 nucleotides upstream from the *tk* gene which is required for quantitative synthesis of the *tk* mRNA *in vivo*. Analysis of the rabbit β-globin gene (Grosveld and Flavell, 1981; Dierks *et al.*, 1981) and the human β-globin gene (Mellon *et al.*, 1981) similarly define control regions which reside 50 to 100 nucleotides upstream from transcription start sites essential for expression in either transient or stable gene transfer experiments. The globin and *tk* gene retain a conserved derivative of the CCAAT homology but the precise role of this element in transcription remains uncertain. Furthermore, the sea urchin histone *H2A* gene (Grosschedl and Birnstiel, 1980b) as well as the SV40 early gene (Benoist and Chambon, 1981) reveal essential elements even farther upstream which maintain quantitative control over the levels of transcription.

This somewhat complex set of observations seems to indicate that promoter control of eukaryotic genes is compound: Physically distinct subsets of nucleotide sequences may serve functionally distinct roles in the transcription process. The TATAA element may serve to dictate the specificity of transcription initiation. A more complex array of upstream elements likely to differ among different genes or sets of genes may modulate the frequency of transcription initiation. The complexity of these elements may reflect the complex regulation exhibited by eukaryotic genes. The observation that such control signals are split also suggests evolutionary mechanisms by which regulatory circuits may be constructed. Shuffling of regulatory elements in the genome, perhaps in a manner suggested for exon shuffling (Gilbert, 1978), may bring genes under the influence of multiple new controls characteristic of many animal cell genes.

In transformed cells, *tk* gene transcription results in a steady level of 5–10 copies of *tk* mRNA in the cell cytoplasm. Infection by herpesvirus bearing a deletion of the *tk* structural gene results in a 5- to 10-fold increase in the levels of *tk* mRNA. If we assume that this phenomenon results from enhanced transcription, the data are most compatible with the synthesis of an early viral protein which acts in *trans* to modulate *tk* transcription. In accord with this conclusion, the extent of induction we observe varies directly with the multiplicity of infection. Thus, regulatory products encoded by the virus are recognized by elements within the *tk* gene even when integrated within the host chromosome. Analysis of induction in 5' deletion mutants further suggests that the recognition sequences reside quite close to the structural gene, either overlap or are interposed among promoter sequences required to maintain constitutive levels of *tk* mRNA.

The *tk* gene integrated in the host cell chromosome is maintained in a nucleosome structure. We observe, however, that sites within the transcriptional control region are exquisitely sensitive to endonucleolytic attack. Hypersensitive sites have been identified in 5' flanking DNA of *Drosophila* heat shock genes (Wu, 1980), β-globin (Stalder *et al.*, 1980; McGhee *et al.*, 1981), histone genes (Samal *et al.*, 1981), conalbumin genes (Kuo *et al.*, 1979; and SV40 and polyoma minichromosomes (Waldeck *et al.*, 1978; Scott and Wigmore, 1978; Saragosti *et al.*, 1980). Furthermore, the specific sensitivity of sites 5' to the β-globin genes correlates with the developmental and tissue-specific expression of these genes (Stalder *et al.*, 1980; McGhee *et al.*, 1981). Hypersensitive sites in *tk* DNA reside within the sequences essential for transcription. It is tempting to assume that this susceptibility reflects a conformation in DNA which is accessible to recognition by transcriptional control factors or perhaps polymerase itself.

References

Benoist, C., and Chambon, P. (1981). *Nature (London)* **290**, 304–309.

Corden, J., Wasylyk, B., Buchwalder, A., Sassone-Corsi, P., Kedinger, D., and Chambon, P. (1980). *Science (Washington, D.C.)* **209**, 1406–1413.

Dierks, P., Wieringa, B., Marti, D., Reiser, J., van Ooyen, A., Meyer, F., Weber, H., and Weissman, C. (1981). *ICN-UCLA Symp. Mol. Cell. Biol.* (in press).

El Kareh, A., Ostrander, M., and Silverstein, S. (1981). *In* "NATO Advanced Study Course on Mammalian Cell Genetics" (T. Caskey, ed.) (in press).

Ghosh, P. K., Lebowitz, P., Frisque, F. J., and Gluzman, Y. (1981). *Proc. Natl. Acad. Sci. U.S.A.* **78**, 100–104.

Gilbert, W. (1978). *Nature (London)* **271**, 501.

Gluzman, Y., Sambrook, J., and Frisque, R. (1980). *Proc. Natl. Acad. Sci. U.S.A.* **77**, 3898–3902.

Graham, F. L., and van der Eb, A. J. (1973). *Virology* **52**, 456–467.

Grosschedl, R., and Birnstiel, M. L. (1980a). *Proc. Natl. Acad. Sci. U.S.A.* **77**, 1432–1436.

Grosschedl, R., and Birnstiel, M. L. (1980b). *Proc. Natl. Acad. Sci. U.S.A.* **77**, 7102–7106.

Grosveld, G. C., and Flavell, R. A. (1981). *Nature (London)* (in press).

Gurdon, J. B., and Brown, D. D. (1978). *Dev. Biol.* **67**, 346–356.

Hu, S.-L., and Manley, J. (1981). *Proc. Natl. Acad. Sci. U.S.A.* **78**, 820–824.

Kressman, A., Clarkson, S., Telford, J., and Birnstiel, M. (1977). *Cold Spring Harbor Symp. Quant. Biol.* **42**, 1077–1082.

Kuo, M. T., Mandel, J. L., and Chambon, P. (1979). *Nucleic Acids Res.* **7**, 2105–2113.

Leiden, J. M., Buttyan, R., and Spear, P. G. (1976). *J. Virol.* **20**, 413.

Lin, S. S., and Munyon, W. (1974). *J. Virol.* **14**, 1199.

Maxam, A., and Gilbert, W. (1980). *Methods Enzymol.* **65**, 499–560.

McGhee, J. D., Wood, W. I., Dolan, M., Engel, J. D., and Felsenfeld, G. (1981). *Cell* (in press).

McKnight, S. L. (1980). *Nucleic Acids Res.* **8**, 5949–5964.

McKnight, S. L., and Gavis, E. R. (1980). *Nucleic Acids Res.* **8**, 5931–5948.

McKnight, S. L., Gavis, E. R., Kingsbury, R., and Axel, R. (1981). *Cell* **25**, 385–398.

Mellon, P., Parker, V., Gluzman, Y., and Maniatis, T. (1981). *Cell* (in press).

Myers, R. M., Rio, D. C., Robbins, A. K., and Tjian, R. (1981). *Cell* **25**, 273–284.

Preston, C. M. (1979). *J. Virol.* **29**, 275.

Rio, D., Robbins, A., Myers, R., and Tjian, R. (1980). *Proc. Natl. Acad. Sci. U.S.A.* **77**, 5706–5710.

Samal, B., Worcel, A., Louis C., and Schedl, P. (1981). *Cell* **23**, 401–409.

Saragosti, S., Moyne, G., and Yaniv, M. (1980). *Cell* **20**, 65–73.

Scott, W. A., and Wigmore, D. J. (1978). *Cell* **15**, 1511–1518.

Smiley, J. (1980). *Nature (London)* **285**, 333.

Stalder, J., Larsen, A., Engel, J. D., Dolan, M., Groudine, M., and Weintraub, H. (1980). *Cell* **20**, 451–460.

Waldeck, W., Fohring, B., Chowdhury, K., Gruss, P., and Sauer, G. (1978). *Proc. Natl. Acad. Sci. U.S.A.* **75,** 5964–5968.

Wasylyk, B., Derbyshire, R., Guy, A., Molko, D., Roget, A., Teoule, R., and Chambon, P. (1980). *Proc. Natl. Acad. Sci. U.S.A.* **77,** 7024–7028.

Wu, C. (1980). *Nature (London)* **286,** 854–860.

27

Nuclear Structure and DNA Organization

BARRY NELKIN, DREW PARDOLL, SABINA ROBINSON,
DON SMALL, AND BERT VOGELSTEIN

I. Introduction

Among the many themes discussed at this symposium, three have arisen recurrently. The first is that there is some change in the genome in the cancer cell, whether that change be due to mutation, recombination, amplification, or insertion of foreign sequences. The second is that there is a change in the structural elements that package the genome. In interphase, this is manifest to the pathologist as the pleomorphic size and shape of the nucleus; during mitosis, it is manifest as an abnormal number and arrangement of the chromosomes. Third, there are changes in gene expression associated with cancer progression. One wonders how the changes in the DNA are related to the changes in the structural elements that package it. To that end, we have been studying the way in which chromatin structural elements are involved in the organization of specific DNA sequences in the nucleus.

There are at least three hierarchical levels involved in structure of chro-

TUMOR CELL HETEROGENEITY
441

matin. At a basic level, the DNA is wound around histone cores to form nucleosomes (*1,2*). The nucleosomes, in turn, are apparently packed in an orderly fashion into solenoids or superbeads (*3-6*). At yet a higher level of organization, these structures are arranged in the nucleus as supercoiled loops, each containing approximately 10^5 base pairs of DNA (*7-12*).

Most of the evidence linking eukaryotic chromosome structure to gene function has been adduced at the nucleosomal level. Active genes in chromatin are more sensitive to treatment with DNase I and micrococcal nuclease (*13-15*). This nuclease sensitivity has been shown to be in part due to the association of specific nonhistone proteins with nucleosomes containing active genes (*16,17*). In addition, DNA sequences surrounding active genes have been shown to be exquisitely nuclease sensitive (*18,19*).

Little information is as yet available on the role of the two supranucleosomal levels of DNA organization in nuclear function. We have been examining the arrangement of genes within supercoiled loops of DNA. These loops of DNA can be directly visualized in eukaryotic nuclei after 2 *M* NaCl extraction of the histones (and perhaps other proteins), which are responsible for compaction of the DNA *in situ* (*12*). In Fig. 1, such an extracted nucleus is shown. There is a central residual nucleus surrounded by a halo of DNA. The central residual nucleus is similar in composition to the nuclear matrix that has been isolated from nuclei after treatment with nucleases and high salt (*20,21*). This matrix has been described as a general structural feature underlying the nucleus in a wide variety of eukaryotes (*22-26*). The residual nucleus (which will henceforth be referred to as the nuclear matrix) has the same size and shape as the nucleus

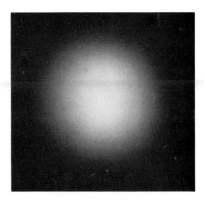

Fig. 1. Visualization of loops of DNA anchored to a central nuclear matrix. Nuclei from 3T3 cells were extracted sequentially with nonionic detergent in isotonic solution and then with a solution containing 2 *M* NaCl. The supercoiled loops were then stained with DAPI, and subsequently relaxed by exposure to 260 nm ultraviolet light. The central sphere is the nuclear matrix, anchoring the loops of DNA.

from which it was made. The halo of DNA surrounding it is actually composed of a series of supercoiled loops. This has been shown biochemically using the intercalating agent ethidium bromide (12).

The diameter of the halo (approximately 12 μm) is consistent with a loop size of approximately 70,000 base pairs. Similarly sized loops have been shown to be anchored to a central chromosome scaffold in metaphase chromosomes (27). By indirect means, the looped organization of DNA has been shown in numerous other cell types (7-11,28). Hence, the organization of DNA into a series of supercoiled loops seems to be a general feature of eukaryotic nuclear structure throughout the cell cycle.

II. Supercoiled Loops and DNA Replication

These loops of DNA, anchored to the nuclear matrix, are not stationary organizational elements. Rather, they have been shown to be mobile during DNA replication and perhaps during other nuclear processes. The most direct evidence for this is provided by autoradiography (12,29).

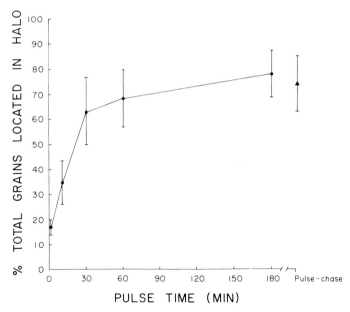

Fig. 2. Autoradiographic demonstration of the association of newly replicated DNA with the nuclear matrix. 3T3 cells were pulsed with [³H]thymidine for various time intervals, then extracted with buffers containing high salt. Means and standard deviations are shown; 25 structures were assessed for each point. (From reference 12, with permission.)

TABLE I

Comparison of Replicon Length and Supercoiled Loop Lengths in Various Nuclei

Organism	Supercoiled loop length[a] (bp) (fluorescence microscopy)	Replicon length[b] (bp) (fiber autoradiography)
Human	75,000	69,000
Drosophila	36,000	40,000
Physarum	36,000	37,500

[a] The supercoiled loop length was measured as the halo diameter of matrix-halo structures in the presence of ethidium bromide (*12*). Loops were relaxed by a 10 second treatment with ultraviolet illumination in the fluorescence microscope. In a variety of mammalian cells, the loops have been measured as 60,000–90,000 bp (B. Vogelstein, unpublished).

[b] The average replicon lengths as assessed by fiber autoradiography were obtained from published data (*82–84*).

When matrix-halo structures such as that shown in Fig. 1 are prepared from cells pulse-labeled with [^{3}H]thymidine, and subsequently autoradiographed, a distinct distribution of the newly labeled DNA is observed. With short pulse times most of the autoradiographic grains are located over the nuclear matrix; with longer pulse times, the grains (representing newly replicated DNA) gradually move from the matrix out into the halo region (Fig. 2). Since these results are from a logarithmically growing population of cells, the data indicate that fixed replication complexes exist within the nuclear matrix, and that the loops of DNA are reeled through these complexes as they are replicated; each loop may function as an individual replicon. The fact that the sizes of the loops are the same as the sizes of the replicons in diverse cells is consistent with this model of eukaryotic DNA replication (Table I).

III. Supercoiled Loops and Gene Expression

Several observations suggest that the loop anchorage sites might also function in gene expression: (1) Miller *et al.* (*30*) and Herman *et al.* (*31*) showed that essentially all the rapidly labeled RNA remains associated with the nuclear matrix after a salt extraction which removed over 90% of the nuclear protein. It has been shown that the hnRNA is bound to the nuclear matrix through a few specific proteins (*32*). (2) Some small molecular weight RNAs have shown to be quantitatively associated with the nuclear matrix (*33,34*). These RNAs have been postulated to be involved in RNA processing by base pairing with sequences at the borders of introns (*35,36*). (3) It has been shown that high affinity binding sites for steroid hormones are located on the nuclear matrix in target tissues (*37-*

40). In these tissues, steroid hormones modulate gene expression at the level of transcription (41,42).

To investigate the involvement of the nuclear matrix in the mechanics of control of gene expression, we have analyzed the nature of the DNA that is closely associated with the matrix anchorage points. We reasoned that if some of the machinery involved in gene expression were located within the nuclear matrix, then the DNA sequences to be expressed might be bound to these elements.

To assess this possibility, the following approach has been used. Nuclei are subjected to 2 M NaCl treatment to remove histones and most other nuclear proteins. The resultant nuclear matrices are then exposed to DNase I to randomly cleave the DNA; this treatment progressively releases DNA from the loops. The extent of the DNase I cleavage can be monitored by fluorescence microscopy of the nuclear matrices (Fig. 1). The halo gradually shrinks in size and then disappears completely with progressive DNase I treatment. As more DNA is released from the loops, the residual DNA attached to the nuclear matrix is progressively more enriched in sequences close to the loop attachment points. This matrix-associated DNA can be recovered by low speed centrifugation.

Using this approach, we initially isolated nuclear matrix-associated DNA from rat liver nuclei (43). C_0t hybridization analysis, using [^{125}I]rRNA (18 S + 28 S) as a probe, demonstrated substantial enrichment of ribosomal RNA genes in nuclear matrix-associated DNA (Fig. 3). This experiment suggested that active ribosomal genes might be associated with the nuclear matrix. However, alternative explanations for the association of rDNA with the nuclear matrix were possible. For example, it is possible that the nucleolus has a different structure than the rest of the genome. This structure could necessitate more extensive nuclease treatment to release DNA from the rDNA containing loops.

To further address the role of the nuclear matrix in gene expression, matrix-associated DNA from SV40 transformed 3T3 cells (cell line SVB203) was isolated (44). These cells have two copies of the SV40 genome tandemly integrated per haploid genome (45), and they actively transcribe the SV40 sequences. Matrix preparations from these cells were obtained containing 3.5% or 9.0% of the total cellular DNA. These DNAs, along with reference total cellular DNA, were extracted and cleaved with the restriction endonuclease HindIII. Equal amounts of these DNA samples were electrophoresed, transferred to nitrocellulose sheets (46), and hybridized with SV40 DNA labeled (47) with ^{32}P (5–10 × 10^7 dpm/μg). This provides a quantitative assay of the relative amount of SV40 DNA sequences in each DNA preparation (44). Figure 4 shows that the nuclear matrix DNA preparations are enriched in SV40 sequences relative to total DNA. Moreover, the preparation containing 3.5% of the

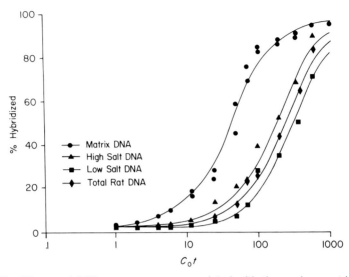

Fig. 3. Ribosomal DNA sequences are associated with the nuclear matrix in rat liver cells. Rat liver nuclei were extracted with a low ionic strength buffer, treated with DNase I, and then extracted with 2 M NaCl. DNA was purified from matrix, low salt extract, high salt extract, and total rat liver nuclei. Hybridization with [^{125}I](18 S + 28 S)rRNA was performed in 70% formamide, 0.2 M sodium phosphate (*85*) to the indicated C_0t values. (From reference *43*, with permission.)

total cellular DNA is more enriched in SV40 sequences than is the preparation containing 9.0% of the total cellular DNA. This finding implies that the transcribed SV40 sequences are close to the loop anchorage points. This experiment was repeated with two other SV40 transformed 3T3 cell lines with similar results (*44*). As a control, matrix and total cellular DNA samples from SVB203 cells were digested with *Hind*III, electrophoresed, transferred, and hybridized as before, except that cloned mouse β-globin cDNA was used as a hybridization probe. In this case, no enrichment of the globin sequence was seen in matrix DNA preparations.

The results with SV40 lend further credence to the possibility of an association between active genes and the nuclear matrix. However, alternative explanations exist. It is possible that the association of SV40 genes with the matrix is due to the transforming capacity of these genes. In addition, sequences near the SV40 origin of replication bind specifically to T antigens (*48*). If SV40 T antigen is found in the matrix of SV40 transformed cells, as is the case in polyoma (*49*) and SV40 productively infected cells (*50*), then preferential SV40 association with the nuclear matrix might be due to its binding to T antigen.

We next asked whether a gene transcribed in one cell type is associated

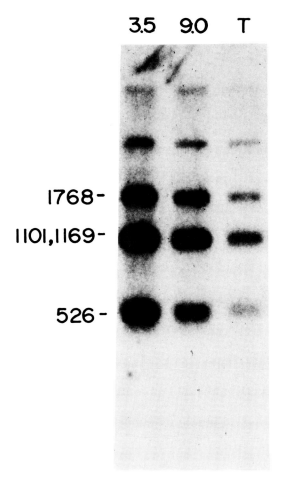

Fig. 4. Nuclear matrix DNA from SV40 transformed cells is enriched in SV40 sequences. Nuclei from SVB203, a 3T3 cell line transformed with SV40, were extracted with 2 *M* NaCl, and then treated with DNase I. Equal amounts of total cellular DNA and DNA from matrix preparations containing 9.0 or 3.5% of the total cellular DNA were digested with restriction endonuclease *Hind*III, electrophoresed, transferred to nitrocellulose filters, hybridized with [³²P]SV40 DNA, and autoradiographed.

with the nuclear matrix in that cell type, but not in a cell type in which the gene is not transcribed. Chicken ovalbumin is transcribed in 90% of the cells in the laying hen oviduct (*51*), but it is not transcribed in chicken liver (*52*). Matrix preparations were made from hen oviduct cells and hen liver cells. The DNA from these preparations was purified and cleaved with the restriction endonuclease *Hinf*1. Equal amounts of total nuclear DNA, or DNA from hen oviduct matrix or hen liver matrix, were then electrophoresed through agarose and transferred to nitrocellulose. ^{32}P-labeled chicken globin or ovalbumin cDNA sequences (cloned in plasmids) were used as hybridization probes for these filters. In these filter hybridization analyses with the ovalbumin probe, five fragments could be detected (53). Four of these are the fragments expected from the ovalbumin gene map [a 1650 bp fragment from the 5' end, 550 and 410 bp fragments from the middle, and a 790 bp fragment from the 3' end of the gene (54)]; the fifth fragment, 2800 bp, is probably from the related X or Y genes, which are related to the ovalbumin gene and are also transcribed in hen oviduct cells (55,56). All these fragments are preferentially associated with the nuclear matrix in oviduct, but not in liver cells (Figs. 5 and 6). Furthermore, the enrichment is higher in DNA from the matrix preparation containing less of the total nuclear DNA (Fig. 5). In several experi-

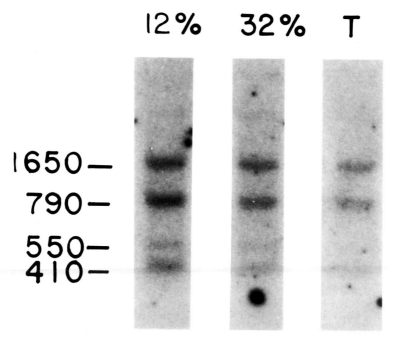

Fig. 5. The ovalbumin gene is preferentially associated with the nuclear matrix of hen oviduct cells. Nuclei were isolated from laying hen oviduct, extracted with 2 M NaCl, and then treated with DNase I. Nuclear matrix preparations containing 32 or 12% of the total cellular DNA were recovered by centrifugation. Equal amounts of DNA from these preparations and from total cellular DNA were digested with the restriction endonuclease HinfI, electrophoresed, transferred to nitrocellulose filters, hybridized with ^{32}P-labeled, cloned ovalbumin cDNA, and autoradiographed. (From reference 53, with permission.)

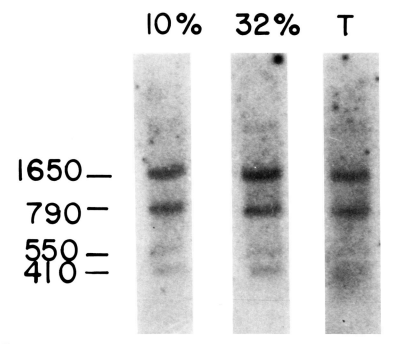

Fig. 6. The ovalbumin gene is not preferentially associated with the nuclear matrix of chicken liver cells. DNA from nuclear matrices of hen liver cells was treated as described in the legend to Fig. 5. (From reference *53*, with permission.)

ments of this type, it has been found that the majority of the ovalbumin gene sequences (up to 60%) are associated with nuclear matrix DNA fractions that contain 10–15% of the total nuclear DNA. These results provide substantial evidence that active genes are associated with the nuclear matrix.

As a technical control for these experiments, the content of chicken globin genes was also assessed in the matrix DNA fractions. The same matrix DNA preparations (cleaved with the same restriction enzyme) that contained elevated concentrations of the ovalbumin gene were *not* enriched for the inactive globin gene (*53*).

In addition to DNA sequences present in one or a few copies per genome, eukaryotic DNA contains sequences present in multiple (10^2–10^7) copies per genome (*57*). While some of these sequences have well-characterized functions, the function of most of these sequences is unknown. Among the functions proposed for these sequences are roles in maintenance of the structure of chromosomes, in mitosis, and in transcriptional regulation (*58-61*).

One of the DNA sequences that has been proposed as a possible regulatory sequence is an interspersed, highly repeated sequence in human DNA (*62*). This sequence, known as the *Alu* family sequence, was found to be transcribed in hnRNA (*63*), and has since been found in the vicinity of numerous transcribed genes (*64-66*). It also serves as an RNA polymerase III promoter *in vitro* (*67*), and it appears to be transcribed by RNA polymerase III *in vivo* (*68*). Since we had found other transcribed sequences closely associated with the nuclear matrix, we also examined the proximity of the *Alu* family sequence to the nuclear matrix.

Matrix and total cellular DNAs were prepared from human A549 cells. Several complementary techniques were used to assay the concentration of *Alu* family sequence in each DNA preparation. First, aliquots of each DNA sample were nick translated and hybridized to excess DNA from an *Alu* family sequence cloned in pBR322 (BLUR8, kindly provided by P. Deininger) and immobilized on nitrocellulose filters. Table II shows that

TABLE II

Quantitation of the *Alu* Family Sequence Content of Human Matrix DNAs

DNA	Relative enrichment	
	Mean	Range

A. Based on densitometry of gels containing *Mbo*I digests of the indicated matrix preparations.

Total nuclear	1.00	
Matrix 31.9%	1.92	
Matrix 12.2%	2.42	
Matrix 7.1%	1.52	

B. Based on hybridization of nick translated *Alu* family sequence DNA (in BLUR 8 plasmid) to total nuclear and matrix DNAs immobilized on nitrocellulose filters. The mean and range for three hybridizations per matrix preparation is indicated.

Total nuclear	1.00	0.95–1.05
Matrix 31.9%	1.85	1.80–2.40
Matrix 12.2%	1.98	1.75–2.40
Matrix 7.1%	1.48	1.30–1.60
Matrix 1.3%	1.62	1.40–1.90

C. Based on hybridization of nick translated total and matrix DNAs to *Alu* family sequence DNA immobilized on nitrocellulose filters. The range of values for three hybridizations per matrix preparation is indicated.

Total nuclear	1.00	0.96–1.08
Matrix 3.9%	1.67	1.55–1.83
Matrix 1.8%	2.20	2.15–2.25
Matrix 0.4%	1.91	1.85–1.98

human nuclear matrix DNA is enriched in *Alu* family sequences. In a converse approach, equal aliquots of the matrix and total cellular DNA preparations were immobilized on nitrocellulose filters, and excess nick translated BLUR8 DNA was used as a hybridization probe. This experiment also demonstrated significant enrichment of *Alu* family sequences in nuclear matrix DNA (Table II). Finally, total cellular and matrix DNAs were digested with *Mbo*I, an enzyme which cleaves the consensus *Alu* family sequence in two places, leaving a 180 bp fragment *(69)* which can be visualized in polyacrylamide gels. As shown in Table II, this 180 bp band is more intense in matrix DNA samples, indicating enrichment of *Alu* family sequences. Thus, by all three methods it is found that some *Alu* family sequence members are closely associated with the nuclear matrix.

Using similar techniques, we have also examined other repeated sequences for their association with the nuclear matrix. Among these are mouse and monkey satellite sequences. Matrix DNA and total cellular DNA was isolated from mouse Friend erythroleukemia (FEL) cells. After the DNA is digested with *Bst*NI, the mouse satellite can be seen as a 245 bp monomer and multimers thereof *(70-72)*. It is evident from Fig. 7 that nuclear matrix from FEL cells is substantially enriched in satellite sequences. Densitometry of the satellite band reveals that this enrichment is up to 2.6-fold. Since the satellite occupies 8–10% of the mouse genome *(70,73)*, one may infer that at least 20–26% of mouse matrix DNA was composed of satellite sequences. Similar results were obtained whether or not the FEL cells were induced to produce hemoglobin, or using SV40 transformed 3T3 cells. On the other hand, the African green monkey satellite sequence is preferentially depleted from matrix DNA isolated from Vero cells (Fig. 8).

It is clear from the above results that the organization of DNA in supercoiled loops in eukaryotic nuclei is strikingly nonrandom. From the results of the experiments examining ribosomal RNA, SV40, ovalbumin, and *Alu* family sequence genes, it seems likely that sequences transcribed by all three mammalian RNA polymerases are in close association with the loop anchorage sites on the nuclear matrix. Consistent with this possibility is the recent finding *(74)* that DNA sequences complementary to whole nuclear RNA are enriched in DNA associated with the nuclear cage (a structure similar to the nuclear matrix).

Several possibilities for the control of this arrangement exist. It is, of course, tempting to assume that genes are transported to the nuclear matrix when they are activated. These active genes would either be attached to the nuclear matrix in a relatively stable fashion or reeled through the matrix as they are transcribed, much as DNA is reeled through the matrix as it is replicated. However, active gene localization at the base of loops

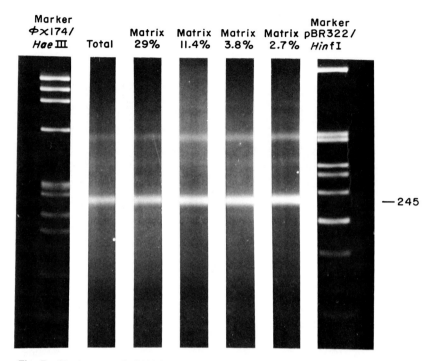

Fig. 7. Nuclear matrix DNA is enriched in mouse satellite sequences. Nuclei from FEL cells were extracted with 2 *M* NaCl and treated with DNase I, as described in the legend to Fig. 4. The DNA was purified and then digested with restriction endonuclease *Bst*NI. Equal amounts of restricted cellular DNA and DNA from nuclear matrix preparations containing 29, 11.4, 3.8, or 2.7% of total cellular DNA were electrophoresed through 4% polyacrylamide and visualized with ethidium bromide fluorescence. (From reference *86*, with permission.)

cannot account for the enrichment of mouse satellite DNA, since those genes are not transcribed (*75*). A model which accounts for these gene arrangements is presented in Fig. 9. In this model, all the DNA in the nucleus is arranged in supercoiled loops anchored to the nuclear matrix. In every cell of any given cell type, each gene has a specified position within its loop. However, the loops in an individual nucleus are of various sizes, and the loop size is determined by the DNA sequences contained therein.

From this model, it can clearly be seen that there are two ways for a DNA sequence to be preferentially associated with the nuclear matrix after nuclease treatment. Some sequences, represented by gene *A* in Fig. 9, will be enriched due to their location at the bases of their loops. Transcribed sequences are bound to the matrix through transcriptional complexes (or other means) and thus operationally form the bases of the DNA

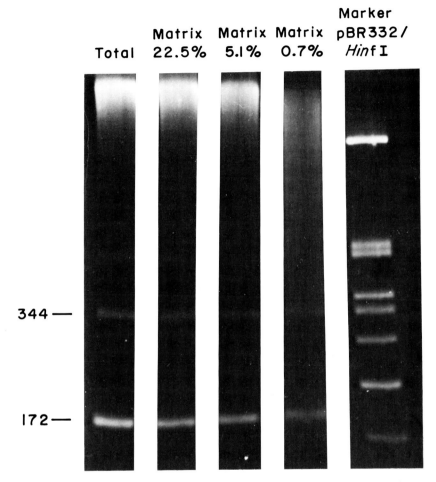

Fig. 8. Nuclear matrix DNA is preferentially depleted in African green monkey α-satellite sequences. Nuclei from Vero cells were extracted with 2 *M* NaCl and treated with DNase I, as described in the legend to Fig. 4. The DNA was purified and digested with restriction endonuclease *Hind*III. Equal amounts of restricted total cellular DNA and DNA from nuclear matrix preparations containing 22.5, 5.1, or 0.7% of the total cellular DNA were electrophoresed through a 7% polyacrylamide gel and visualized by ethidium bromide fluorescence. (From reference *86,* with permission.)

loops in which they reside. Other sequences, represented by gene *B* in Fig. 9, will appear to be preferentially associated with the nuclear matrix due to their position in a loop of smaller than average size. These small loops would require more DNase I per unit length to release them from the nuclear matrix. The multiple tandem copies of mouse satellite DNA are presumably enriched in the matrix DNA fractions because they are

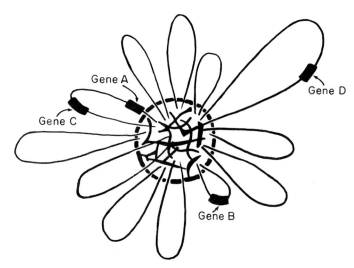

Fig. 9. A model of gene arrangement with respect to supercoiled loops and the nuclear matrix. A histone depleted nucleus in G1 phase of the cell cycle is depicted with the DNA loops extended and anchored to the central nuclear matrix. Gene *A* is associated with the nuclear matrix because it resides at the base of a loop. Gene *B* is associated with the nuclear matrix because it resides in a loop smaller than the average. Gene *C* is impoverished in matrix DNA because it lies at the end of a loop. Gene *D* is impoverished because it lies within a loop larger than the average. (From reference *86*, with permission.)

arranged in loops shorter than the average. Conversely, the African green monkey satellite is depleted in the matrix DNA because it is arranged in loops larger than the average. Variability in loop length has been seen directly by electron microscopy of chromosome scaffolds (*27*).

IV. Supercoiled Loops and Cancer

Going back to our original question, then, we again ask how nuclear structural elements are related to the changes in DNA seen in the cancer cell. Although these investigations are in their infancy, there are several observations that suggest a link between the looped organization of DNA and the changes in DNA that occur in cancer.

First, it has been found in several laboratories that carcinogens preferentially react with elements at the bases of the loops. These carcinogens include benzo[*a*]pyrene (*76,77*) and the nitrosoureas (*78*). This interaction may be related to the finding by Hartwig and co-workers that the superhelical density of supercoiled loops in transformed cells is significantly higher than in normal cells (*79*).

Second, tumor promotion may exert its effects by altering the normal relationship between replicon origins and loops of DNA. Normally, replicon origins are at the base of a DNA loop at the beginning of S phase; during S phase these loops are reeled through the matrix so that the origins end up at the periphery of a loop (80). This may prevent a replicon from being replicated more than once in each cell cycle. Tumor promoters, however, may somehow alter the arrangement of origins within supercoiled loops, thereby allowing multiple rounds of replication within one S phase (81).

Finally, the amplification of certain DNA sequences that occurs in tumor cells does not involve simply the amplification of the affected gene itself; rather, the whole loop on which the gene resides can be amplified. The best example of this is in the amplification of the dihydrofolate reductase (DHFR) gene observed with methotrexate treatment. In Chinese hamster cells resistant to methotrexate, the entire 135,000 bp loop in which the DHFR gene resides is amplified, and the loop probably maintains the parental organization of sequences (J. Hamlin, personal communication). This amplification of loops, of course, may be related to the abnormal replication of loops induced by tumor promoters noted above.

V. Conclusion

In conclusion, the DNA of the eukaryotic nucleus is arranged into approximately 50,000 loops, each 30,000–100,000 base pairs in length. These loops are not stationary, but move through the nucleus as they are replicated and each loop seems to function as an individual replicon. Genes have specific orientations with respect to the loop–matrix axis, and this orientation can change with cell differentiation. The looped organization of DNA seems to be involved in several of the genetic processes occurring in cancer. We hope that further study of this organization will lead to a better understanding of these processes.

Acknowledgments

This work was supported by NIH grants CA-06973 and CA-31053, NIH training grants CA-09243 and CA-07309, and a gift from the Bristol-Myers Co.

References

1. Felsenfeld, G. (1978). *Nature (London)* **271**, 115.
2. Kornberg, R. D. (1977). *Ann. Rev. Biochem.* **46**, 931.

3. Finch, J. T., and Klug, A. (1976). *Proc. Natl. Acad. Sci. U.S.A.* **73**, 3966.
4. Worcel, A., and Benjayati, C. (1977). *Cell* **12**, 83.
5. Renz, M., Nehls, P., and Hozier, J. (1977). *Proc. Natl. Acad. Sci. U.S.A.* **74**, 1879.
6. Stratling, W. H., Muller, V., and Zentgraf, H. (1978). *Exp. Cell Res.* **117**, 301.
7. Cook, P. R., and Brazell, I. A. (1975). *J. Cell Sci.* **19**, 261.
8. Ide, T., Nakane, M., Anzai, K., and Andoh, T. (1975). *Nature (London)* **258**, 445.
9. Benyajati, C., and Worcel, A. (1976). *Cell* **9**, 393.
10. Pinon, R., and Salts, Y. (1977) *Proc. Natl. Acad. Sci. U.S.A.* **74**, 2850.
11. Hartwig, M. (1978). *Acta Biol. Med. Ger.* **37**, 421.
12. Vogelstein, B., Pardoll, D. M., and Coffey, D. S. (1980). *Cell* **22**, 79.
13. Weintraub, H., and Groudine, M. (1976). *Science (Washington, D.C.)* **193**, 848.
14. Garel, A., and Axel, R. (1976). *Proc. Natl. Acad. Sci. U.S.A.* **73**, 3966.
15. Senear, A. W., and Palmiter, R. D. (1981). *J. Biol. Chem.* **256**, 1191.
16. Levy-Wilson, B., and Dixon, G. H. (1979) *Proc. Natl. Acad. Sci. U.S.A.* **76**, 1682.
17. Weisbrod, S., and Weintraub, H. (1979). *Proc. Natl. Acad. Sci. U.S.A.* **76**, 630.
18. Wu, C., Bingham, P. M., Livak, K. J., Holmgren, R., and Elgin, S. C. R. (1979). *Cell* **16**, 797.
19. Stalder, J., Larson, A., Engel, J. D., Dolan, M., Groudine, M., and Weintraub, H. (1980). *Cell* **20**, 451.
20. Berezney, R., and Coffey, D. S. (1974). *Biochem. Biophys. Res. Commun.* **60**, 1410.
21. Peters, K. E., and Comings, D. E. (1980). *J. Cell Biol.* **86**, 135.
22. Hodge, L. D., Mancini, P., Davis, F. M., and Heywood, P. J. (1977). *Cell Biol.* **72**, 192.
23. Long, B. W., Huang, C. Y., and Pogo, A. O. (1979). *Cell* **18**, 1079.
24. Herlan, G., and Wunderlich, F. (1976). *Cytobiologie* **13**, 291.
25. Mitchelson, K. R., Bekers, A. G. M., and Wanka, F. J. (1979). *Cell Sci.* **39**, 247.
26. Poznanovic, G., and Sevaljevic, L. (1980). *Cell Biol. Int. Rep.* **4**, 701.
27. Paulson, J. R., and Laemmli, U. K. (1977). *Cell* **12**, 817.
28. Razin, S. V., Mantieva, V. L., and Georgiev, G. P. (1979). *Nucleic Acids Res.* **7**, 1713.
29. McCready, S. J., Godwin, J., Mason, D. W., Brazell, I. A., and Cook, P. R. (1980). *J. Cell Sci.* **46**, 365.
30. Miller, T. E., Huang, C.-Y., and Pogo, A. O. (1978). *J. Cell Biol.* **76**, 675.
31. Herman, R., Weymouth, C., and Penman, S. (1978). *J. Cell Biol.* **78**, 663.
32. Van Eekelen, C. A. G., and Van Venrooij, W. J. (1981). *J. Cell Biol.* **88**, 554.
33. Zieve, G., and Penman, S. (1976). *Cell* **8**, 19.
34. Miller, T. E., Huang C.-Y., and Pogo, A. O. (1978). *J. Cell Biol.* **76**, 692.
35. Lerner, M., Boyle, J., Mount, S., Wolin, S., and Steitz, J. A. (1980). *Nature (London)* **283**, 220.
36. Rogers J., and Wall, R. (1980). *Proc. Natl. Acad. Sci. U.S.A.* **77**, 1877.
37. Barrack, E. R., Hawkins, E. F., Allen, S. L., Hicks, L. L., and Coffey, D. S. (1977). *Biochem. Biophys. Res. Commun.* **79**, 829.
38. Agutter, P. S., and Burchall, K. (1979). *Exp. Cell Res.* **124**, 45.
39. Hardin, J. W., and Clark, J. H. (1979). *J. Cell Biol.* **83**, 252a.
40. Barrack, E. R., and Coffey, D. S. (1980). *J. Biol. Chem.* **255**, 7265.
41. Gorski, J., and Gannon, F. (1976). *Annu. Rev. Physiol.* **38**, 425.
42. O'Malley, B. W., Roop, D. R., Lai, E. C., Nordstrom, J. L., Catterall, J. F., Swaneck, G. F., Colbert, D. A., Tsai, M.-J., Dugaiczyk, A., and Woo, S. L. C. (1979). *Recent Prog. Horm. Res.* **35**, 1.
43. Pardoll, D., and Vogelstein B. (1980). *Exp. Cell Res.* **128**, 466.
44. Nelkin, B. D., Pardoll, D., and Vogelstein, B. (1980). *Nucleic Acids Res.* **8**, 5623.
45. Ketner, G., and Kelley, T. J. (1980). *Mol. Biol.* **144**, 163.
46. Southern, E. M., (1975). *J. Mol. Biol.* **98**, 503.
47. Rigby, P. W. J., Dieckman, M., Rhodes, C., and Berg, P. J. (1977). *Mol. Biol.* **113**, 237.

48. Reed, S. I., Ferguson, J., Davis, R. W., and Stark, G. R. (1975). *Proc. Natl. Acad. Sci. U.S.A.* **72**, 1605.
49. Buckler-White, A. H., Humphrey, G. W., and Pigiet, V. (1980). *Cell* **22**, 3.
50. Deppert, W. (1978). *J. Virol.* **26**, 165.
51. Palmiter, R. D. (1973). *J. Biol. Chem.* **248**, 8260.
52. Ono, T., and Getz, M. (1980). *J. Dev. Biol.* **75**, 481.
53. Robinson, S., Nelkin, B., and Vogelstein, B. (1982). *Cell* **28**, 99.
54. O'Hare, H., Breathnach, R., Benoist, C., and Chambon, P. (1979). *Nucleic Acids Res.* **7**, 321.
55. Royal, A., Garapin, A., Cami, B., Perrin, F., Mandel, J. L., LeMeur, M., Bregegegre, F., Gannon, F., LePennec, J. P., Chambon, P., and Kourilsky, P. (1979). *Nature (London)* **279**, 125.
56. Lawson, G. M., Tsai, M.-J., and O'Malley B. W. (1980). *Biochem.* **19**, 4403.
57. Britten, R. J., and Kohne, D. E. (1968). *Science (Washington, D.C.)* **161**, 529.
58. Appels, R., and Peacock, W. J. (1978). *Int. Rev. Cytol.*, Suppl. 8, p. 70.
59. Britten, R. J., and Davidson, E. H., (1969). *Science (Washington, D.C.)* **165**, 349.
60. Walker, P. M. B. (1971). *Prog. Biophys. Mol. Biol.* **23**, 145.
61. Jelinek, W. R., Toomey, T. P., Leinwand, L., Duncan, C. H., Biro, P. A., Choudary, P. V., Weissman, S. M., Rubin, C. M., Houck, C. M., Deininger, P. L., and Schmid, C. W. (1980). *Proc. Natl. Acad. Sci. U.S.A.* **77**, 1398.
62. Houck, C. M., Rinehart, F. P., and Schmid, C. W. (1979). *J. Mol. Biol.* **132**, 289.
63. Jelinek, W., Evans, R., Wilson, M., Salditt-Georgieff, M., and Darnell, J. E. (1978). *Biochemistry* **17**, 2776.
64. Duncan, C., Biro, P. A., Choudary, P. V., Elder, J. T., Wang, R. R. C., Forget, B. G., deRiel, J. K., and Weissman, S. M. (1979). *Proc. Natl. Acad. Sci. U.S.A.* **76**, 5095.
65. Fritsch, E. F., Lawn, R. M., and Maniatis, T. (1980). *Cell* **19**, 95.
66. Bell, G. I., Pictet, R., and Rutter, W. J. (1980). *Nucleic Acids Res.* **8**, 4091.
67. Pan, J., Elder, J. T., Duncan, C. N., and Weissman, S. M. (1981). *Nucleic Acids Res.* **9**, 117.
68. Haynes, S. R., and Jelinek, W. R. (1981). *Proc. Natl. Acad. Sci. U.S.A.* **78**, 6130.
69. Rubin, C. M., Houck, C. M., Deininger, P. L., Friedmann, T., and Schmid C. W. (1980). *Nature (London)* **284**, 372.
70. Southern, E. M. (1975). *J. Mol. Biol.* **94**, 51.
71. Horz, W., Hess, I., and Zachau, H. G. (1974). *Eur. J. Biochem.* **45**, 501.
72. Horz, W., and Zachau, H. G. (1977). *Eur. J. Biochem.* **73**, 383.
73. Waring, M., and Britten, R. J. (1966). *Science (Washington, D.C.)* **154**, 791.
74. Jackson, D. A., McCready, S. J., and Cook. P. R. (1981). *Nature (London)* **292**, 552.
75. Flamm, W. G., Walker, P. M. B., and McCallum, M. (1969). *J. Mol. Biol.* **40**, 423.
76. Hemminki, J., and Vainio, H. (1979). *Cancer Lett. (Shannon, Irel.)* **6**, 167.
77. Matsuura, H., Ueyama, H., Moni, S., and Ueda, K. (1979). *J. Nutr. Sci. Vitaminol.* **25**, 495.
78. Tew, K. D., Wong, A. L., and Schein, P. S. (1981). Submitted for publication.
79. Hartwig, M., Matthes, E., and Arnold, W. (1981). *Cancer Lett. (Shannon, Irel.)* **13**, 153.
80. Hunt, B. F., and Vogelstein, B. (1981). *Nucleic Acids Res.* **9**, 349.
81. Varshavsky, A. (1981). *Cell* **25**, 561.
82. Hand, R. (1977). *Hum. Genet.* **37**, 5.
83. Funderud, S., Andreassen, R., Haugli, F. (1979). *Nucleic Acids Res.* **6**, 1417.
84. Blumenthal, A. B., Kriegstein, H. J., and Hogness, D. S. (1973). *Cold Spring Harbor Symp. Quant. Biol.* **38**, 205.
85. Vogelstein, B., and Gillespie, D. H. (1977). *Biochem. Biophys. Res. Commun.* **75**, 1127.
86. Small, D., Nelkin, B., and Vogelstein, B. (1982). *Proc. Natl. Acad. Sci. U.S.A.* **79** (in press).

PART VI

Perspectives

28

What Viruses Tell Us about Tumorigenesis

WALLACE P. ROWE

I. Introduction

When the bacteriophages were first studied, their importance was seen in the possibility that they could be used as therapeutic agents to cure bacterial diseases. As we all know, this expectation was not realized; but instead, the basic research on their replication, genetics, and cellular interactions led to molecular genetics and much of the present revolution in biology.

It is a useful analogy to consider tumor virology as being in the course of a similar evolution. Initially touted as important because of their possibly providing a simplistic answer to the cause and prevention of cancer, viruses have instead become a major source of knowledge and techniques for analyzing the nature and cellular basis of malignancy.

Although this analogy is valid in many ways, it must be stressed that in the case of the tumor viruses, the initial stage of disappointment was only relative to the excessive expectations. Tumor viruses are not laboratory artifacts, but are major causes of naturally occurring tumors, not only in animal systems but in a few instances in man as well. Retrovirus-induced leukemias of fowl, cattle, and cats are of major importance in agriculture and veterinary medicine, as are lymphomas of chickens caused by the Marek's disease herpesvirus. Lymphomas due to herpesviruses and retroviruses occur in monkeys, and virus-induced papillomas are widespread among mammals. In man, EB virus induces Burkitt lymphomas and Asiatic nasopharyngeal carcinoma, and there is strong evidence for retroviral etiology of cutaneous T cell lymphomas. Involvement of herpes 2 in the etiology of cervical carcinoma remains a distinct possibility, and there is a strong suspicion that cytomegalovirus could be an etiologic factor in the remarkable wave of Kaposi's sarcoma cases in homosexuals. The importance of hepatitis B virus in hepatocellular carcinoma is also clear.

The input of virology to tumor biology and general cell biology is at many levels. As blocks of genes that are small enough to be sequenced completely, that code for a variety of phenotypically recognizable effects, that can be easily inserted into a wide variety of host cells, and that can be mutagenized precisely *in vitro*, viruses offer many of the same opportunities for the study of eukaryotic gene regulation and expression that the bacteriophages offer for prokaryotes. Tumor viruses in particular offer remarkable opportunities for genetic and biochemical analysis of the regulation of cell phenotypes associated with malignancy.

II. Interactions between Viral and Host Cell Genomes

In large part, current basic research in tumor virology can be seen as studies of the genetic interactions between viral and host cell genomes, and as attempts to identify both the viral component (genetic sequence or gene product) that is the proximal trigger of cell transformation, and the cellular component with which it interacts. These studies are proceeding rapidly with both RNA and DNA tumor viruses, as exemplified by retroviruses and papovaviruses, respectively.

Retroviruses are a large, diverse, and complex group of viruses found in a wide variety of vertebrate hosts. Some are carried as endogenous, chromosomal proviruses that are part of the normal genetic makeup of a species, while others are maintained in nature by horizontal spread. As agents that are comparable to lysogenic bacteriophages, the endogenous retroviruses provide a unique set of host genes that in some ways are subject to normal cell regulation, but in other ways are more diverse and dynamic than other gene systems.

In the mouse, the chromosomal DNA contains multiple copies of the genomes of several families of retroviruses: C-type or leukemia viruses;

B-type or mammary tumor viruses; and "A particles," which are defective viruses expressed in certain tumors and in early embryogenesis. The endogenous C-type virus sequences are of several types, closely related to one another; these are distantly related to the C-type viruses and related genomic sequences of other mammals. The two major types of murine leukemia viruses (MuLVs) are the ecotropic viruses, which are strains that can infect mouse cells from without; and the xenotropic viruses, which can replicate in cell cultures of certain heterologous vertebrates but are unable to penetrate and replicate in mouse cells. Some mice are lacking the ecotropic virus genomes, but all carry xenotropics. Ecotropic genomes are usually in low abundance, there being one to ten copies per haploid genome in the ecotropic-positive strains, while the xenotropic genomes are present in several dozen copies. Some of the endogenous C-type genomes are defective, but a surprisingly high proportion have the length and internal organization of infectious genomes, even in strains of mice that rarely express infectious virus. Some of these genomes are expressed during embryogenesis or in particular differentiated cell types, but little is known of their control. The major MuLV proteins, the envelope and core proteins, can be expressed in certain tissues in a noncoordinate manner; and various ones of these have been characterized as a thymic differentiation alloantigen (Gix), as major glycoprotein components of normal mouse serum and epididymal fluid, and as tumor antigens. Whether the subgenomic expressions of MuLV genomes are from few or many of the endogenous loci, from differential expression of portions of the same genome, from different loci in different cell types, and if they are expressed preferentially from complete or defective genomes are still unanswered questions.

Retroviruses are involved in oncogenesis by several distinct genetic mechanisms. Thymic lymphomas, the best known retroviral malignancy in mice, occur in animals with a high level of ecotropic MuLV infection. This high expression develops in mice carrying highly inducible endogenous ecotropic virus genomes, along with a permissive allele of the *Fv-1* gene, a host gene that regulates the efficiency of ecotropic virus infection of mouse cells. As the ecotropic viruses spread through the mouse, genetic recombination takes place between their genomes and the endogenous xenotropic-related sequences in the cell DNA. Certain of these recombinants with substitution of xenotropic envelope sequences in the viral envelope gene acquire a dual eco-xeno envelope glycoprotein that confers on the virus the ability to infect both mouse and heterologous species cells. They also gain, for reasons that are unclear, the ability to produce foci of cytopathic changes in a mink lung cell culture line, a unique property of much technical usefulness that was responsible for the initial designation of this class of viruses as MCF, for "mink cell focus-forming" viruses. Most important, the MCF viruses of thymic origin also acquire, by recombination, a different 3' terminal repeat region, which is the portion of the viral genome that contains the promoter signals. The thymic MCF viruses have the ability to infect thymocytes, which ecotropic viruses cannot do, and are able to induce thymic lymphoma on passage to the appropriate strains of mice. Otherwise stated, one type of retroviral oncogenesis involves the production of new tissue-specific variants by virus–virus recombination between exogenous and endogenous viral sequences. The molecular mechanism of thymocyte transformation is not known, but may be one of the two mechanisms discussed below.

While there is every reason to conclude that MCF viruses are an essential part of the etiological chain of spontaneous viral thymomagenesis, the role of MCF viruses in other forms of hematopoietic malignancy is less clear. There is indirect evidence to indicate that generation of an MCF virus is important for induction of erythroblastosis by the Friend leukemia helper virus, and the constant presence of MCF viruses in spontaneous B-cell (reticulum cell) neoplasms of high-virus mice suggests a role in this disease also.

A second mechanism of retroviral carcinogenesis also involves genetic recombination into an ecotropic viral genome, in this case of nonviral host cell sequences. Most of the rapidly transforming retrovirus variants, such as sarcoma, myeloblastosis, and Abelson B-cell lymphoma viruses, as well as the multitropic MC-29 avian tumor virus, are of this type. These variants generally are defective, the genome containing cell sequences in place of a large portion of the internal coding region, with intact terminal repeats. The cell DNA sequences from which these hybrid genomes derive are highly conserved genes; they are present throughout the animal kingdom and must represent genes for key cell functions whose unregulated expression induces malignant transformation in particular differentiated cell types. The nature of the gene products of these *onc* genes, the basis for the cell specificity of their transforming capacity, and the degree of their expression in various types of human malignancy are problems of the utmost importance in oncology. Some, but not all, of these *onc* gene proteins have been identified as having protein kinase activity, and the nature of the cellular substrate is under active investigation in a number of laboratories.

In both the virus–virus and virus–cell recombinant retroviruses, it is likely that the functional genomes that we detect are only the tip of the iceberg. Recombination may well be occurring at high frequency between replicating ecotropic viruses and other genetic elements in the cell, but only those rare genomes that create a new tissue host range or that stimulate proliferation of the cells they infect come to our attention and can be isolated.

The third mechanism of retroviral oncogenesis is the "promoter insertion" model. In this model, the terminal repeat region of an infecting virus can act as a promoter for a cell gene in the vicinity of its integration site. Since integration appears to be essentially random, some cells will by chance have an *onc* gene turned on, with resulting malignant transformation. An extension of this idea is that the endogenous, nonexpressed retroviral genomes could also function as inappropriate promoters of neighboring genes. This could be envisioned as happening *in situ*, i.e., in the gene region where the viral genes are in the germ line, or following transposition of viral genomes by infection or transposon-type movement between or within cells.

The DNA tumor virus systems are in many respects very different from the retrovirus systems. With the DNA viruses one does not see the emergence of rapidly transforming variants or variants with highly specific tropisms for particular differentiated cell types; there is no evidence of their carrying cell-derived "onc" genes even though defective papovavirus genomes can contain host sequences. Rather, the normal viral gene products required for replication of the virus are the basis of their oncogenicity. The T antigens of papovaviruses, which are the early gene products of the virus, are expressed constitutively in transformed cells; and their expression is clearly correlated with the transformed state. The function of some of the T antigens is to bind to a specific region of the viral DNA and thereby switch off transcription of the early T antigen-coding genes and switch on DNA replication and late gene transcription. It can well be imagined that the continued presence of large amounts of such a regulatory element could have profound effects on cell behavior. With molecularly cloned genomes subjected to site-specific mutagenesis, the genetic analysis of their binding to DNA, their initiation of DNA synthesis, and their effects on viral and cellular transcription should yield information of major importance for cell biology.

Strikingly, the middle T antigen of polyoma virus, which is the protein most clearly associated with polyoma tumorigenesis, has a protein kinase activity like many of the retroviral "onc" gene products. Mutagenesis within the polyoma middle T coding region can produce an increase or decrease in transforming ability; undoubtedly such mutants will facilitate eventual recognition of the cellular target of middle T transformation, based on increased or decreased ability to be bound by the mutants.

III. Viral Polypeptide–Cell Protein Interactions

Another property of a T antigen, SV40 large T, is of exceptional interest in cancer biology. In transformed cells, this T antigen was found to be complexed to a normal cell protein of 48,000 to 50,000 daltons. Subsequently, this 50,000-MW protein has been found in a variety of nonviral tumors, in normal rodent embryos, and complexed to an EB virus antigen in Burkitt lymphoma cells. This clearly is a candidate for being a molecule with profound importance for cell regulation.

In this regard, it seems likely that many viruses will be found to synthesize polypeptides that complex with normal cell enzymes to change their substrate specificity or reaction rate to favor viral synthesis; such a strategy would be a highly efficient use of a small amount of genomic information. Indeed, it is likely that one of the major bases of the great host and tissue specificity of viral infections is the presence or availability of such target host polypeptides. Finding these polypeptides, by using their association with viral peptides, may allow identification of important cell differentiation markers and functions, as well as possible transformation-specific proteins like the 50,000. Just as the capturing of an *onc* gene by a retrovirus provides a highly selective way of identifying a key cellular element, the recognition of cell molecules physically associated with viral transformation proteins can be another strategy for finding the proximal targets of oncogenicity.

IV. Genetic Analysis of Tumorigenesis in Mice

Another area of oncology where tumor viruses are of much importance is in the genetic analysis of tumorigenesis in mice. Despite the power of mouse genetics in providing model systems for the study of biological problems, it has not yet progressed far in the area of inherited predisposition to nonviral tumors. Retroviruses are both the basis of this deficiency and the possible key to further progress. Retroviruses have interfered with the development of the field in two ways. First, the dramatic high-incidence tumor systems, leukemias and mammary tumors, turned out to be retroviral diseases, so that the genetic analysis of their occurrence, while of profound importance for understanding retroviruses and their biological significance, could not be extrapolated to the generality of cancer. Second, the ubiquity of retroviruses and the complexity of their expression have made it very difficult to determine whether or not a given genetic effect involves retrovirus expression. Only when the genes that primarily affect retroviral infection have been clarified and appropriate congenic mouse strains bred will the field of mouse cancer genetics be able to reach its full potential.

In contrast to this rather pessimistic assessment, I think there is much to gain from genetic studies of mouse tumorigenesis by the highly cell lineage-specific variant retroviruses such as erythroblastosis and T and B cell lymphoma viruses, again provided the basic antiviral genes have been understood and equalized. The ability to induce tumors in particular cell types with high efficiency and specificity, as well as to recombine and mutagenize the inducing virus *in vivo*, provides unique opportunities to study cell regulation and oncogenesis and their genetic control.

V. Summary

In summary, tumor virology seems to be bridging the gap between the elegance and precision of basic bacteriophage and bacterial genetic expression and the staggering complexity of eukaryotic cells. We are seeing phenomena such as genetic recombination, lysogeny, induction, transduction, insertional mutagenesis, polar mutational effects, host range changes, and phenotypic conversion in our day-to-day studies of vertebrate cells and tumors. The identification of candidate "cancer genes" and elucidation of their mechanism of action are proceeding rapidly, and virologists are adding progressively to the list of human tumors in which viruses play a major determinative role. One cannot but feel the imminence of profound insights into tumorigenesis.

![chapter number 29](stylized numeral 29)

The Concept of DNA Rearrangement in Carcinogenesis and Development of Tumor Cell Heterogeneity

ANDREW P. FEINBERG AND DONALD S. COFFEY

I. Introduction

The purpose of this chapter is to address the origin of tumor cell heterogeneity and to propose a concept that it is the end result of a rearrangement of the linear order of the DNA molecule within the genome. It is believed that this rearrangement process is initiated during the early phases of carcinogenesis.

It is now well-established that many human cancers manifest visible chromosomal rearrangements that represent gross changes in large segments of DNA contained within one or more chromosomal bands (1). Although these translocations of chromosomal bands are not observed in all cancer cells, they nevertheless raise the possibility that a more subtle or microarrangement of DNA might be occurring beyond the resolution of our present chromosomal banding techniques, which are now limited to observations made at the light microscopic level. Even at this low level of resolution, it is not known how far back in the progression from a normal cell to a cancer cell one can place evidence for chromosomal rearrangement. In this regard, we have analyzed published case histories of patients with genetic disorders that predispose to cancer to determine the types of chromosomal rearrangements that have been reported in the *nontumor* cells of these patients. The presence in patients predisposed to cancer of an increased tendency for chromosomal rearrangements in nontumor cells cannot prove that this increases the probability that specific DNA rearrangements that cause cancer may ensue. However, these chromosomal rearrangements might nevertheless indicate that DNA rearrangement may occur even before clinical cancer appears. Thus, in these patients, there may be an abnormality of the process that governs the normal order of DNA within the genome. The rearrangements that have been documented in nontumor cells of patients predisposed to cancer indicate that the phenomenon of DNA rearrangement is not merely the result of a cell being a cancer cell.

We are also proposing that DNA rearrangement progresses to further genetic instability and culminates in the development of tumor cell heterogeneity, so that a cancer is composed of a wide variety of cells of varying genetic compositions (see Sections II and III). Chromatin structure may be involved in the process of DNA rearrangement and instability; the association of DNA with specific structural elements of the nucleus is discussed in relation to these concepts (see Section IV).

II. Tumor Cell Heterogeneity

It now seems apparent that the rapid development of therapeutic resistance probably accounts for the major limitation in controlling the more common forms of human solid tumors. It was long believed that much of this therapeutic resistance was the result of adaptation at the cellular level, wherein enzymes were induced rapidly within the cell to alter transport or processing of the drug or to repair or protect the cancer cell from the specific effects of a particular therapeutic modality. In contrast, more recent evidence indicates that therapeutic resistance may result in most cases from tumor cell heterogeneity, in which preexisting drug resistant subpopulations of cells (clones) are selected for continued growth by not having responded to the treatment (2). How then might tumor cell hetero-geneity arise, wherein a single primary tumor may be composed of a wide variety of tumor cells with different properties and varying degrees of therapeutic sensitivity? Is the development of tumor cell heterogeneity a genetic phenomenon that reflects a variety of changes in the genome in the different types of cells? Alternatively, could the heterogeneity result merely from cellular adaptation, which is defined as epigenetic variations in cellular regulatory or control phenomena that are *not* the result of ge-netic changes that alter the DNA? Obviously, tumor cell heterogeneity may involve the development of a variety of different tumor cells within the cancer that can arise from both genetic and nongenetic (epigenetic) phenomena. For example, variations in the circulation and microenviron-ment within a single tumor mass would result in cells receiving different amounts of perfusion and nourishment. Furthermore, tumor cells in con-tact with different host elements located within the tumor might be ex-pected to display variations in their expressions and responses. Both types of environmental variation can produce cellular heterogeneity that does not result from genetic changes. However, a more permanent form of tumor cell heterogeneity would result from changes in the cellular ge-netic elements that could result in part from inherent genetic instability or increased rates of cellular mutation. Nowell has described the features of this type of genetic progression (3). If these genetic changes continued within the tumor, they would ultimately provide the cancer with a wide variety of different clones of tumor cells that could be selected for growth advantage by any number of changes in the tumor environment that are induced by therapeutic treatment or imposed by the host. Survival of the fittest cells coupled with the most optimal growth properties would select a population of cells for continuing growth. The various processes that could lead to tumor cell heterogeneity are summarized in the schematic in Fig. 1.

Several recent animal tumor models have implicated genetic instability as a major mechanism for the development of subclones of tumor cells that express variation in tumor properties (4–5). Since tumor cell hetero-geneity is becoming central to so many areas of oncology, such as hormo-nal response (6), metastatic patterns (7), immunological properties (8), and radiation and drug sensitivity (7,9,10), it would seem that the cause of this phenomenon of cellular heterogeneity may be related to the funda-mental nature of carcinogenesis. Indeed, the controversy (genetic versus epigenetic) surrounding the explanation of the basic causes of therapeutic resistance and the factors producing tumor cell heterogeneity is very simi-lar to that involving the mechanism of carcinogenesis. In both controver-sies the arguments narrow to a selection between epigenetic and genetic mechanisms. An apparent paradox has thus been developing, since evi-

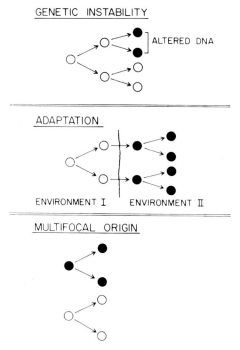

Fig. 1. Three different models for the development of tumor cell heterogeneity. Black and white circles indicate tumor cells with different properties.

dence has been accumulating for both the genetic and epigenetic approaches in explaining both carcinogenesis and tumor cell heterogeneity. Often when an area of research is faced with apparently paradoxical positions, the conflict is resolved by the development of another hypothesis that encompasses the essence of both arguments; the concept of DNA rearrangement would appear to be just such a resolving hypothesis.

III. Carcinogenesis

A. The Genetic–Epigenetic Paradox

The popular concept that carcinogenesis is a mutational phenomenon originated in 1914 with Boveri, who proposed that chromosomal changes in cancer cells enhance cell proliferation (*11*). The idea that cancer arises from *genetic* changes has received its greatest support from the following observations: (1) Cancer cells beget cancer cells. (2) Mutagenic agents such as chemical carcinogens and radiation appear to induce cancer by direct perturbation of DNA (*12*). (3) Animals can be bred to have an increased incidence of spontaneous cancers. (4) Some human Mendelian disorders, such as xeroderma pigmentosum and Bloom's syndrome, are associated with an increased incidence of cancer (*13*). (5) Chromosomal and genetic aberrations can often be observed within cancer cells, and specific chromosomal rearrangements are consistently seen in some types of cancer (*1*). (6) Some viruses that insert genetic elements into cellular DNA are capable of transforming the host cell. (7) DNA from cancer cells or chemically transformed cells can be used to transform normal cells (*14*).

In contrast, the most cogent arguments that carcinogenesis may be a nonmutational, *epigenetic* phenomenon are based in part on the following observations: (1) Some cancer cells appear to be reversible to an apparently normal state. Experiments with teratocarcinomas have clearly demonstrated that these tumor cells, when placed in the normal blastocyst of rodents, can be redirected to normal differentiation (*15–18*). The chimeric mice derived from this procedure possess normal somatic cells and competent germ cells which were derived from the original tumor cells, indicating that tumor cells may retain the capacity for apparently normal totipotent differentiation (*19*). Earlier, it was shown that the Lucké renal adenocarcinoma of the frog can be reversed by transplanting a tumor nucleus into the cytoplasm of an enucleated frog egg, thereby producing a tadpole (*20–21*). Also, crown galls can be reverted to a normal growth state when transplanted onto stems of normal plants (*22–23*). However, the crown gall and Lucké tumor are plasmid or virus induced, and in the case of the Lucké tumor, the experimental methods have been challenged (*19*) although recently confirmed (*24*). Normal differentiation of malignant cells can also be induced *in vitro,* as measured by morphology, electrical activity, or histochemical markers in neuroblastoma (*25*) and murine (*26–27*) and human leukemia (*28*) or by tumorgenicity and growth in soft agar in human colon cancer (*29*). Similar reversion is thought to occur rarely *in vivo* in human neuroblastoma (*30–31*) and leukemia (*31*), and progeny cells of squamous cell carcinoma cells have been shown by radiolabeling to differentiate into benign squamous cells (*32*). These examples of reversibility require the reestablishment of normal genetic expression and control. (2) Often, the measured frequency of point mutation on exposure to chemical carcinogens or UV light is less than, and the time of latency greater than, that of transformation by these agents (*33–34*). This may suggest a nonmutational basis for transformation; however, these observations vary with the experimental system and are controversial (*35*). Even so, reversal from a malignant to a normal phenotype, when it occurs at all, must occur at a frequency much higher than is seen in point mutation, since even a single tumor cell can be induced to give rise to normal progeny cells (*16*). (3) Cancer can be viewed as the expression of normal cellular functions at the wrong time. Most if not all of the characteristics of cancer cells such as continued proliferation, expression of embryonic markers, and invasion of other tissues can be seen in normal cells at some time during development. In addition, normal cells have been transformed by transplantation to an ectopic site (*36–39*). Many malignant properties are expressed by normal cells that are treated with chemical promoters; when the promoter is withdrawn the cells revert to a normal state (*40*).

The above evidence, taken together, suggests that both mutational (genetic) and nonmutational (epigenetic) factors may be involved in the etiology of cancer. One might argue that there are many types of cancer and that a variety of mechanisms may be responsible for their induction. On the other hand, the broad spectrum of etiological and biological factors may be explained by a generalized hypothesis, asuch as potentially reversible DNA rearrangement, that could encompass both the genetic and apparently epigenetic observations.

B. DNA Rearrangement in Carcinogenesis

The concept of chromosomal rearrangement as a normal aspect of phenotypic expression was introduced in 1911 by Morgan, who proposed that an equal exchange between homologous chromosomes during meiosis could explain genetic linkage (*41*). McClintock, in 1950, discovered that genetic rearrangement affects phenotypic expression in the seeds of maize during development by movement of transposable genetic controlling elements (*42*). Such transposable elements have subsequently been observed in both prokaryotes and eukaryotes (*43*). The extent of DNA rearrangement in the normal differentiation of mammalian cells has not been determined. However, the development of antibody diversity associated with the formation of specific immunoglobulins, which occurs during the differentiation of B lymphocytes, results from DNA deletions (*44–47*), which in effect rearrange the DNA.

The possible role of DNA rearrangement in cancer was first noted by Temin, who suggested that tumor proviruses might act similarly to transposable elements, and that their location at specific sites in the host genome might modify cellular expression and lead to cancer (*48*). Tumor viruses can change the linear order of the DNA by insertion into the host genome, and recent experimental evidence supports the hypothesis that a specific DNA arrangement or proviral DNA within the host genome leads to cancer in two animal tumor virus systems (*49–51*). Many cytogenetic studies show that consistent chromosomal rearrangements are often found in cancer cells, and from these studies, it has been suggested that DNA rearrangement may lead to cancer (52–55). Any DNA rearrangement could be preserved during subsequent cellular replication and would appear as a genetic or mutational event. In addition to point mutations, gross chromosomal aberrations or sister chromatid exchanges can also be induced by most carcinogenic agents (56–58). DNA repair disorders that predispose to cancer also manifest chromosomal rearrangements (1,59, 60). Thus, if specific DNA rearrangements are shown to cause cancer, these carcinogenic rearrangements may be the genetic events attributed to mutation.

Reversal of the DNA arrangement in a tumor cell, in order to restore the original linear order of DNA existing in normal cells, may underlie the apparent reversibility of cancer in several systems. DNA rearrangement could account for the high frequency of reversal, in these systems, from the malignant state to the normal state. For example, a transposable element that controls the mating type of yeast (61) can cause interconversion between two phenotypic states after a single cell division (62). The high frequency of transformation of normal cells on exposure to carcinogens also might be explained by DNA rearrangement rather than by point mutation (35,63). Thus, DNA rearrangement provides a potential unifying mechanism to encompass both genetic and apparently epigenetic factors in carcinogenesis. The linear order of DNA segments could be rearranged by transpositions, insertions, deletions, or inversions, although in the case of deletions, reversibility would not seem possible unless the deleted segment were episomal.

There is as yet no direct evidence that any form of DNA rearrangement within a single somatic cell causes human cancer. Indirect evidence for genetic rearrangement in human carcinogenesis is derived from cancer cytogenetics. Nonrandom chromosomal rearrangements were first observed in chronic myelogenous leukemia cells (64), and other rearrangements have now been identified in a wide variety of cancers (1,52,65). However, at present, it is not known whether the rearrangements seen in the chromosomes of cancer cells cause the malignant state or result from it.

An alternative indirect argument for DNA rearrangement rather than point mutation as a cause of human cancer is derived from Cairns' recent genetic epidemiological study (63). Cairns examined published data on mortality from fatal internal cancers among patients with two inherited disorders that predispose to cancer, Bloom's syndrome and xeroderma pigmentosum. He points out that patients with xeroderma pigmentosum show a markedly deficient capacity to repair DNA damage caused by UV light, and that the resulting mutations are associated only with skin cancer and not with fatal internal cancers. In contrast, patients with Bloom's

TABLE I

Reported DNA Rearrangements in Nontumor Cells in Genetic Disorders That Predispose to Cancer

Syndrome	Cytogenetic type of DNA rearrangement in nontumor cells									Change in ploidy		References
	Trans-location	Marker chromosome	Dicentric	Chromatid interchange	Ring chromosome	Sister chromatid exchange	Inversion	Interstitial deletion	Gap, break or terminal deletion	Aneuploidy	Polyploidy	
Chromosomal instability												
Bloom's syndrome	+[a]		+[a]	+[a]		+[a]			+[a]			79–84,164–165
Xeroderma pigmentosum		+[a]	+[a]	+[b]		+[b]			+[b]	+[a]	+[a]	1, 59, 163
Fanconi's anemia		+[a]	+[a]	+[a]	+[a]		+[a]		+[a]	+[a]	+[a]	
Ataxia telangiectasia	+[a]		+[a]	+[a]	+[a]		+[a]		+[a]	+[a]	+[a]	
Congenital chromosomal anomalies												
Down's syndrome	+[c]	+[c]	+[b,c]		+[b]				+[b]	+[c]		166–178
Gonadal dysgenesis	+[c]	+[c]	+[c]		+[c]		+[c]		+[c,d]	+[c]		166, 179
Klinefelter's syndrome	+[c]	+[c]					+[c]			+[c]		166, 179
13-deletion syndrome	+[c]				+[c]	+[a]		+[c]				180–182
AGR triad	+[c]							+[c]		+[c]		183–185

					References
Other genetic disorders					
Dyskeratosis congenita		+[b]	+[a]		66–69
Acute lymphocytic leukemia (familial)	+[a]	+[a,c]		+[e]	186–187
Renal cell carcinoma (familial)	+[c]				102
Medullary thyroid carcinoma (familial)	+[a]	+[a]	+[a]		187–188

[a] Occurring spontaneously in cultured somatic cells.
[b] Inducible in somatic cells by chemical agents or radiation, significantly more frequently than in control cells.
[c] Karyotypic anomaly in those patients with the abnormality.
[d] Gonadoblastoma occurs more frequently in patients with an intact Y chromosome (189).
[e] In obligate carrier.

syndrome, whose cells manifest an increase in DNA rearrangements, demonstrate a markedly increased mortality from the common fatal internal cancers. From his analysis, Cairns concludes that for people without these disorders the main source of mutagenic lesions in DNA is UV light which produces nonfatal skin cancer, and that genetic rearrangements, rather than chemical mutagens, cause most internal human cancers (63).

C. Reported Chromosomal Rearrangements in Nontumor Cells of Patients with Genetic Disorders That Predispose to Cancer

An analysis of the published case histories of genetic disorders that predispose to cancer was performed to determine the cytogenetic types and chromosomal locations of chromosomal rearrangements reported in the *nontumor cells* of patients with these disorders. Nontumor cells were chosen in order to determine whether these rearrangements might precede clinical cancer rather than result from the cancer per se. A rearrangement was defined as a change in the linear order of chromosomal segments. In Table I, disorders showing spontaneous or inducible rearrangements occurring in somatic cells are listed as chromosomal instability disorders. Some other disorders that predispose to cancer show characteristic germ cell-derived karyotypic anomalies which predispose to cancer. In other genetic disorders that predispose to cancer, too few observations of chromosomal rearrangement have yet been made to permit definitive classification.

It is well known that the classical chromosomal instability disorders, Bloom's syndrome, ataxia telangiectasia, Fanconi's anemia, and xeroderma pigmentosum all manifest an increased incidence of cancer (1). This observation also holds true for the recently described, but not yet generally accepted, chromosomal instability disorders, viz., dyskeratosis congenita (66–69), incontinentia pigmenti (70,71), basal cell nevus syndrome (72–74), glutathione reductase deficiency anemia (75,76), Kostmann's agranulocytosis (77), and Mibelli's porokeratosis (78). Interestingly, karyotypic or inducible chromosomal rearrangements may be a more common finding than is generally recognized in some congenital chromosomal anomalies that predispose to cancer. For example, most cases of Down's syndrome are caused by trisomy 21, which is not strictly speaking a rearrangement as defined here. However, translocations and other rearrangements are also seen (79), and cells from Down's syndrome patients have been reported to shown an increased susceptibility to X-ray or chemically induced chromosomal aberrations (80–84).

There are additional individual cases reported to indicate that chromosomal rearrangements in nontumor cells may be a feature of other genetic disorders that increase the incidence of cancer, such as the following: Gardner's syndrome (addendum to 85,86); Werner's syndrome (87–91); Chediak–Higashi syndrome (92,93); Sipple's syndrome (94); familial polyposis coli (86); Peutz–Jeghers' syndrome (86); and tuberous sclerosis (95). It remains to be determined whether there is a *significant* increase in chromosomal rearrangements in patients with these and other genetic disorders that predispose to cancer; however, we believe they may be more common than is generally realized.

Although the chromosomal rearrangements seen in these disorders vary widely by cytogenetic type and include both stable chromosomal anomalies and acquired somatic cell rearrangements (Table I), they do show some interesting similarities in chromosomal location (Table II). The observation has been made, in the case of four genetic disorders that predispose to cancer, that the site of rearrangement in nontumor cells is the same region as that involved in nonrandom rearrangements in a variety of noninherited cancers (96–101,103). The first is ataxia telangiectasia, in which nontumor cells show spontaneous translocations on the long arm of chromosome 14 similar to those seen in a variety of lymphomas (98). Second, a family with hereditary renal cell carcinoma possesses an inherited karyotypic translocation from the short arm of chromosome 3 to the long arm of chromosome 8 (102), sites of nonrandom rearrangement in many patients with lymphoproliferative malignancies and some patients with mixed salivary gland tumors (96,100). Third, patients with a congenital karyotypic deletion within chromosome 13 are predisposed to retinoblastoma; retinoblastoma cells from patients without this karyotypic anomaly have shown a similar deletion (97,99,103). Fourth, patients with a karyotypic deletion in the short arm of chromosome 11 are predisposed to Wilms' tumor, and a similar deletion has been observed in Wilms' tumor cells from patients without this congenital karyotype (101).

The present analysis shows that such an association can be made in patients with eight additional disorders. Thus, patients with genetic disorders that predispose to cancer have shown chromosomal rearrangements in *nontumor* cells on the *same* chromosomal arms as those that characterize cancer cell rearrangements (Table II). In some cases, these rearrangements are in close proximity to those observed in tumors. As with the four disorders for which such an association has been made previously (96–101,103), the type of cancer that patients with the genetic disorders listed here develop include lymphoproliferative malignancies as well as solid tumors. Although nonrandom chromosomal rearrangements in tumor cells have been reported primarily in leukemias and lymphomas, Mi-

TABLE II

Comparison of DNA Rearrangements in Cancer Cells and in Nontumor Cells Genetically Predisposed to Cancer

Chromosomal arm involved in rearrangement	Noninherited cancers in which nonrandom chromosomal rearrangement has been established[a]	(bands)	Inherited disorders in which chromosomal rearrangement in nontumor cells has been reported	(bands)	References
1q	Lymphoproliferative malignancies	(1q25-41)	Familial acute lymphocytic leukemia[b]	(1q25,1q32)	187
			Fanconi's anemia[b]		190
			Gonadal dysgenesis[c]		169, 191
			Bloom's syndrome[b]		192
			Xeroderma pigmentosum[b]		193
3p	Mixed salivary gland tumor	(3p25)	Familial renal cell carcinoma[c]	(3p21)	102; association discussed in ref. 100
			Gonadal dysgenesis[c]	(3p11)	167
5q	Preleukemia	(5q14-qter)	Fanconi's anemia[b]	(5q31)	194
	Acute nonlymphocytic leukemia		Klinefelter's syndrome[c]	(5q21,5q32)	166
			Gonadal dysgenesis[c]		195
7q	Acute nonlymphocytic leukemia	(7q22)	Gonadal dysgenesis[c]	(7q11,7q22)	166
			Familial medullary thyroid carcinoma[b]	(7q22)	187
8q	Lymphoproliferative malignancies	(8q22)	Familial renal cell carcinoma[c]	(8q24)	102; association discussed in refs. 96, 100
	Mixed salivary gland tumor	(8q21)			

9q	Chronic myelogenous leukemia	(9q34)	Fanconi's anemia[b]		163
11p	Wilms' tumor	(11p13)	AGR triad[c]	(11p13)	Association discussed in ref. 101
13q	Retinoblastoma	(13q14)	13-deletion syndrome[c]	(13q14)	Association discussed in refs. 97, 99, 103
14q	Lymphomas including Burkitt's	(14q32)	Ataxia telangiectasia[b]	(14q12,14q32)	Association discussed in ref. 98
	Ovarian papillary cystadenocarcinoma	(14q24)	Down's syndrome[c]		79
15q	Acute promyelocytic leukemia	(15q26)	Gonadal dysgenesis[c]		173
17q	Acute promyelocytic leukemia	(17q22)	Familial medullary thyroid carcinoma[b]	(17q23)	187
21q	Acute myeloblastic leukemia	(21q22)	Down's syndrome[c]		79
			Fanconi's anemia[b]		194
			Gonadal dysgenesis[b]	(21q11 or 21)	196
22q	Chronic myelogenous leukemia	(22q11)	Gonadal dysgenesis[c]	(22q13)	197
	Meningioma				

[a] See reviews (1, 52, 65).
[b] Clonal abnormality in cultured cells.
[c] Karyotypic anomaly.

telman has found that rearrangements in solid tumors may occur on the same chromosomes as those rearranged nonrandomly in leukemias (52).

Until many more cytogenetic observations are made of patients with these disorders, one cannot know if the associations reported in Table II are random or nonrandom. However, Table II supports the observation that specific rearrangements similar to those seen in some cancers, or regional instability on the same chromosomal arms, may begin to occur in nontumor cells of patients with genetic disorders that predispose to cancer even before clinical cancer appears. An analysis of a wide variety of genetic disorders that predispose to cancer shows chromosomal rearrangements in nontumor cells of these patients similar to those that appear nonrandomly in cancer patients (Tables I and II), suggesting that DNA rearrangement may precede the development of clinical cancers. Direct confirmation of this observation will require cytogenetic studies of patients with the more than 200 genetic disorders that predispose to cancer, particularly of the cancer-prone tissues of these patients.

The proposed model of DNA rearrangement in human carcinogenesis is summarized in Fig. 2. Both genetic disorders and external carcinogens may set in motion DNA rearrangements that ultimately lead to a carcinogenic arrangement. Most carcinogens studied do cause gross chromosomal aberrations or sister chromatid exchanges (56–58), and as illustrated here, many patients with genetic disorders, whether they are chromosomal instability disorders or congenital chromosomal anomalies, share some form of DNA rearrangement in their nontumor cells that would alter the linear order of DNA segments within the genome. Interestingly, many of the rearrangements seen in these cells involve the same chromosomal segments rearranged nonrandomly in a variety of cancers. If some carcinogenic rearrangements were potentially reversible, they might explain the apparent reversibility of several experimental and animal cancers, which forms one of the principal epigenetic arguments for carcinogenesis.

It is important to note that the rearrangements seen in the nontumor cells of patients with the disorders we have studied may not themselves be sufficient for carcinogenesis. Age, tissue differences, carcinogen exposure and susceptibility, and genetic predisposition all may play an important role in the progression to a carcinogenic DNA arrangement and might explain the differences in tissue susceptibility to cancer. For example, xeroderma pigmentosum patients, who show chromosomal fragility in both lymphocytes and fibroblasts on exposure to UV light, may commonly develop only skin cancer simply because only their skin is exposed to this agent. On the other hand, intrinsic tissue differences may play an important role in the heritable colorectal cancer syndromes, since chromosomal changes are seen commonly in culture only in those tissues pre-

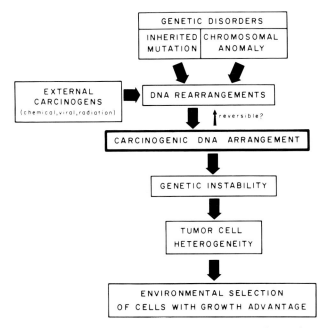

Fig. 2. A schematic of the concept of DNA rearrangement in carcinogenesis and the development of tumor cell heterogeneity. DNA rearrangement is set in motion by genetic disorders or external carcinogens and leads to specific carcinogenic arrangements. If the carcinogenic arrangement produces genetic instability, a variety of tumor cells could be formed with different genetic compositions. Environmental factors within the host would select those clones with the most optimal growth properties.

disposed to cancer (*104,105*). Viral infection may enhance the development of cancer in ataxia telangiectasia, since the development of cytogenetically abnormal clones with a proliferative advantage in culture is enhanced by viral agents (*106*). In addition, immune deficiency may facilitate the development of cancer in ataxia telangiectasia and Bloom's syndrome.

Some patients with cancer do not necessarily possess the chromosomal rearrangements characteristic of that cancer, and thus the causal nature of these rearrangements in carcinogenesis may be challenged. For example, these rearrangements may represent fragile loci perturbed secondarily by the cancer (1). However, as the resolution of cytogenetic techniques is improving, the fraction of apparently cytogenetically normal cancer patients is shrinking (*107,108*). These chromosomal rearrangements are seen grossly at the light microscopic level, and DNA rearrangements occurring at the molecular level may not be detectable by current cytogenetic methods. For example, sister chromatid exchange may be 100 times more sensitive an indicator of rearrangements that occur than are gross chromosomal aberrations (58,109), and chemically detected rearrangements, seen in excess in Bloom's syndrome cells (110), may be 10 times more sensitive an indicator of rearrangement than sister chromatid exchange (57,111,112). Thus, many DNA rearrangements could occur without visual detection by current cytogenetic methods. Ultimately, the link between structural aberrations seen cytogenetically and DNA rearrangement at the molecular level will require an understanding of chromosomal structural organization.

The concept summarized in Fig. 2 is consistent with two other observations in oncology. The first is Knudson's two-step hypothesis of carcinogenesis in genetic disorders, which explains the early appearance and multiple foci of familial versus sporadic cancers of several types, and which may correspond to the two stages of chemical carcinogenesis. Patients with an inherited predisposition to cancer are thought to be born with one mutation in the germ line, and to develop a second mutation in some somatic cells (113–115). There is some support for Knudson's hypothesis from observations of biochemical markers in familial medullary thyroid carcinoma (116). In Fig. 2, this first mutation would represent a Mendelian mutation or germ cell chromosomal anomaly, and the second mutation would in fact correspond to a carcinogenic DNA arrangement arising in somatic cells.

The second observation consistent with Fig. 2 is that of specific DNA arrangements in some animal viral tumors. It has recently been shown that the avian leukosis virus provirus integrates adjacent to and causes enhanced expression of a cellular gene, leading to neoplastic transformation (50,51). Whether this type of carcinogenic DNA arrangement is responsible for nonviral human cancers is unknown, but sequences homologous to animal viral oncogenes have been cloned from human DNA (117). More recently, the enhanced expression of cellular oncogenes has been observed in human lymphomas (118) and tumor cell lines (119). Klein has proposed that in B lymphocyte-derived tumors, specific observed chromosomal translocations may bring the immunoglobulin gene region under the influence of such a promoter (55). In Fig. 2, the joining of a promoter sequence to a cellular oncogene in viral carcinogenesis would be the carcinogenic DNA arrangement.

In summary, observations from several areas of oncology have been used in this chapter to link genetic, epigenetic, and cytogenetic aspects of cancer. As observed at the cytogenetic level, DNA rearrangement may be more common in cancer-prone tissues than has generally been realized. If DNA rearrangement is a common pathway to cancer, as hypothesized here, one would predict that biochemical examination of DNA from cancer-prone and malignant cells should demonstrate specific carcinogenic DNA arrangements. Since transposable elements can induce mutation at a high frequency (120), it is tempting to speculate that such rearrangements, if shown to exist, would lead to genetic instability and ultimately progress to a state of tumor cell heterogeneity.

IV. Nuclear Structure and Function

There is increasing evidence that chromatin structure may be involved directly in DNA function. Our understanding of chromatin structure has progressed from the nucleosomal bead concept of DNA–histone interactions to the view of higher-order arrangements of the packed DNA into supercoiled loops of DNA attached to a residual nuclear skeleton termed the nuclear matrix (121–123). As the concept of DNA rearrangement develops, it is important to understand these events at the molecular level, and this will undoubtedly involve nuclear structural elements. At present there is limited information regarding the role of nuclear structural elements in forming specific chromosomal bands, and in DNA replication and transcription. However, there is increasing evidence that the nuclear matrix serves an important function in these processes. In this section we will attempt to review these nuclear structural concepts with regard to their potential role in the process of DNA rearrangement.

For many years, it was believed that the nuclear membrane maintained the structural integrity of the eukaryotic nucleus. High molarity salt solutions (1 M NaCl) were used first by Zbarsky and Georgiev (124–127) and later by Busch and colleagues (128,129) to extract the majority of DNA and chromatin from the nucleus. This treatment left a relatively intact lipid-containing nuclear membrane that encompassed the nucleus, which still contained residual internal structures. The later development of mild nonionic detergents (Triton X-100) made it possible to extract the nuclear membrane lipid components. Thus, a series of extractions of nuclei with detergent, hypotonic, and hypertonic solutions could remove over 98% of the total nuclear phospholipid DNA and RNA, and 90% of the nuclear proteins (130,131); these residual chromatin-depleted nuclear ghosts still maintained their spherical and structural integrity. Electron microscopy of this insoluble skeleton structure revealed a matrix network or scaffolding system that was composed on its periphery of residual elements of the nuclear membrane and nuclear pore complexes, surrounding an internal fibrillar network that extended from the periphery to residual elements of the nucleolus. This residual nuclear framework structure was first isolated from rat liver nuclei and was characterized and termed the nuclear matrix (130,131). The nuclear matrix represented only 5–10% of the total nuclear protein, and yielded a few major polypeptide bands on sodium dodecyl sulfate polyacrylamide gel electrophoresis (131). The prominent protein fractions are free of histones and have apparent molecular weights of 60,000–70,000, and by partial tryptic digest fingerprinting techniques, appear to be related structurally (131,132). In addition, there are several clusters of minor polypeptides of approximately 50,000 and 100,000 to 200,000 (131).

The nuclear matrix appears to play a central role in the structural organization and function of both DNA and nuclear RNA. DNA appears to be attached to the matrix and is organized in supercoiled loops, each containing 30,000–100,000 base pairs, and each loop is anchored at its base to the matrix. During replication, these loops of DNA appear to be reeled through fixed sites for DNA synthesis that are attached to the matrix (121, 122). Actively transcribed genes are enriched on the matrix (133–135), and it has been suggested that RNA may also be synthesized at fixed sites on the nuclear matrix (136). RNP particles are part of the matrix, and hnRNA and snRNA are associated almost exclusively with the matrix (137–141). Thus, the nuclear matrix appears to play a central role in DNA replication and transcription and may be involved in DNA processing and transport. The nuclear matrix structure also contains specific binding sites for steroid hormones (142). For a recent review of nuclear matrix functions, see ref. 143. DNA arrangement with respect to the nuclear matrix may be important in many nuclear functions, which may be mediated by DNA loop topology (123).

One of the hallmarks of cancer pathology is the concomitant development of tumor agressiveness and changes in cell morphology. The nuclei become enlarged and invaginated and have a pleiomorphic structure which is reflected in both the nucleolus and in changes in the packing of the chromatin. Since the matrix determines the shape of the nucleus, such gross physical changes must involve the nuclear matrix in at least a passive way.

When gross chromosomal rearrangements of DNA occur in cancer, they would appear to require concomitant involvement of the nuclear matrix component to which the loops are attached (Fig. 3), since the higher-order topology of bands appears to be preserved when several bands are translocated as a group from one chromosome to another. At present, it is not known what constitutes the chromosomal core structure and bands. However, some nuclear matrix proteins from the interphase nucleus do appear in the condensed metaphase chromosome (144,145). It has been

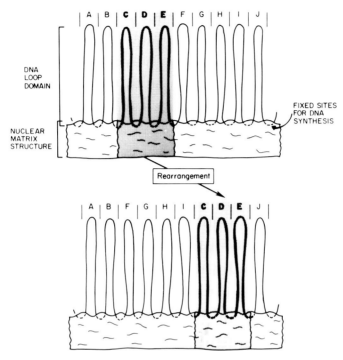

Fig. 3. DNA rearrangements may involve the concomitant movement of the nuclear matrix component to which supercoiled loop domains are attached.

reported recently that carcinogens bind to the nuclear matrix (*146–148*), and the nuclear matrix also appears to be the site of attachment of the polyoma viral transformation (T) antigen (*149*). Zbarsky has reported changes in the nuclear matrix in tumor cells (*150*). The nuclear matrix contains the fixed sites for DNA replication (*121*), and the site of DNA replication may be the locus of sister chromatid exchange (*151*), a form of rearrangement induced by many carcinogens. It is interesting that cells from patients with Bloom's syndrome, which predisposes to both chromosomal rearrangements and cancer, show slow "movement" of the replicating fork (*152*), which appears to be located on the nuclear matrix. We do not know if the nuclear matrix is involved actively in carcinogenesis. However, matrix-associated loops of DNA could resemble transposable elements (*123*).

In summary, we propose that the nuclear matrix is an important site for the control of DNA structure and function and that the matrix and the attachment of loop domains may be important elements in the process of DNA rearrangement.

V. Overview

The concept of DNA rearrangement in carcinogenesis proposed in this chapter and by Ruth Sager (*153*) and others (*35,48,52,53,55,63,154*) is a potentially important hypothesis to resolve many aspects of cancer, including genetic and epigenetic characteristics and genetic instability leading to a final state of tumor cell heterogeneity. The classical cytogenetic studies reviewed by Sandberg (*155*) and Nowell (*156*) clearly demonstrate that segments of DNA do rearrange, as witnessed by movement of chromosomal bands in the formation of specific marker chromosomes. Whether these chromosomal changes represent cause or effect in cancer has not been resolved. However, these chromosomal rearrangements appear to be related to the development of genetic instability and tumor cell heterogeneity. Tumor cell heterogeneity in several animal models appears to be the result of genetic instability, as exemplified by the studies of Isaacs (*4*) and Fidler (*157*). Baylin (*158*), Nadler (*159*), and Tropé (*160*) present convincing evidence for tumor cell heterogeneity in human cancers, and the therapeutic implications have been emphasized by Calabresi (*161*) and Goldie (*162*).

Although DNA rearrangement in human cancer is an attractive hypothesis, only limited evidence has been accumulated at present to support this concept. The recent studies of Astrin and colleagues may provide the most tangible evidence that an oncogene has been activated in a human cancer (*118*). This activation may have been accomplished by the specific arrangement of a promoter sequence next to an endogenous oncogene. We must now await a more direct test of the hypothesis that DNA rearrangement is an initial and paramount event in all forms of carcinogenesis and that tumor cell heterogeneity is the result of ensuing genetic instability. Tumor cell heterogeneity has proved to be a devastating problem in the control of cancer, and this symposium has provided a forum to discuss new concepts that may help to resolve this enigma.

References

1. Sandberg, A. A. (1980). "The Chromosomes in Human Cancer and Leukemia." Elsevier North-Holland, Amsterdam.
2. Skipper, H. E. (1978). "Cancer Chemotherapy," Vol. 1. Southern Research Inst., Birmingham, Alabama.
3. Nowell, P. C. (1976). *Science (Washington, D.C.)* **194**, 23–28.
4. Isaacs, J. T. (1982). This volume, Chapter 7.
5. Cifone, M. A., and Fidler, I. J. (1981). *Proc. Natl. Acad. Sci. U.S.A.* **78**, 6949–6952.
6. Isaacs, J. T., and Coffey, D. S. (1981). *Cancer Res.* **41**, 5070–5075.
7. Fidler, I. J. (1978). *Cancer Res.* **38**, 2651–2660.

8. Kerbel, R. S. (1979). *Nature (London)* **280**, 358–360.
9. Heppner, G. H., Dexter, D. L., DeNucci, T., Miller, F. R., and Calabresi, P. (1978). *Cancer Res.* **38**, 3758–3763.
10. Tropé, C. (1975). *Neoplasma* **22**, 171–180.
11. Boveri, T. (1914). "Zur Frage der Entstehung Maligner Tumoren." Fischer, Jena.
12. Barrett, J. C., Tsutsui, T., and Ts'o, P. O. P. (1978). *Nature (London)* **274**, 229–232.
13. Ponder, B. A. J. (1980). *Biochim. Biophys. Acta* **605**, 369–410.
14. Weinberg, R. A. (1981). *Biochim. Biophys. Acta* **651**, 25–35.
15. Brinster, R. L. (1974). *J. Exp. Med.* **140**, 1049–1056.
16. Illmensee, K., and Mintz, B. (1976). *Proc Natl. Acad. Sci. U.S.A.* **73**, 549–553.
17. Mintz, B., and Illmensee, K. (1975). *Proc. Natl. Acad. Sci. U.S.A.* **72**, 3585–3589.
18. Papaioannou, V. E., McBurney, M. W., Gardner, R. L., and Evans, M. J. (1975). *Nature (London)* **258**, 70–73.
19. Mintz, B., and Fleischmann, R. A. (1981). *Adv. Cancer Res.* **34**, 211–278.
20. McKinnell, R. G. (1979). *Int. Rev. Cytol., Suppl.* **9**, 179–188.
21. McKinnell, R. G., Deggins, B. A., and Labat, D. D. (1969). *Science (Washington, D.C.)* **165**, 394–396.
22. Braun, A. C. (1959). *Proc. Natl. Acad. Sci. U.S.A.* **45**, 932–938.
23. Braun, A. C., and Wood, H. N. (1976). *Proc. Natl. Acad. Sci. U.S.A.* **73**, 496–500.
24. Mizell, M., DiBerardino, M. A., Friesendorf, D. G., and Hoffner, N. J. (1981). *Annu. Meet. Am. Soc. Microbiol. Abstr.* **81**, 235.
25. Kimhi, Y., Palfrey, C., Spector, I., Barak, Y., and Littauer, U. Z. (1976). *Proc. Natl. Acad. Sci. U.S.A.* **73**, 462–466.
26. Filbach, E., Landau, T., and Sachs, L. (1972). *Nature New Biol.* **237**, 276–278.
27. Friend, C., Scher, W., Holland, J. G., and Sato, T. (1971). *Proc. Natl. Acad. Sci. U.S.A.* **68**, 378–382.
28. Paran, M., Sachs, L., Barak, Y., and Resnitzky, P. (1970). *Proc. Natl. Acad. Sci. U.S.A.* **67**, 1542–1549.
29. Dexter, D. L., and Hazer, J. C. (1980). *Cancer* **45**, 1178–1184.
30. Cushing, H., and Wolbach, S. B. (1927). *Am. J. Pathol.* **3**, 203–216.
31. Everson, T. C., and Cole, W. H. (1966). "Spontaneous Regression of Cancer." Saunders, Philadelphia, Pennsylvania.
32. Pierce, G. B., and Wallace, C. (1971). *Cancer Res.* **31**, 127–134.
33. Barrett, J. C., and Ts'o, P. O. P. (1978). *Proc. Natl. Acad. Sci. U.S.A.* **75**, 3297–3301.
34. Chan, G. L., and Little, J. B. (1978). *Proc. Natl. Acad. Sci. U.S.A.* **75**, 3363–3366.
35. Straus, D. S. (1981). *J. Natl. Cancer Inst.* **67**, 233–241.
36. Furth, J., and Sobel, H. (1947). *J. Natl. Cancer Inst.* **8**, 7–16.
37. Gateff, E. (1978). *Biol. Rev.* **53**, 123–168.
38. Solter, D., Skreb, N., and Damjanov, I. (1970). *Nature (London)* **227**, 503–504.
39. Stevens, L. C. (1970). *Dev. Biol.* **21**, 364–382.
40. Weinstein, I. B., Yamasaki, H., Wigler, M., Lee, L.-S., Fisher, P. B., Jeffrey, A., and Grunberger, D. (1979). In "Carcinogens: Identification and Mechanisms of Action" (A. C. Griffin, and C. R. Shaw, eds.), pp. 399–418. Raven, New York.
41. Morgan, T. H. (1911). *Science (Washington, D.C.)* **34**, 384.
42. McClintock, B. (1950). *Proc. Natl. Acad. Sci. U.S.A.* **36**, 344–355.
43. Calos, M. P., and Miller, H. (1980). *Cell* **20**, 579–595.
44. Early, P., Huang, H., Davis, M., Calame, K., and Hood, L. (1980). *Cell* **19**, 981–992.
45. Max, E. E., Seidman, J. G., and Leder, P. (1979). *Proc. Natl. Acad. Sci. U.S.A.* **76**, 3450–3454.
46. Sakano, H., Huppi, K., Heinrich, G., and Tonegawa, S. (1979). *Nature (London)* **280**, 288–294.

47. Sakano, H., Maki, R., Kurosawa, Y., Roeder, W., and Tonegawa, S. (1980). *Nature (London)* **286,** 676–683.
48. Temin, H. M. (1980). *Perspect. Biol. Med.* **14,** 11–26.
49. Blair, D. G., Oskarsson, M., Woud, T. G., McClements, W. L., Fischinger, P. J., and Vande Woude, G. G. (1981). *Science (Washington, D.C.)* **212,** 941–943.
50. Hayward, W. S., Neel, B. G., and Astrin, S. M. (1981). *Nature (London)* **290,** 475–480.
51. Neel, B. G., Hayward, W. S., Robinson, H. L., Fang, J., and Astrin, S. M. (1981). *Cell* **23,** 323–334.
52. Mitelman, F., and Levan, G. (1978). *Hereditas* **89,** 207–232.
53. Rowley, J. D. (1977). *In* "Chromosomes Today" (A. De La Capelle, and M. Sorsa, eds.), Vol. 6, pp. 345–355. Elsevier North-Holland, Amsterdam.
54. Sager, R. (1979). *Nature (London)* **282,** 447–448.
55. Klein, G. (1981). *Nature (London)* **294,** 313–318.
56. Ishidate, M., Jr., and Odashima, S. (1977). *Mutat. Res.* **48,** 337–354.
57. Latt, S. A., Schreck, R. R., Loveday, K. S., Dougherty, C. P., and Shuler, C. F. (1980). *Adv. Hum. Genet.* **10,** 267–331.
58. Perry P., and Evans, H. J. (1975). *Nature (London)* **258,** 121–125.
59. Friedberg, E. C., Ehmann, U. K., and Williams, J. I. (1979). *Adv. Radiat. Biol.* **8,** 85–174.
60. German, J. (1972). *Prog. Med. Genet.* **8,** 61–101.
61. Hicks, J. B., Strathern, J. N., and Klar, A. J. S. (1979). *Nature (London)* **282,** 478–483.
62. Hicks, J. B., and Herskowitz, I. (1976). *Genetics* **83,** 245–258.
63. Cairns, J. (1981). *Nature (London)* **289,** 353–357.
64. Nowell, P. C., and Hungerford, D. A. (1960). *Science (Washington, D.C.)* **132,** 1497.
65. Rowley, J. D. (1980). *Annu. Rev. Genet.* **14,** 17–39.
66. Burgdorf, W., Kurvink, K., and Cervenka, J. (1977). *J. Med. Genet.* **14,** 256–257.
67. Carter, D. M., Pan, M., Gaynor, A., McGuire, J. S., and Sibrack, L. (1979). *J. Invest. Dermatol.* **73,** 97–101.
68. Morrison, J. G. L. (1974). *S. Afr. Med. J.* **48,** 223–225.
69. Scoggins, R. B., Prescott, K. J., Asher, G. H., Blaylock, W. K., and Bright, R. W. (1974). *Clin. Res.* **19,** 409.
70. Cantu, J. M., del Castillo, V., Jimenez, M., and Ruiz-Barquin, E. (1973). *Ann. Génét.* **16,** 117–119.
71. DeGrouchy, J., Bonnette, J., Brussieux, J., Roidot, M., and Begin, P. (1972). *Ann. Génét.* **15,** 61–65.
72. Happle, R., and Kupferschmid, A. (1972). *Hummangenetik* **15,** 287–288.
73. Happle, R., Mehrle, G., Sander, L. Z., and Höhn, H. (1971). *Arch. Dermatol. Forsch.* **241,** 96–114.
74. Yunis, J. J., and Gorlin, R. J. (1963). *Chromosoma* **14,** 146–153.
75. Hampel, K. E., Löhr, G. W., Blume, K. G., and Rüdiger, H. W. (1969). *Humangenetik* **7,** 305–313.
76. Schroeder, T. M., and Kurth, R. (1971). *Blood* **37,** 96–112.
77. Matsianiotis, N., Kiossoglou, K. A., Karpouzas, J., and Anastasea-Vlachou (1966). *Lancet* **2,** 104.
78. Taylor, A. M. R., Harnden, D. G., and Fairburn, E. A. (1973). *J. Natl. Cancer Inst.* **51,** 371–378.
79. Penrose, L. S., and Smith, G. F. (1966). "Down's Anomaly." Little, Brown, Boston, Massachusetts.
80. Countryman, P. I., Heddle, J. A., and Crawford, E. (1977). *Cancer Res.* **37,** 52–58.
81. Higurashi, M., and Conen, P. E. (1972). *Pediatr. Res.* **6,** 514–520.

82. Lambert, B., Hansson, K., Bui, T. H., Funes-Cravioto, F., and Lindsten, J. (1976). *Ann. Hum. Genet.* **39**, 293–303.
83. O'Brien, R. L., Poon, P., Kline, E., and Parker, J. W. (1971). *Int. J. Cancer* **8**, 202–210.
84. Sasaki, M. S., Tonomura, A., and Matsubara, S. (1970). *Mutat. Res.* **10**, 617–633.
85. Kopelovich, L., and Sirlin, S. (1980). *Cancer* **45**, 1108–1111.
86. Utsunomiya, J. (1977). *In* "Pathophysiology of Carcinogenesis in Digestive Organs." *Proc. Int. Symp. Princess Takamatsu Cancer Res. Fund, 7th, 1976.* Univ. Park Press, Baltimore, Maryland.
87. Cerimele, G., Scappaticci, S., Danesino, C., and Sanna, E. (1979). *J. Invest. Dermatol.* **72**, 289.
88. Epstein, C. J., Martin, G. M., Schultz, A. L., and Motulsky, A. G. (1966). *Medicine* **45**, 177–221.
89. Hoehn, H., Bryant, E. M., Au, K., Norwood, T. H., Boman, H., and Martin, G. M. (1975). *Cytogenet. Cell Genet.* **15**, 282–298.
90. Nordenson, I. (1977). *Hereditas* **87**, 2–5.
91. Salk, D., Au, K., Hoehn, H., and Martin, G. M. (1981). *Cytogenet. Cell Genet.* **30**, 92–107.
92. Rosenzajn, A. L., Radnai, J., Tatarski, A., and Benderlei, A. (1969). *Isr. J. Med. Sci.* **5**, 1087.
93. Say, B., Tunçbilek, Yamak, B., and Balci, S. (1970). *J. Med. Genet.* **7**, 417–421.
94. VanDyke, D. L., Jackson, C. E., and Babu, V. R. (1981). *Clin. Res.* **29**, 37A.
95. Suzuki, Y. (1977). *Brain Nerve* **29**, 537–542.
96. Evans, H. J. (1981). *In* "Genes, Chromosomes, and Neoplasia" (F. E. Arrighi, P. N. Rao, and E. Stubblefield, eds.), pp. 511–527. Raven, New York.
97. Hashem, N., and Khalifa, Sh. (1975). *Hum. Hered.* **25**, 35–49.
98. Hecht, F., and Kaiser-McCaw, B. (1981). *In* "Cancer" (J. H. Burchenal, and H. F. Oettgen, eds.), Vol. 1, pp. 433–444. Grune & Stratton, New York.
99. Knudson, A. G., Jr. (1981). *In* "Genes, Chromosomes, and Neoplasia" (F. E. Arrighi, P. N. Rao, and E. Stubblefield, eds.), pp. 453–462. Raven, New York.
100. Mark, J., Dahlenfors, R., Ekedahl, C., and Stenman, G. (1980). *Cancer Genet. Cytogenet.* **2**, 231–242.
101. Kaneko, Y., Celida Egues, M., and Rowley, J. D. (1981). *Cancer Res.* **41**, 4577–4578.
102. Cohen, A. J., Li, F. P., Berg, S., Marchetto, D. J., Tsai, S., Jacobs, S. C., and Brown, R. S. (1979). *N. Engl. J. Med.* **301**, 592–595.
103. Balaban-Malenbaum, G., Gilbert, F., Nichols, W. W., Hill, R., Shields, J., and Meadows, A. T. (1981). *Cancer Genet. Cytogenet.* **3**, 243–250.
104. Danes, B. S. (1978). *Cancer* **41**, 2330–2334.
105. Danes, B. S. (1976). *Cancer* **38**, 1983–1988.
106. Jean, P., Richer, C.-L., Murer-Orlando, M., Luu, D. H., and Joncas, J. H. (1979). *Nature (London)* **277**, 56–58.
107. Rowley, J. D. (1981). *N. Engl. J. Med.* **305**, 164–166.
108. Yunis, J. J., Bloomfield, C. D., and Ensrud, K. (1981). *N. Engl. J. Med.* **305**, 135–139.
109. Latt, S. A. (1974). *Proc. Natl. Acad. Sci. U.S.A.* **71**, 3162–3166.
110. Waters, R., Regan, J. D., and German, J. (1978). *Biochem. Biophys. Res. Commun.* **83**, 536–541.
111. Moore, P. D., and Holliday, R. (1976). *Cell* **8**, 573–579.
112. Rommelaere, J., and Miller-Faurès, A. (1975). *J. Mol. Biol.* **98**, 195–218.
113. Hethcote, H. W., and Knudson, A. G., Jr. (1978). *Proc. Natl. Acad. Sci. U.S.A.* **75**, 2453–2457.
114. Knudson, A. G., Jr. (1971). *Proc. Natl. Acad. Sci. U.S.A.* **68**, 820–823.

115. Knudson, A. G., Jr., and Strong, L. C. (1972). *J. Natl. Cancer Inst.* **48**, 313–324.
116. Baylin, S. B., Hsu, S. H., Gann, D. S., Smallridge, R. C., and Wells, S. A., Jr. (1978). *Science (Washington, D.C.)* **199**, 429–431.
117. Martin, M. A., Bryan, T., Rasheed, S., and Khan, A. S. (1981). *Proc. Natl. Acad. Sci. U.S.A.* **78**, 4892–4896.
118. Rovigatti, U. G., Rogler, C. E., Neel, B. G., Hayward, W. S., and Astrin, S. M. (1982). This volume, Chapter 20.
119. Eva, A., Robbins, K. C., Andersen, P. R., Srinivasan, A., Tronick, S. R., Reddy, E. P., Ellmore, N. W., Galen, A. T., Lautenberger, J. A., Pasas, T. S., Westin, E. H., Wong-Staal, F., Gallo, R. C., and Aaronson, S. A. (1982). *Nature (London)* **295**, 116–119.
120. Green, M. M. (1980). *Annu. Rev. Genet.* **14**, 109–120.
121. Pardoll, D. M., Vogelstein, B., and Coffey, D. S. (1980). *Cell* **19**, 527–536.
122. Vogelstein, B., Pardoll, D. M., and Coffey, D. S. (1980). *Cell* **22**, 79–85.
123. Feinberg, A. P., and Coffey, D. S. (1982). *Proc. 1981 Wistar Symp. Nucl. Env. Nucl. Matrix, 2nd.* (G. G. Maul, ed.), Liss, New York (in press).
124. Zbarsky, I. B., and Debov, S. S. (1948). *Dokl. Akad. Nauk S.S.S.R.* **63**, 795–798.
125. Zbarsky, I. B., and Georgiev, G. P. (1959). *Biochim. Biophys. Acta* **32**, 301–302.
126. Georgiev, G. P., and Chentsov, J. S. (1962). *Exp. Cell Res.* **27**, 570–572.
127. Zbarsky, I. B., Dmitrieva, N. P., and Yermolayeva, L. P. (1962). *Exp. Cell Res.* **27**, 573–576.
128. Narayan, K. S., Steele, W. J., Smetana, K., and Busch, H. (1967). *Exp. Cell Res.* **46**, 65–77.
129. Steele, W. J., and Busch, H. (1963). *Biochim. Biophys. Acta* **129**, 54–67.
130. Berezney, R., and Coffey, D. S. (1974). *Biochim. Biophys. Res. Commun.* **60**, 1410–1417.
131. Berezney, R., and Coffey, D. S. (1977). *J. Cell Biol.* **73**, 616–637.
132. Shaper, J. H., Pardoll, D. M., Kaufmann, S. H., Barrack, E. R., Vogelstein, B., and Coffey, D. S. (1979). *Adv. Enzyme Regul.* **17**, 213–248.
133. Pardoll, D. M., and Vogelstein, B. (1980). *Exp. Cell Res.* **128**, 466–470.
134. Nelkin, B. D., Pardoll, D. M., and Vogelstein, B. (1980). *Nucleic Acids Res.* **8**, 5623–5633.
135. Robinson, S., Nelkin, B. D., and Vogelstein, B. (1982). *Cell,* **28**, 99–106.
136. Jackson, D. A., McCready, S. J., and Cook, P. R. (1981). *Nature (London)* **292**, 552–555.
137. vanEekelen, C. A. G., and vanVenrooij, W. J. (1981). *J. Cell Biol.* **88**, 554–563.
138. Herman, R., Weymouth, L., and Penman, S. (1978). *J. Cell Biol.* **78**, 663–674.
139. Berezney, R., and Coffey, D. S. (1977). *J. Cell Biol.* **73**, 616–637.
140. Miller, T. E., Huang, C.-Y., and Pogo, A. O. (1978). *J. Cell Biol.* **76**, 675–691.
141. Miller, T. E., Huang, C.-Y., and Pogo, A. O. (1978). *J. Cell Biol.* **76**, 692–704.
142. Barrack, E. R., and Coffey, D. S. (1980). *J. Biol. Chem.* **255**, 7265–7275.
143. Barrack, E. R., and Coffey, D. S. (1982). *Recent Prog. Horm. Res.* **38** (in press).
144. Matsui, S., Antoniades, G., Basler, J., Berezney, R., and Sandberg, A. A. (1981). *J. Cell Biol.* **91**, 60a.
145. Peters, K. E., Okada, T. A., and Comings, D. E. (1981). *J. Cell Biol.* **91**, 72a.
146. Blazsek, I., Vaukhonen, M., and Hemminski, K. (1979). *Res. Commun. Chem. Pathol. Pharmacol.* **23**, 611–626.
147. Hemminki, K., and Vainio, H. (1979). *Cancer Lett.* **6**, 167–173.
148. Ueyama, H., Matsuura, T., Numi, S., Nakayasu, H., and Ueda, K. (1981). *Life Sci.* **29**, 655–661.
149. Buckler-White, A. J., Humphrey, G. W., and Pigiet, V. (1980). *Cell* **22**, 37–46.

150. Zbarsky, I. B. (1981). *Mol. Biol. Rep.* **7**, 139–148.
151. Kato, H. (1980). *Cancer Genet. Cytogenet.* **2**, 69–78.
152. Hand, R., and German, J. (1975). *Proc. Natl. Acad. Sci. U.S.A.* **72**, 758–762.
153. Sager, R. (1982). This volume, Chapter 25.
154. Echols, H. (1981). *Cell,* **25**, 1–2.
155. Sandberg, A. A. (1982). This volume, Chapter 23.
156. Nowell, P. C. (1982). This volume, Chapter 22.
157. Fidler, I. J. (1982). This volume, Chapter 9.
158. Baylin, S. B. (1982). This volume, Chapter 2.
159. Nadler, L. M. (1982). This volume, Chapter 4.
160. Tropé, C. (1982). This volume, Chapter 10.
161. Calabresi, P. (1982). This volume, Chapter 12.
162. Goldie, J. H. (1982). This volume, Chapter 8.
163. Ray, J. H., and German, J. (1981). *In* "Genes, Chromosomes, and Neoplasia" (F. E. Arrighi, P. N. Rao, and E. Stubblefield, eds.), pp. 351–378. Raven, New York.
164. Berg, J. M., Gardner, H. A., Gardner, R. J. M., Goh, E. G., Markovic, V. D., Simpson, N. E., and Worton, R. G. (1980). *J. Med. Genet.* **17**, 144–155.
165. Dekaban, A. S., Bender, M. A., and Economos, G. E. (1963). *Cytogenetics* **2**, 61–75.
166. Canki, N., and Dutrillaux, B. (1979). *Hum. Genet.* **47**, 261–268.
167. Carpenter, N. J., Say, B., and Browning, D. (1980). *J. Med. Genet,* **17**, 216–221.
168. Cohen, M. M., Capraro, V. J., and Takagi, N. (1962). *Ann. Hum. Genet.* **30**, 313–323.
169. Cooper, H. L., and Hernits, R. A. (1963). *Am. J. Hum. Genet.* **15**, 465–475.
170. Daniel, A., Saville, T., and Southall, D. B. (1979). *J. Med. Genet,* **16**, 278–284.
171. Khodr, G. S., Cadena, G. D., Ong, T. C., and Siler-Khoder, T. M. (1979). *Am. J. Dis. Child.* **133**, 277–282.
172. Laca, Z., Ivanovic, M., Dramusic, V., and Moric-Petrovic, S. (1979). *Hum. Genet.* **49**, 237–241.
173. Laszlo, J., Gaal, M., and Bosze, P. (1976). *Clin. Genet.* **9**, 61–70.
174. Málková, J., Michalová, K., Chrz, R., Kobilková, J., Matlik, K., and Stàrka, L. (1975). *Humangenetik* **27**, 251–253.
175. Nielsen, J., and Friedrich, U. (1971). *Clin. Genet.* **3**, 52–58.
176. Piazzi, M. J., Teixeira, A. C., Amari, M. F., Netto, A. S., and Marçallo, F. A. (1977). *Obstet. Gynecol.* **50**, 35S–38S.
177. Shapiro, L. R., Graves, Z. R., Warburton, D., and Huss, H. A. (1978). *In* "Birth Defects," Original Article Series, Vol. 14, No. 6C (R. L. Summit, and D. Bergsma, eds.), pp. 167–170. Liss, New York.
178. Ying, K. L., Ives, E. J., and Stephenson, O. D. (1977). *Clin. Genet.* **11**, 402–408.
179. Isurugi, K., Imao, S., Hirose, K., and Aoki, H. (1977). *Cancer* **39**, 2041–2047.
180. Riccardi, V. M., Hittner, H. M., Francke, V., Pippin, S., Holmquist, G. P., Kretzer, F. L., and Ferrell, R. (1979). *Clin. Genet.* **15**, 332–345.
181. Turleau, C., Cabanis, M.-O., and de Grouchy, J. (1980). *Ann. Génét.* **23**, 169–170.
182. Yunis, J. J., and Ramsay, N. K. C. (1978). *Am. J. Dis. Child.* **132**, 161–163.
183. Hittner, H. M., Riccardi, V. M., and Francke, U. (1979). *Ophthalmology* **86**, 1173–1183.
184. Ladda, R., Atkins, L., Littlefield, J., Neurath, P., and Marimuthu, K. M. (1974). *Science (Washington, D.C.)* **185**, 784–787.
185. Riccardi, V. M., Sujansky, E., Smith, A., and Francke, U. (1978). *Pediatrics* **61**, 604–610.
186. Hinkes, E., Crandall, B. F., Weber, F., and Craddock, C. G. (1973). *Blood* **41**, 259–263.

187. Sasaki, M. S., Tsunematsu, Y., Utsunomiya, J., and Utsumi, J. (1980). *Cancer Res.* **40,** 4796–4803.
188. Hsu, T. C., Pathak, S., Samaan, N., and Hickey, R. C. (1981). *JAMA, J. Am. Med. Assoc.* **246,** 2046–2048.
189. Simpson, J. L., and Photopulos, G. (1976). *In* "Birth Defects," Original Article Series, Vol. 12, No. 1 (D. Bergsma, ed.), pp. 15–50. Liss, New York.
190. Harnden, D. G. (1977). *In* "Human Genetics" (S. Armendares, and R. Lisker, eds.), pp. 355–366. Excerpta Medica, Amsterdam.
191. Philip, J., Frydenberg, O., and Sele, V. (1965). *Cytogenetics* **4,** 329–339.
192. Rauh, J. L., and Soukup, S. W. (1968). *Am. J. Dis. Child.* **116,** 409–413.
193. German, J., Gilleran, T. G., Setlow, R. B., and Regan, J. D. (1973). *Ann. Génét.* **16,** 23–27.
194. Auerbach, A. D., Wolman, S. R., and Chaganti, R. S. K. (1980). *Cytogenet. Cell Genet.* **28,** 265–270.
195. Mann, J. D., and Higgins, J. A. (1974). *Am. J. Hum. Genet.* **26,** 416.
196. Kallio, H. (1973). *Acta Obstet. Gynecol. Scand. Suppl.* **24,** 1–78.
197. Palmer, C., Nance, W., Cleary, R., and Dexter, R. (1973). *Am. J. Hum. Genet.* **25,** 57A.

Index

A

Abelson murine leukemia virus
  generation, 215
  transformed cell
    growth factor, low molecular weight,
      215, 216
    transformation defective mutant, 208
    transforming growth factor, 206, 208,
      215–217
ACTH, see Adrenocorticotropic hormone
Actin, intracellular organization, tumorgenicity, 287
Actinomycin D, DLD-1 colon carcinoma,
  186, 187
Adenocarcinoma
  Lucké, reversion, 5, 473
  lung, monoclonal antibody phenotype,
    43
  murine mammary, tumor subpopulation
    model, 227
  prostatic, Dunning R-3327-H
    androgen sensitivity, 103, 107
    chromosomal change, 109
    fast growing anaplastic, 109, 110
    fluctuation analysis, 105–107
    genetic instability, 108, 109
    growth curve, 102
    histological properties, 103, 104
    hormone therapy, growth response,
      102, 103
    karyotype, 108
    origin, 102
    relapse, 103
  Walker 256, in vitro drug effect, 152
  13762, clonal instability, 93
Adhesiveness, metastatic cell, 132
Adrenocortical tumor, mouse, gene ampli-
  fication, 400
Adrenocorticotropic hormone, small cell
  lung cancer, 41, 42

Ah receptor, polycyclic aromatic hydrocarbon binding, 268
Albinism, genetic basis, 242
Ames test
  chemical carcinogenic potential, 412
Amethopterin, see also Methotrexate
  colon cancer drug sensitivity heteroge-
    neity, 159
  stomach cancer drug sensitivity hetero-
    geneity, 162
Amine precursor uptake and decarboxylation system, see APUD
Amino acid analysis, transforming growth
  factor, 211
Anchorage independence
  carcinogen dose dependency, 306
  latency time, carcinogen altered cell, 303
Anchorage-dependent phenotype acquisition, 293
Androgen ablation, prostatic cancer therapy, 100, 101
Androgen sensitivity, Dunning R-3327-H
  tumor, 107, 109, 111
Aneuploidy
  tumor evolution, 359, 360
  tumor, human, 385–387
Anguidine, LX-1 lung carcinoma, 187, 188
Antibody
  hybridoma, binding specificity, tumor
    associated antigen, 314
  tumor growth stimulation, 75
Antibody binding test, radiolabeled, 313,
  314
Antigen
  anti-murine embryonic liver, prepara-
    tion, 87
  carcinoembryonic
    calcitonin ratio, medullary thyroid car-
      cinoma, 23
    carcinogenic marker, 5
    cell differentiation, 195, 196